MATHEMATICS FOR MEDICAL AND CLINICAL LABORATORY PROFESSIONALS

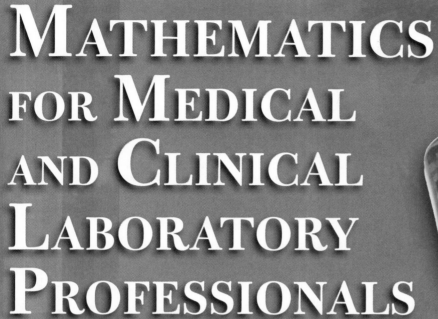

MATHEMATICS FOR MEDICAL AND CLINICAL LABORATORY PROFESSIONALS

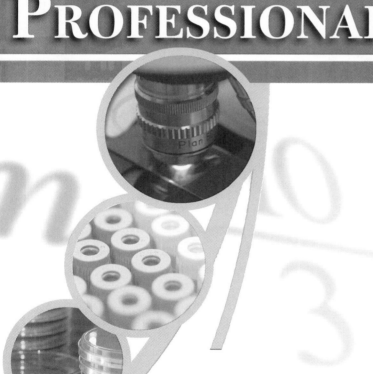

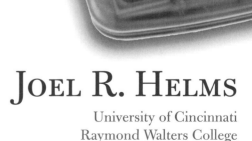

JOEL R. HELMS

University of Cincinnati
Raymond Walters College
Blue Ash, Ohio

DELMAR
CENGAGE Learning™

Australia • Brazil • Japan • Korea • Mexico • Singapore • Spain • United Kingdom • United States

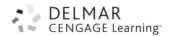
DELMAR
CENGAGE Learning

Mathematics for Medical and Clinical Laboratory Professionals

Joel R. Helms

Vice President, Career and Professional Editorial: Dave Garza

Director of Learning Solutions: Matthew Kane

Senior Acquisitions Editor: Sherry Dickinson

Managing Editor: Marah Bellegarde

Product Manager: Laura J. Wood

Editorial Assistant: Jennifer Waters

Vice President, Career and Professional Marketing: Jennifer McAvey

Marketing Director: Wendy Mapstone

Marketing Manager: Michele McTighe

Marketing Coordinator: Scott Chrysler

Production Director: Carolyn Miller

Production Manager: Andrew Crouth

Content Project Manager: Brooke Greenhouse

Senior Art Director: Jack Pendleton

For product information and technology assistance, contact us at **Cengage Learning Customer & Sales Support, 1-800-354-9706**

For permission to use material from this text or product, submit all requests online at **www.cengage.com/permissions**
Further permissions questions can be emailed to **permissionrequest@cengage.com**

Library of Congress Control Number: 2007942055

ISBN-13: 978-1-4354-0040-5

ISBN-10: 1-4354-0040-2

Delmar
Executive Woods
5 Maxwell Drive
Clifton Park, NY 12065
USA

Cengage Learning is a leading provider of customized learning solutions with office locations around the globe, including Singapore, the United Kingdom, Australia, Mexico, Brazil, and Japan. Locate your local office at **www.cengage.com/global**

Cengage Learning products are represented in Canada by Nelson Education, Ltd.

To learn more about Delmar, visit **www.cengage.com/delmar**

Purchase any of our products at your local bookstore or at our preferred online store **www.cengagebrain.com**

Notice to the Reader

Publisher does not warrant or guarantee any of the products described herein or perform any independent analysis in connection with any of the product information contained herein. Publisher does not assume, and expressly disclaims, any obligation to obtain and include information other than that provided to it by the manufacturer. The reader is expressly warned to consider and adopt all safety precautions that might be indicated by the activities described herein and to avoid all potential hazards. By following the instructions contained herein, the reader willingly assumes all risks in connection with such instructions. The publisher makes no representations or warranties of any kind, including but not limited to, the warranties of fitness for particular purpose or merchantability, nor are any such representations implied with respect to the material set forth herein, and the publisher takes no responsibility with respect to such material. The publisher shall not be liable for any special, consequential, or exemplary damages resulting, in whole or part, from the readers' use of, or reliance upon, this material.

Printed in the United States of America
2 3 4 5 6 7 16 15 14 13 12

CONTENTS

APPENDIX C: **PERTINENT FORMULAS**   303

APPENDIX D: **WEST NOMOGRAM**   307

APPENDIX E: **ANSWERS TO ODD-NUMBERED QUESTIONS**   309

DEDICATION

To my wife, Erin, and my children, Kelsey, Brianne, Deirdre, Corey, Michael, and Sean.

To Tom and Karen Rehak.

To the medical laboratory technology students in the United States Navy.

Thank you to Stephen Eliason, M.D., for his review, comments, and suggestions.

PREFACE

Mathematics for Medical and Clinical Laboratory Professionals is designed to give students the mathematical foundation necessary to be successful in basic medical math courses as well as in courses that follow in the health and clinical laboratory science curriculums. The mathematical concepts, calculations, and theories taught in entry-level math courses in the health sciences curriculums are included, along with the essential tools needed to ensure that students develop a strong preliminary knowledge of advanced content. With its step-by-step approach, *Mathematics for Medical and Clinical Laboratory Professionals* is also perfect for clinical lab professionals looking for a refresher of mathematical concepts.

Conceptual Approach

Written by a mathematician, this text provides a fresh perspective on old concepts by using an understandable, systematic, and sensible approach. Instead of simply stating mathematical rules, the text first explains the rules. Once the structure of a rule is understood, the absorption of mathematical concepts related to that rule becomes that much stronger. This serves as an important tool in mastering the more advanced mathematical content in the text, including dilutions, factors and titers, charting data, and chemistry and logarithms, among others. While math can be a difficult topic to grasp, *Mathematics for Medical and Clinical Laboratory Professionals* addresses each unique user's needs by providing easy-to-follow learning tools for the student, instructor, and clinical lab professional alike.

Organization of Content

The text is divided into 12 chapters along with five appendices. The first two chapters provide a review of basic mathematical concepts and procedures. Each subsequent chapter focuses on a specific topic, including solutions, hematology, and urinalysis and renal clearance, among others. Each chapter begins with an introduction and is divided into subsections that discuss important components of each chapter's topic in a way that is both manageable for the student learner and easily accessible for the instructor or clinical lab professional. The appendices include a table of Greek symbols, the periodic table of the elements, and pertinent formulas used in the laboratory.

Features

- With *hundreds of practice problems* throughout the text, including *practice problems at the end of each section,* users learn to actively apply important concepts while the concepts are still fresh in their minds.

- *End-of-chapter test questions* provide a final review of all materials learned throughout each chapter.

- *Answers to all odd-numbered questions* (Appendix E) allow users to quiz themselves and allow instructors to utilize even-numbered problems as homework, class assignments, or test questions.

- *Step-by-step examples* throughout each section detail every part of a mathematical equation to ensure that a user can clearly visualize how a solution is formed and aid the instructor in teaching difficult mathematical concepts.

- *Key terms* are bolded in the text and defined in a *glossary* to emphasize importance and provide a quick reference guide.

- *Notes boxes* point out useful facts and tips.

- *End-of-chapter summaries* organize all important rules and equations in one place for easy review.

- *Using Your Calculator boxes* teach users how to perform complex equations on a calculator in addition to learning them on paper.

- Chapter 10 contains a *technology feature* that guides users through a step-by-step process of graphing data in Microsoft Excel.

- Important mathematical rules and equations are indicated in color throughout the text.

For the Student

Student Solution Manual to Accompany Mathematics for Medical and Clinical Laboratory Professionals ISBN 1-4354-0041-0

This manual contains step-by-step solutions to every odd-numbered problem in the text, including practice problems and chapter tests. The manual allows students to further understand how to correctly work a math problem by using the step-by-step analysis to learn from their mistakes, whether in the classroom or at home.

For the Instructor

Instructor Solution Manual to Accompany Mathematics for Medical and Clinical Laboratory Professionals ISBN 1-4354-0042-9

This manual contains step-by-step solutions to all problems in the text, including practice problems and chapter tests. Coupled with the text, it provides instructors with numerous easy-to-use teaching tools that work together to enhance a student's overall learning experience. For example, after assigning even-numbered problems for homework, instructors can use the step-by-step examples in the text to first show students how to properly use a formula or rule. Then they can use the solution manual to help struggling students understand how to calculate a correct answer for each assigned problem.

REVIEWERS

We would like to thank the following content reviewers:

Brian Abela, M.S.
West Hills Community College, Lemoore
Lemoore, CA

Gordon A. DeSpain, M.A.
San Juan College
Farmington, NM

Barbara H. Estridge, MT (ASCP), CLS (NCA)
Auburn University
Auburn, AL

Keith Kuchar
College of DuPage
Glen Ellyn, IL

Michele Benjamin Lesmeister, M.A.
Renton Technical College
Renton, WA

Mary Marlin, B.A.
West Virginia Northern Community College
Weirton, WV

David A. Palkovich, M.S.
Oklahoma City Community College
Oklahoma City, OK

Mary Phillips, B.S.Ed.
Lancaster General College of Nursing and Health Sciences
Lancaster, PA

Dr. Ed Smith, Ed.D.
Roane State Community College
Oak Ridge, TN

Robert Ulmer, M.Ed.
Santa Fe Community College
Union County, FL

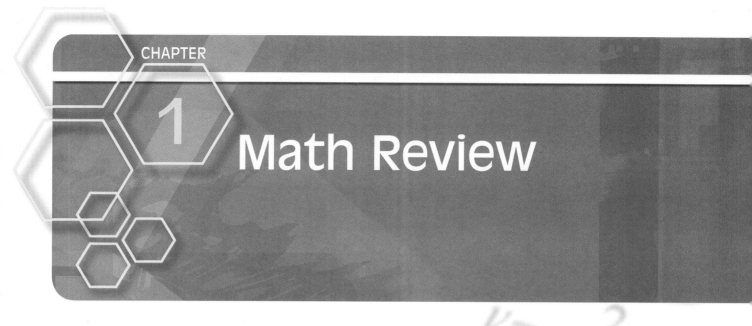

Math Review

CHAPTER 1

INTRODUCTION

In this chapter we review basic operations with integers, fractions, percents, and decimals. These topics lay the foundation for the rest of the book. Being proficient with integers, fractions, percents, and decimals is essential to doing well in the remaining chapters.

1.1 – OPERATIONS WITH INTEGERS

Adding Integers

To add integers we must first remember that the negative sign means the opposite of a number. Thus, the opposite of 3 is -3. Moreover, we know the opposite of -3 must be positive 3. Mathematically, the opposite of -3 would be notated as $-(-3)$. But as we just discussed, we know this must equal positive 3. Therefore, $-(-3) = 3$. A good way to think about these types of numbers is to associate them with money. For example, the opposite of having \$3 is owing \$3. When evaluating the sum of two numbers, think of money. For example,

$$3 + (-3) = 0 .$$
$$\uparrow \qquad \uparrow$$
$$\text{Have} \quad \text{Owe}$$

This equation is true because if you have \$3 and you owe \$3, you have no money left after paying what you owe.

1

RULES FOR ADDING TWO INTEGERS
- If the two integers being added have the same sign, the sign of the answer will have the same sign as the two integers being added.
- If the two integers being added have different signs, the sign of the answer will have the sign attached to the larger integer.

EXAMPLE 1-1: Evaluate the following.

a) $-5 + 3 = -2$

If you owe 5 and have 3, after you pay the 3 you have, you still owe 2. Notice the sign of the larger integer, 5, is negative; thus, the answer will be negative.

b) $-2 + (-4) = -6$

If you owe 2 and then owe 4 more, in total you owe 6. Notice that the two integers have the same sign; thus, the answer will have the same sign as well.

c) $5 + (-3) = 2$

If you have 5 and owe 3, after you pay the 3 you owe you still have 2 left. Notice the sign of the larger integer, 5, is positive; thus, the answer will be positive.

Subtracting Integers

As noted previously, the negative sign means the opposite. So we can think of -3 as "the opposite of having \$3," which is owing \$3. Therefore, subtraction can be thought of in the same way as we discussed addition.

$$3 - 3 = 0 \text{ is the same as } 3 + (-3) = 0$$

$\uparrow$

Opposite of having

Because subtraction is the same as *adding* the opposite, the rules for subtraction are the same as those for adding.

EXAMPLE 1-2: Evaluate the following.

a) $-5 - 4 = -9$

If you owe 5 and owe 4 more, in total you owe 9. Notice the sign of each integer is negative and thus the answer must be negative.

b) $6 - 8 = -2$

If you have 6 and owe 8, after you pay the 6 you have, you still owe 2. Notice the sign of the larger integer, 8, is negative; thus, the answer must be negative.

c) $-4 + 3 = -1$

If you owe 4 and have 3, after you pay the 3 you have, you still owe 1. Notice the sign of the larger integer, 4, is negative and thus the answer must be negative.

d) $-8 - (-5)$

First note that $-(-5)$ is $+5$. Rewriting we have $-8 + 5$, and $-8 + 5 = -3$.

e) $-7 - 4 - (-2)$

First, write $-(-2)$ as $+2$, yielding $-7 - 4 + 2$. Adding these we get an answer of -9.

Multiplying Integers

Let's begin by remembering exactly what multiplication means. Recall that multiplication is nothing more than repeated addition.

So $(3)(4) = 12$ because this actually means add 4 three times.

$$(3)(4) = 4 + 4 + 4 = 12$$

With this in mind, we now consider multiplication of positive and negative numbers. Most students at this level already have it ingrained in their mind that a positive times a negative equals a negative. Why? We answer that by analyzing $(3)(-4)$.

$(3)(-4) = -12$ because this actually means add -4 three times, which is precisely -12.

$$(3)(-4) = (-4) + (-4) + (-4) = -12$$

Before we consider multiplying a negative times a negative, let's take a closer look at the number -3. This can also be represented by (-3). All we did was put parentheses around -3. So this still means the opposite of 3. But $-(3)$ also means the opposite of 3. Therefore (-3) is the same as $-(3)$. With this in mind, we can rewrite the multiplication problem

$$(-3)(-4)$$

as

$$-(3)(-4).$$

Now this can be thought of as the opposite of 3 times -4 since the negative sign out in front means the opposite. But we know that 3 times -4 equals -12 and the opposite of -12 is positive 12. So our conclusion is that a negative times a negative equals a positive.

> **RULES FOR MULTIPLYING TWO INTEGERS**
> - A *positive* times a *positive* equals a *positive*.
> - A *negative* times a *positive* equals a *negative*.
> - A *positive* times a *negative* equals a *negative*.
> - A *negative* times a *negative* equals a *positive*.

EXAMPLE 1-3: Evaluate the following.

a) $(5)(-6)$

We know a positive times a negative equals a negative. Therefore, the answer is -30.

b) $(-7)(-5)$

We know a negative times a negative equals a positive. Therefore, the answer is 35.

c) $(-2)(8)$

We know a negative times a positive equals a negative. Therefore, the answer is -16.

d) $(-2)(-4)(-3)$

We know a negative times a negative equals a positive. Therefore, $(-2)(-4) = 8$, but $(8)(-3)$ equals a negative. Therefore, the answer is -24.

Dividing Integers

The rules for division are the same as those for multiplication. This is because when we evaluate a division problem, all we really need to do is look at it as a multiplication problem. In other words, division is really multiplication in disguise. For example, $6 \div 3 = 2$ because 3 divides into 6 two times. But we can also look at $6 \div 3$ as a multiplication problem. To see this we write $6 \div 3$ in long division format:

$$3 \overline{)6} \, .$$

Here the question really involves multiplication: What number multiplied by 3 equals 6? Clearly the answer is 2.

Now why does $6 \div (-3) = -2$? To answer this question, we again look at this as a long division problem.

$$-3 \overline{)6}$$

To get the answer, we must figure out what number multiplied by -3 equals positive 6. As discussed in our study of multiplication, we know the answer is -2 because $(-2)(-3) = 6$. Therefore,

$$-3 \overline{)\, 6 \,}^{-2} \, .$$

What about $-6 \div (-3)$? Again we look at this in long division format.

$$-3\overline{)-6}$$

To answer the question, we need to determine what number times -3 equals -6. We know the answer is positive 2 because $(2)(-3) = -6$. Therefore, $-6 \div (-3) = 2$ because

$$-3\overline{)-6}^{\,2}\,.$$

Before we do a few examples, recall that a fraction also implies division. That is, $6 \div 3$ can be written as $\frac{6}{3}$, and both of these are equal to 2.

> **RULES FOR DIVIDING TWO INTEGERS**
> - A *positive* divided by a *positive* equals a *positive*.
> - A *negative* divided by a *positive* equals a *negative*.
> - A *positive* divided by a *negative* equals a *negative*.
> - A *negative* divided by a *negative* equals a *positive*.

EXAMPLE 1-4: Evaluate the following.

a) $\frac{-20}{-5}$

   The answer is 4 because a negative divided by a negative is a positive.

b) $\frac{-12}{2}$

   The answer is -6 because a negative divided by a positive is a negative.

c) $\frac{15}{-3}$

   The answer is -5 because a positive divided by a negative is a negative.

NOTE

The fraction $\frac{-10}{2}$ is the same as $\frac{10}{-2}$, which is the same as $-\frac{10}{2}$. All three are equal to -5. The point is, given a negative fraction, the negative sign can go in the numerator (top) or the denominator (bottom) or out in front. This fact comes in handy, especially when adding and subtracting fractions, which is the topic of the next section.

Division Involving Zero

Most students are familiar with the fact that zero divided by any number is zero. Why is this so? To answer this we begin by analyzing the specific case of why $\frac{0}{6} = 0$. Remember from our previous discussions that $\frac{0}{6}$ as a long division problem would be written as $6\overline{)0}$. We must determine what number multiplied by 6 equals zero. The answer is zero because any number multiplied by zero is equal to zero. Therefore:

> Zero divided by *any* number is equal to zero.

Next we analyze why any number divided by zero is undefined. We examine the specific case of why $\frac{6}{0}$ is undefined. In long division format, this is written as $0\overline{)6}$. We must determine what number multiplied by zero equals 6. There is no number we know of because any number multiplied by zero equals zero. Hence, it is undefined. Therefore:

> Any number divided by zero is undefined.

PRACTICE PROBLEMS: Section 1.1

Add or subtract the following.

1. 3 – 8
2. –4 – 6
3. –7 + 4
4. –6 – (–5)
5. 8 – (–3)
6. –18 + 12
7. 24 – 30
8. 11 – 21

9. –20 – 30
10. 16 – (–7)
11. 15 – (–3)
12. –4 + 3 – (–5)
13. 3 – 8 + 2
14. –7 – (–8) – 12
15. –38 – (–21)
16. –28 – 28

17. –45 + 50
18. 40 – (–20)
19. –7 – (–2)
20. 6 – 8
21. –5 – 10
22. –3 – (–1)
23. 15 – 22 + 10
24. –8 – (–8) – (–12) – 5

Multiply the following.

25. $5 \times (-4)$

26. $-8(-9)$

27. $(-6)7$

28. -2×-20

29. 9×9

30. $7 \times (-8)$

31. $-5(-5)$

32. -8×8

33. $(-2)(-7)$

34. $(-5)(4)$

35. $8(-3)$

36. $(-5)(6)$

37. $4 \times (-5) \times (-2)$

38. $-2(-5)(-3)$

Divide the following.

39. $10 \div (-5)$

40. $-12 \div (-6)$

41. $-20 \div 4$

42. $\frac{-30}{-15}$

43. $\frac{-45}{9}$

44. $\frac{60}{-12}$

45. $\frac{-32}{-4}$

46. $\frac{-70}{10}$

47. $\frac{40}{-5}$

48. $\frac{-64}{-8}$

49. $\frac{-20}{-2}$

50. $\frac{-12}{-4}$

51. $\frac{25}{-5}$

52. $\frac{-30}{3}$

53. $\frac{0}{12}$

54. $\frac{4}{0}$

1.2 – FRACTIONS

In a fraction the **denominator** is the bottom number and the **numerator** is the top number. To add or subtract fractions, we need a common denominator. However, when we multiply or divide fractions, we *do not* need common denominators.

> Common denominators *are* necessary when *adding* or *subtracting* fractions. Common denominators *are not* necessary when *multiplying* or *dividing* fractions.

Multiplying Fractions

When multiplying fractions simply multiply the top numbers, also called *numerators,* and multiply the bottom numbers, also called *denominators.* Common denominators are not necessary when multiplying fractions.

For example, $\frac{3}{8} \times \frac{5}{7} = \frac{3 \times 5}{8 \times 7} = \frac{15}{56}$.

If given the fraction $\frac{14}{21}$, you can reduce it as follows:

$$\frac{14}{21} = \frac{7 \times 2}{7 \times 3} = \frac{7}{7} \times \frac{2}{3} = 1 \times \frac{2}{3} = \frac{2}{3} = \frac{2}{3}.$$

In this example the 7s reduce to a value of 1. Often students say the 7s *cancel*. Next we reduce by *cross canceling* before we multiply.

In the following example, 5 cross cancels with 30. In other words, 5 divides into 5 one time and 5 divides into 30 six times. This is why there is a little 1 by the 5 and a little 6 by the 30. Likewise, 4 cross cancels with 12 since 4 divides into 4 one time and 4 divides into 12 three times.

$$\frac{5}{12} \times \frac{4}{30} = \frac{\cancel{5}^{1}}{\cancel{12}^{3}} \times \frac{\cancel{4}^{1}}{\cancel{30}^{6}} = \frac{1 \times 1}{3 \times 6} = \frac{1}{18}$$

One situation that often throws students is multiplying a whole number by a fraction. The best way to handle this is to think of the whole number as a fraction (over 1). For example,

$$12 \times \frac{3}{4} = \frac{12}{1} \times \frac{3}{4} = \frac{\cancel{12}^{3}}{1} \times \frac{3}{\cancel{4}^{1}} = \frac{3 \times 3}{1 \times 1} = \frac{9}{1} = 9.$$

Adding and Subtracting Fractions

When adding or subtracting fractions, once the denominators are the same, simply add/subtract the numerators (top numbers) and place this value over the common denominator. An example of adding is

$$\frac{1}{7} + \frac{3}{7} = \frac{1+3}{7} = \frac{4}{7}.$$

An example of subtracting is

$$\frac{3}{11} - \frac{5}{11} = \frac{3-5}{11} = \frac{-2}{11} = -\frac{2}{11}.$$

If the denominators are not the same, first modify the fractions so they have common denominators. Following is an example of adding fractions with unlike denominators.

$$\frac{1}{6} + \frac{3}{8}$$

Because the denominators are not the same, the next step is to determine the **least common denominator**, or LCD. Before we do that, recall that the LCD is the smallest number that both denominators divide into evenly (without a remainder).

NOTE

The LCD is the least common multiple.

If it is not clear that 24 is the LCD in the following example, to determine the LCD begin by writing down the multiples of each denominator. The LCD (or least common multiple) will be the first common number.

| Multiples of 6: | 6 | 12 | 18 | 24 | 30 |
| Multiples of 8: | 8 | 16 | 24 | 32 | 40 |

The LCD is 24 because 24 is the first common number. Now multiply each fraction by an appropriate fraction to change it to an equivalent fraction with a denominator of 24. Therefore, $\frac{1}{6}$ must be multiplied by $\frac{4}{4}$, and $\frac{3}{8}$ must be multiplied by $\frac{3}{3}$.

$$\left(\frac{4}{4}\right)\frac{1}{6} + \frac{3}{8}\left(\frac{3}{3}\right) = \frac{4}{24} + \frac{9}{24} = \frac{4+9}{24} = \frac{13}{24}$$

EXAMPLE 1-5: Evaluate the following.

a) $\frac{2}{9} + \frac{1}{3}$

The LCD is 9: $\frac{2}{9} + \frac{1}{3}\left(\frac{3}{3}\right) = \frac{2}{9} + \frac{3}{9} = \frac{5}{9}$.

b) $\frac{5}{6} - \frac{3}{8}$

The LCD is 24: $\left(\frac{4}{4}\right)\frac{5}{6} - \frac{3}{8}\left(\frac{3}{3}\right) = \frac{20}{24} - \frac{9}{24} = \frac{11}{24}$.

c) $\frac{2}{5} + \frac{1}{3}$

The LCD is 15: $\left(\frac{3}{3}\right)\frac{2}{5} + \frac{1}{3}\left(\frac{5}{5}\right) = \frac{6}{15} + \frac{5}{15} = \frac{11}{15}$.

d) $\frac{1}{3} - \frac{2}{9}$

The LCD is 9: $\left(\frac{3}{3}\right)\frac{1}{3} - \frac{2}{9} = \frac{3}{9} - \frac{2}{9} = \frac{1}{9}$.

e) $\frac{2}{3} - \frac{1}{8}$

The LCD is 24: $\left(\frac{8}{8}\right)\frac{2}{3} - \frac{1}{8}\left(\frac{3}{3}\right) = \frac{16}{24} - \frac{3}{24} = \frac{13}{24}$.

Dividing Fractions

For division, the rule is invert the second fraction and multiply.

$$\text{For example, } \frac{2}{15} \div \frac{4}{9} = \frac{2}{15} \times \frac{9}{4} = \frac{\cancel{2}^{1}}{\cancel{15}^{5}} \times \frac{\cancel{9}^{3}}{\cancel{4}^{2}} = \frac{1 \times 3}{5 \times 2} = \frac{3}{10}.$$

$$\uparrow$$
$$\text{Invert}$$

EXAMPLE 1-6: Simplify the following and express as a fraction.

a) $\dfrac{3}{7} \times \dfrac{28}{9}$

First, reduce: $\dfrac{\cancel{3}^{1}}{\cancel{7}^{1}} \times \dfrac{\cancel{28}^{4}}{\cancel{9}^{3}} = \dfrac{4}{3}$ (later we discuss how to write this as a mixed number).

b) $\dfrac{5}{6} \div \left(-\dfrac{15}{36}\right)$

This is the same as $\dfrac{5}{6} \times \left(-\dfrac{36}{15}\right)$. Reducing the 6 with the 36 and the 5 with the 15, we get $\dfrac{\cancel{5}^{1}}{\cancel{6}^{1}} \times \left(-\dfrac{\cancel{36}^{6}}{\cancel{15}^{3}}\right) = -\dfrac{6}{3} = -2$.

c) $\dfrac{1}{4} \times 20 \times 30$

This is equivalent to $\dfrac{1}{4} \times \dfrac{20}{1} \times \dfrac{30}{1} = \dfrac{20 \times 30}{4 \times 1 \times 1} = \dfrac{600}{4} = 150$.

d) $\dfrac{2}{3} \times 9 \div \dfrac{1}{4}$

First, rewrite 9 as a fraction: $\dfrac{2}{3} \times \dfrac{9}{1} \div \dfrac{1}{4}$.

Next, apply the rule for division, which is invert and multiply: $\dfrac{2}{3} \times \dfrac{9}{1} \times \dfrac{4}{1}$.

Last, simplify: $\dfrac{2}{\cancel{3}^{1}} \times \dfrac{\cancel{9}^{3}}{1} \times \dfrac{4}{1} = \dfrac{2 \times 3 \times 4}{1 \times 1 \times 1} = 24$.

Writing Fractions as Decimals

As previously discussed, we know a fraction means division. Therefore, fractions can also be written as decimals. For example, $\dfrac{1}{5}$ can be written as a decimal by dividing:

$$\dfrac{1}{5} \text{ is the same as } 5\overline{)1.0}\,; \text{ dividing we find } 5\overline{)1.0}^{\,0.2}.$$

Therefore, $\dfrac{1}{5} = 0.2$.

Similarly, $\frac{3}{4} = 0.75$. (We could also get this by typing 3 divided by 4 into the calculator.)

We discuss decimals in more detail in the next section.

EXAMPLE 1-7: Write the following fractions as decimals.

a) $\frac{4}{5}$

In long division format, $\frac{4}{5}$ is $5\overline{)4.0}^{\,0.8}$. Therefore, $\frac{4}{5} = 0.8$.

We could have easily typed this into our calculator to obtain this result.

b) $\frac{3}{4}$

In long division format, we have $4\overline{)3.00}^{\,0.75}$. Therefore, $\frac{3}{4} = 0.75$.

Unit Rates

A **unit fraction** is a fraction that has a 1 in the numerator. However, in many applications we want the denominator to have a 1. For example, if a car can travel 280 miles per 8 gallons of gasoline, we usually want to break this down so we know how many miles the car can travel on 1 gallon of gasoline. Thus, we want to write $\frac{280 \text{ miles}}{8 \text{ gallons}}$ as a fraction in which the denominator is 1. To accomplish this divide 280 by 8 to get 35. Therefore, $\frac{280 \text{ miles}}{8 \text{ gallons}} = \frac{35 \text{ miles}}{1 \text{ gallon}}$. This is called a **unit rate**.

EXAMPLE 1-8: A person receives 36 for every fours of work. Write this as a unit rate.

Thirty-six dollars every four hours can be expressed as $\frac{\$36}{4 \text{ hours}}$.

Simplifying we find $\frac{\$\overset{9}{\cancel{36}}}{\underset{1}{\cancel{4}} \text{ hours}} = \frac{\$9}{1 \text{ hour}}$. In words, this is saying "9 dollars per hour."

Improper Fractions and Mixed Numbers

Up to this point, the only type of fraction we have discussed is what is called the **proper fraction**. Proper fractions have a denominator that is larger than the numerator. A fraction whose numerator is larger than the denominator is called an **improper fraction**, such as $\frac{3}{2}$. Notice that all improper fractions are greater than 1. Therefore, we can express all improper fractions as a whole number together with a fraction. Such numbers are called **mixed numbers**, and an example is $5\frac{3}{4}$. This leads us to the question of how to write an improper fraction as a mixed number. This is accomplished by dividing the denominator into the numerator and keeping track of the remainder. For example, to write $\frac{7}{2}$ as a mixed number, note that 2 divides into 7 three times with a remainder of 1. Thus, $\frac{7}{2} = 3\frac{1}{2}$. To write a mixed number as an improper fraction, do the following:

$$3\frac{1}{2} = \frac{2 \times 3 + 1}{2} = \frac{6+1}{2} = \frac{7}{2}.$$

To add or subtract mixed numbers, convert each mixed number into an improper fraction and then add/subtract as illustrated earlier. After you get your result, convert it back to a mixed number.

For example,

$$2\frac{1}{5} + 3\frac{1}{2} = \frac{11}{5} + \frac{7}{2} = \frac{2}{2} \cdot \frac{11}{5} + \frac{5}{5} \cdot \frac{7}{2} = \frac{22}{10} + \frac{35}{10} = \frac{57}{10} = 5\frac{7}{10}.$$

EXAMPLE 1-9: Evaluate the following.

a) $5\frac{1}{4} - 2\frac{1}{3}$

First, write the mixed numbers as improper fractions: $\frac{21}{4} - \frac{7}{3}$. We now see the LCD is 12.

$$\left(\frac{3}{3}\right)\frac{21}{4} - \frac{7}{3}\left(\frac{4}{4}\right) = \frac{63}{12} - \frac{28}{12} = \frac{35}{12} = 2\frac{11}{12}$$

b) $2\frac{5}{8} + 1\frac{1}{2}$

First, write the mixed numbers as improper fractions: $\frac{21}{8} + \frac{3}{2}$. The LCD is 8.

$$\frac{21}{8} + \frac{3}{2}\left(\frac{4}{4}\right) = \frac{21}{8} + \frac{12}{8} = \frac{33}{8} = 4\frac{1}{8}$$

EXAMPLE 1-10: Simplify the following and give your answer as a mixed number: $5\frac{3}{4} \div 3\frac{3}{8}$.

First, write the mixed numbers as improper fractions: $\frac{23}{4} \div \frac{27}{8}$. Now invert and multiply.

$$\frac{23}{\cancel{4}_1} \times \frac{\cancel{8}^2}{27} = \frac{46}{27} \quad \text{and} \quad \frac{46}{27} = 1\frac{19}{27}$$

Simplifying Complex Fractions

EXAMPLE 1-11: Completely simplify the following fractions. Problems involving these types of manipulations arise in many areas such as molarity and normality.

a) $\dfrac{\frac{3}{4}}{\frac{3}{8}}$

    This can be written as $\dfrac{3}{4} \div \dfrac{3}{8} = \dfrac{3}{4} \times \dfrac{8}{3} = \dfrac{24}{12} = 2$.

b) $\dfrac{\frac{3}{4}}{6}$

    This translates to $\dfrac{3}{4} \div 6$, and this is the same as $\dfrac{3}{4} \div \dfrac{6}{1} = \dfrac{3}{4} \times \dfrac{1}{6} = \dfrac{3}{4} \times \dfrac{1}{\cancel{6}^2} = \dfrac{1}{8}$.

c) $\dfrac{\left(\frac{6+12}{4+8}\right)}{2}$

    Simplifying the numerator we get $\dfrac{\frac{18}{12}}{2} = \dfrac{18}{12} \div 2 = \dfrac{18}{12} \times \dfrac{1}{2} = \dfrac{\cancel{18}^9}{12} \times \dfrac{1}{\cancel{2}^1} = \dfrac{9}{12} = \dfrac{3}{4}$.

PRACTICE PROBLEMS: Section 1.2

Add or subtract the following.

1. $\dfrac{5}{8} + \dfrac{2}{8}$

2. $\dfrac{5}{7} - \dfrac{4}{7}$

3. $\dfrac{7}{8} - \dfrac{5}{6}$

4. $\dfrac{1}{12} + \dfrac{3}{8}$

5. $\dfrac{3}{8} + \dfrac{1}{4}$

6. $\dfrac{3}{10} + \dfrac{1}{6}$

7. $\dfrac{2}{3} + \dfrac{1}{6}$

8. $\dfrac{3}{5} - \dfrac{1}{6}$

9. $\dfrac{7}{12} - \dfrac{3}{8}$

10. $\dfrac{1}{9} + \dfrac{2}{3}$

11. $\dfrac{11}{16} - \dfrac{1}{6}$

12. $\dfrac{5}{6} + \dfrac{3}{4}$

13. $2\dfrac{1}{2} - 1\dfrac{1}{3}$

14. $3 + 2\dfrac{7}{12}$

15. $5\dfrac{4}{9} - \left(-2\dfrac{2}{3}\right)$

16. $\dfrac{2}{3} - 2\dfrac{1}{6}$

17. $3\dfrac{3}{4} + \dfrac{1}{2}$

18. $5\dfrac{3}{8} - 4\dfrac{5}{6}$

19. $10\dfrac{1}{3} - 2\dfrac{3}{5}$

20. $6\dfrac{1}{4} - 3\dfrac{1}{2}$

21. $1\dfrac{3}{8} + 2\dfrac{5}{6}$

22. $5\dfrac{3}{4} - 3$

Continues

PRACTICE PROBLEMS: Section 1.2 (continued)

Multiply the following.

23. $\frac{2}{3} \times \frac{1}{5}$

24. $\frac{5}{8} \times \frac{2}{15}$

25. $\frac{3}{7} \times \frac{21}{30}$

26. $-\frac{6}{8} \times \frac{5}{12}$

27. $\frac{2}{9} \times \frac{3}{5}$

28. $\frac{5}{16} \times \frac{4}{5}$

29. $\frac{5}{9} \times \frac{3}{10}$

30. $\frac{1}{4} \times \left(-\frac{6}{8}\right)$

31. $\frac{9}{16} \times \frac{4}{27}$

32. $\frac{3}{5} \times \frac{1}{4}$

33. $3\frac{1}{2} \times 2\frac{1}{4}$

34. $1\frac{2}{3} \times \left(-2\frac{3}{5}\right)$

35. $2\frac{3}{4} \times 4$

36. $\frac{5}{6} \times 2\frac{1}{3}$

37. $2\frac{1}{2} \times 3\frac{4}{5}$

38. $2\frac{3}{4} \times 1\frac{5}{8}$

39. $1\frac{5}{12} \times 2\frac{5}{6}$

40. $3\frac{3}{8} \times 2\frac{2}{5}$

Divide the following.

41. $\frac{2}{3} \div \frac{1}{3}$

42. $\frac{3}{5} \div \frac{9}{15}$

43. $\frac{5}{6} \div \left(-\frac{3}{8}\right)$

44. $\frac{5}{9} \div \frac{10}{3}$

45. $\frac{7}{8} \div \frac{3}{4}$

46. $\frac{1}{2} \div \frac{1}{4}$

47. $\frac{7}{12} \div \frac{21}{36}$

48. $\frac{15}{24} \div \frac{21}{48}$

49. $3\frac{3}{4} \div 2\frac{1}{3}$

50. $9 \div \frac{3}{4}$

51. $\frac{5}{8} \div 10$

52. $3\frac{3}{4} \div 1\frac{1}{4}$

53. $1\frac{5}{8} \div \frac{3}{2}$

54. $-1\frac{1}{2} \div \frac{1}{4}$

55. $3\frac{5}{6} \div 2$

56. $-9 \div 4\frac{3}{8}$

57. $5\frac{5}{8} \div 1\frac{1}{6}$

58. $2\frac{1}{4} \div 6\frac{2}{3}$

Write as a unit fraction or unit rate.

59. $\dfrac{\$1,800}{4 \text{ weeks}}$

60. $\dfrac{720 \text{ square inches}}{5 \text{ square feet}}$

61. $\dfrac{24,000 \text{ cells}}{4 \text{ square millimeters}}$

62. $\dfrac{120 \text{ mL}}{8 \text{ kg}}$

63. $\dfrac{16 \text{ grams}}{80 \text{ liters}}$

64. $\dfrac{9 \text{ feet}}{2 \text{ inches}}$

Simplify the complex fractions.

65. $\dfrac{\frac{5}{8}}{15}$

66. $\dfrac{\frac{2}{3}}{6}$

67. $\dfrac{\frac{1}{2}}{2}$

68. $\dfrac{8}{\frac{2}{3}}$

69. $\dfrac{\frac{5}{12}}{\frac{10}{3}}$

70. $\dfrac{\frac{1}{4}}{\frac{1}{2}}$

71. $\dfrac{\frac{3}{10}}{\frac{1}{5}}$

72. $\dfrac{\frac{9}{2}}{\frac{3}{4}}$

73. $\dfrac{\left(\frac{1}{4}+\frac{5}{6}\right)}{12}$

74. $\dfrac{\left(\frac{5}{6}-\frac{7}{12}\right)}{4}$

75. $\dfrac{\left(1-\frac{3}{4}\right)}{8}$

76. $\dfrac{\left(\frac{5}{9}+\frac{1}{5}\right)}{3}$

77. $\dfrac{\frac{1}{6}+\frac{2}{7}}{\frac{3}{5}-\frac{1}{4}}$

78. $\dfrac{\frac{1}{5}-\frac{1}{7}}{\frac{5}{7}+\frac{1}{10}}$

1.3 – PERCENTS AND DECIMALS

Let's begin by reviewing the different place values in a decimal number. We will use the following number for illustration.

$$23.6789$$

The 2 is in the *tens* position, the 3 is in the *ones* position, the 6 is in the *tenths* position, the 7 is in the *hundredths* position, the 8 is in the *thousandths* position, and the 9 is in the *ten-thousandths* position (and so forth). To see the reason these positions are named the way they are, let's look at a few fractions. First, note that $\frac{6}{10}$ is read as "six-tenths." Now $\frac{6}{10}$ as a decimal is 0.6. Note the six is in the tenths position. Now look at $\frac{7}{100}$. Again, this is read as "seven-hundredths." That is because $\frac{7}{100}$ written as a decimal is 0.07 and notice the 7 is in the hundredths position. The relationship between fractions and decimals is easy to see—they are simply two different notations expressing the same thing.

Percents

Percent is an important concept and is widely used in the laboratory sciences. Percentages are used for calculations associated with solutions and in areas such as clinical chemistry, nursing, hematology, immunology, and biostatistics. Percent means "per 100." Therefore, 40 out of 100 is 40%. Forty percent written as a fraction would be $\frac{40}{100}$. Percents can also be thought of as "parts over whole." Therefore, we can think of $\frac{40}{100}$ as 40 parts per 100 parts, which is precisely 40%. We also know that fractions can be written as decimals; therefore, all decimals can also be written as percents. For example, $\frac{17}{100}$ as a decimal is 0.17; to make this a percent, just multiply by 100%. That is, $\frac{17}{100}$ is equal to 0.17, and 0.17 as a percent is $0.17 \times 100\% = 17\%$. Also notice we could have multiplied as follows: $\frac{17}{100} \times 100\% = 17\%$.

As another example let's write $\frac{1}{2}$ as a percent:

$$\frac{1}{2} = 0.5 \text{, and converting to a percent, } 0.5 \times 100\% = 50\% \text{.}$$

And thus $\frac{1}{2}$ is the same as 0.5, which is the same as 50%.

> Converting a fraction to a percent:
> 1) Write the fraction as a decimal.
> 2) Multiply the decimal by 100%.

EXAMPLE 1-12: Convert the following fractions to percents.

a) $\frac{3}{8}$

$$\frac{3}{8} = 0.375 \text{; converting to a percent, } 0.375 \times 100\% = 37.5\%$$

b) $\frac{4}{5}$

$$\frac{4}{5} = 0.8 \text{; converting to a percent, } 0.8 \times 100\% = 80\%$$

> Converting a mixed number to a percent:
> 1) Write the mixed number as an improper fraction.
> 2) Write the improper fraction as a decimal.
> 3) Multiply the decimal by 100%.

EXAMPLE 1-13: Write the following mixed numbers as percents.

a) $1\frac{2}{5}$

$$1\frac{2}{5} = \frac{5 \times 1 + 2}{5} = \frac{7}{5} = 1.4 = 1.4 \times 100\% = 140\%$$

b) $2\frac{3}{4}$

$$2\frac{3}{4} = \frac{11}{4} = 2.75 = 2.75 \times 100\% = 275\%$$

Relationships among Fractions, Percents, and Decimals

Next we convert percents to decimals. To convert a percent to a decimal, divide by 100%, which is equivalent to moving the decimal to the left two places (and drop the % symbol). For example,

$$40\% = \frac{40\%}{100\%} = 0.40.$$

To convert a percent to a decimal, divide by 100% (and drop the % symbol).

It is important to have a solid understanding of the relationships among percents, decimals, and fractions. Many homework problems involve these concepts, and students are encouraged to work every problem. Understanding these relationships will greatly help you to have a good intuitive understanding of percents. Having an intuitive understanding of percents helps when solving problems involving percents.

EXAMPLE 1-14: Write 0.37 as a fraction.

Because there are two decimal places, we know this is "37 hundredths," which written as a fraction is $\frac{37}{100}$.

To convert a decimal to a percent, just multiply by 100%.

EXAMPLE 1-15: Write the following decimals as percents.

a) 0.246

Simply multiply by 100%, yielding 24.6%.

b) 2.5

Multiplying by 100% gives 250%.

EXAMPLE 1-16: Evaluate the following and express your answer as a percent. Calculations similar to these arise in hematology.

a) $80\% \times \frac{3}{4}$

First, convert $\frac{3}{4}$ to a decimal and then multiply: $80\% \times 0.75 = 60\%$.

b) $\frac{78\%}{27.6}$

$\frac{78\%}{27.6} = 2.8\%$ (All we needed to do was divide.)

c) $\frac{40\% \times (50\% \div 80\%)}{3}$

First, note that when two percents are divided, such as $50\% \div 80\%$, the percent signs cancel, $\frac{50\%}{80\%} = \frac{50}{80}$, and we are left with a fraction that can be written as a decimal without the percent sign: $\frac{50}{80} = \frac{5}{8} = 0.625$.

$$\frac{40\% \times (50\% \div 80\%)}{3} = \frac{40\% \times 0.625}{3} = \frac{25\%}{3} = 8.3\%$$

PRACTICE PROBLEMS: Section 1.3

Write the percents as decimals.

1. 5%

2. 38%

3. 12.9%

4. 2.6%

5. 0.45%

6. 125.2%

7. 8%

8. 0.2%

9. 4.5%

10. 1%

Write the decimals as percents.

11. 0.113

12. 1.56

13. 0.03

14. 0.9

15. 0.4

16. 0.167

17. 1.25

18. 0.08

19. 0.12

20. 0.33

21. 0.009

22. 0.872

Write the fractions or mixed numbers as percents. Round to two decimals when necessary.

23. $\frac{3}{4}$

24. $\frac{3}{8}$

25. $\frac{3}{5}$

26. $\frac{5}{6}$

27. $\frac{7}{11}$

28. $\frac{5}{3}$

29. $\frac{4}{5}$

30. $\frac{1}{2}$

31. $\frac{1}{4}$

32. $\frac{1}{5}$

33. $2\frac{1}{2}$

34. $3\frac{2}{5}$

35. $1\frac{3}{4}$

36. $2\frac{1}{7}$

37. $2\frac{1}{4}$

38. $3\frac{4}{5}$

Evaluate the following expressions containing percents and give your answer as a percent.

39. $15.5\% \times \frac{3}{4}$

40. $25.4\% \times 0.125$

41. $25\% \times \frac{1}{3}$

42. $20\% \times 30\%$

43. $6\% \times 70\%$

44. $\frac{1}{2}\% \times \frac{3}{4}$

45. $\frac{16\%}{2.4}$

46. $\frac{27.4\%}{8.1}$

47. $\frac{36\%}{2.4+1.2}$

48. $\frac{4.3\% \times 1.9\%}{1.2+2.7}$

CHAPTER SUMMARY

- When adding and subtracting signed numbers, it can be helpful to think of money, with positive numbers being money you have and negative numbers being money you owe.
- Multiplying two signed numbers that have the same sign results in a positive number. If the two numbers have different signs, the result will be negative. Likewise, the same applies for division.
- Rules for adding integers:
  - If the two integers have the same sign, the sign of the answer will have the same sign as the two integers.
  - If the two integers have different signs, the sign of the answer will have the sign attached to the larger integer.
- Subtraction is the same as *adding* the opposite, so the rules for subtraction are the same as the rules for adding.
- Rules for multiplication:
  - A *positive* times a *positive* equals a *positive*.
  - A *negative* times a *positive* equals a *negative*.
  - A *positive* times a *negative* equals a *negative*.
  - A *negative* times a *negative* equals a *positive*.
- Rules for division:
  - A *positive* divided by a *positive* equals a *positive*.
  - A *negative* divided by a *positive* equals a *negative*.
  - A *positive* divided by a *negative* equals a *negative*.
  - A *negative* divided by a *negative* equals a *positive*.
- Adding or subtracting fractions requires common denominators. However, common denominators are not needed for multiplying or dividing fractions.
- The least common denominator (LCD) can also be thought of as the least common multiple.
- All fractions can be represented as decimals and all decimals can be represented as fractions.
- Fractions larger than 1 can be expressed as improper fractions; therefore, all improper fractions can also be expressed as mixed numbers.
- When adding, subtracting, multiplying, or dividing mixed numbers, first convert each mixed number to an improper fraction, perform the operation, then convert the answer back to a mixed number if necessary.
- A unit fraction is any fraction that has a 1 in the numerator. In many applications we want the denominator to be 1.
- When simplifying complex fractions, first simplify the numerator and denominator and then perform the division.
- The first decimal place to the right of a decimal is the tenths position, the second is the hundredths, the third is thousandths, and so on.
- Percent means "per 100."

- To convert a decimal to a percent, multiply by 100%.
- To convert a fraction to a percent, first convert the fraction to a decimal and then multiply the decimal by 100%.

CHAPTER TEST

1. Perform the following operations.

    a) $-5 + 4$

    b) $5 - 12$

    c) $-6 - 9$

    d) $4 - (-3)$

    e) $-2 - (-5) - 4$

    f) $(-6)(-9)$

    g) $(3)(-7)$

    h) $(-2)(-3)(-8)$

    i) $\frac{-45}{-9}$

    j) $\frac{12}{-6}$

    k) $(-15) \div 3$

2. Evaluate the following.

    a) $\frac{2}{3} - \frac{5}{6}$

    b) $-\frac{5}{8} + \frac{7}{12}$

    c) $\frac{7}{8} + \frac{5}{9}$

    d) $\left(\frac{5}{9}\right)\left(\frac{3}{10}\right)$

    e) $\left(-\frac{6}{15}\right)\left(\frac{9}{2}\right)$

    f) $\frac{7}{12} \div \frac{14}{36}$

    g) $\left(\frac{3}{5}\right) \div \left(-\frac{9}{10}\right)$

    h) $3\frac{2}{5} - 1\frac{1}{4}$

    i) $4\frac{1}{5} \div 2\frac{3}{10}$

    j) $5\frac{7}{8} \times 2\frac{1}{4}$

3. Write 7% as a decimal.

4. Write 0.29 as a percent.

5. Write $\frac{3}{10}$ as a percent.

6. Write $2\frac{1}{5}$ as a percent.

7. Evaluate $\frac{2}{5} \times 28\%$ and give your answer as a percent.

2

Basic Algebra and Mathematical Essentials

INTRODUCTION

This chapter gives an overview of the essential mathematical topics encountered in the clinical and medical laboratory disciplines. Understanding these topics is important because the operations learned in this chapter, along with those in Chapter 1, will be used over and over throughout the remainder of this book as well as in other courses that follow in the clinical and medical science disciplines. Taking the time to thoroughly learn, master, and understand the topics in this chapter will pay off in the future.

2.1 – SOLVING EQUATIONS

Reciprocals

If the product of two numbers is 1, then the two numbers are said be **reciprocals** of each other. Therefore, the reciprocal of any fraction $\frac{a}{b}$ is defined as $\frac{b}{a}$ because $\frac{a}{b} \times \frac{b}{a} = 1$.

The reciprocal of 6 is $\frac{1}{6}$ because $6 \times \frac{1}{6} = 1$. Likewise, the reciprocal of $\frac{3}{5}$ is $\frac{5}{3}$ because $\frac{3}{5} \times \frac{5}{3} = 1$.

EXAMPLE 2-1: Find the reciprocal of $\frac{1}{7}$.

The reciprocal is 7 because $7 \times \frac{1}{7} = 1$.

Solving Equations

The basic idea behind solving any equation is that whatever is done to one side of the equation must also be done to the other side. The purpose is to maintain the equality. For example, consider the equation $5 = 5$. If we add 2 to just one side (say the left side) and not to the other, we get $7 = 5$, which is clearly not true. But if we add 2 to both sides, we get $7 = 7$ and maintain the equality.

Second, when solving any equation, the goal is to get the variable on one side of the equal sign and the numbers on the other side. To get the variable x by itself, we must get all the numbers on the other side of the equal sign. To accomplish this, for any number on the same side as the variable x, we perform the opposite operation (technically called the inverse operation) on both sides. For example, say we want to solve

$$x + 4 = 7.$$

The 4 is added to x on the left side, so to get the 4 on the right side, the opposite operation must be performed; therefore, to get the solution, we must subtract 4 from both sides.

$$\begin{array}{r} x + 4 = 7 \\ -4 \quad -4 \\ \hline x = 3 \end{array}$$

As another example, let's say we want to solve

$$2x = 10.$$

Notice that x is multiplied by 2. Division is the opposite of multiplication; therefore, we must divide both sides by 2 to solve this equation:

$$\frac{\cancel{2}x}{\cancel{2}} = \frac{10}{2}.$$

The 2s reduce (often we say cancel) on the left side, and we get the solution of $x = 5$.

Now let's consider solving

$$\frac{x}{3} = 8.$$

Notice that x is divided by 3. The opposite of division is multiplication; therefore, to get x by itself, we must multiply both sides by 3.

$$3 \cdot \frac{x}{3} = 8 \cdot 3$$

Simplifying we get

$$\cancel{3} \cdot \frac{x}{\cancel{3}} = 24; \text{ therefore, } x = 24.$$

Let's now solve a problem that involves several operations. Keep in mind that to successfully solve the problem, you must get rid of one number at a time by doing the opposite to both sides until you attain your goal of getting x by itself. For example, solve the following:

$$2x - 6 = 20.$$

First, add 6 to both sides.

$$
\begin{array}{r}
2x - 6 = 20 \\
+6 \;\; +6 \\
\hline
2x = 26
\end{array}
$$

Next, divide both sides by 2.

$$\frac{2x}{2} = \frac{26}{2}$$

Simplifying we get

$$x = 13.$$

Now consider solving an equation in which the number in front of x, called the **coefficient of x**, is a fraction. To solve these types of equations, multiply both sides by the reciprocal of the fraction. For example, to solve

$$\frac{3}{4}x = 12$$

note first that the coefficient of x is a fraction, thus you must multiply both sides by the reciprocal of the coefficient, yielding

$$\frac{4}{3} \cdot \frac{3}{4}x = 12 \cdot \frac{4}{3}.$$

On the left side of the equation, the 3s and 4s reduce to 1, and we are left with $1 \cdot x = x$ (which is exactly what we want). On the right side, we have an end result of 16. Remember, on the right side think of $12 \cdot \frac{4}{3}$ as $\frac{12}{1} \times \frac{4}{3} = \frac{\cancel{12}^{4}}{1} \times \frac{4}{\cancel{3}^{1}} = \frac{4 \times 4}{1 \times 1} = \frac{16}{1} = 16$. Therefore, the solution is

$$x = 16.$$

NOTE

Substituting $x = 16$ into the original equation, we get $\frac{3}{4}(16) = 12$, which is the same as $12 = 12$, which is true. This is how we check to see whether our solution is correct. It is always a good idea to check your answers.

EXAMPLE 2-2: Solve: $\frac{2}{3}x - 1 = 7$

First, add 1 to both sides, yielding

$$\frac{2}{3}x = 8 .$$

Now multiply both sides by $\frac{3}{2}$, yielding

$$x = 8 \times \frac{3}{2} = \frac{8}{1} \times \frac{3}{2} = \frac{24}{2} = 12 .$$

Again, if we substitute $x = 12$ into the original problem, we get $\frac{2}{3}(12) - 1 = 7$.
Simplifying the left-hand side, we get $8 - 1 = 7$, which is the same as $7 = 7$, which is true.

EXAMPLE 2-3: Solve: $15 = \dfrac{\frac{x}{12}}{3}$

To solve this, first multiply both sides by 3.

$$3 \cdot 15 = \dfrac{\frac{x}{12}}{3} \cdot 3$$

Simplifying we get

$$45 = \frac{x}{12} .$$

Multiplying both sides by 12, we get

$$12 \cdot 45 = \frac{x}{12} \cdot 12 ,$$

which gives us a solution of $x = 540$. (Substitute 540 into the original problem to check whether this is truly the solution.)

EXAMPLE 2-4: Solve: $\frac{x}{3} - 2 = 5$

First, add 2 to both sides.

$$\frac{x}{3} = 7$$

Because x is divided by 3, multiply both sides by 3 giving

$$(3)\frac{x}{3} = 7(3) .$$

Simplifying we get

$$x = 21 .$$

The Distributive, Commutative, and Associative Properties

The **distributive property** states that $a(b + c) = ab + ac$.

The a has been distributed to the b and the c. This can be visualized as

$$a(\overbrace{b + c)} = ab + ac.$$

EXAMPLE 2-5: Solve: $2(x - 4) = 20$

First, apply the distributive property to the left-hand side, yielding

$$2x - 2 \cdot 4 = 20,$$

which is equivalent to

$$2x - 8 = 20.$$

Adding 8 to both sides yields

$$2x = 28.$$

Dividing both sides by 2 yields $x = 14$.

EXAMPLE 2-6: Solve: $3(x + 4) - x = 36$

First, distribute the 3 onto the x and the 4, yielding

$$3x + 12 - x = 36.$$

Simplifying the left-hand side by adding the $3x$ and the $-x$ gives us

$$2x + 12 = 36.$$

Subtracting 12 from both sides gives

$$2x = 24.$$

Dividing both sides by 2, we find

$$x = 12.$$

EXAMPLE 2-7: Solve: $\frac{3(x-5)}{4} = 10$

First, simplify the numerator by distributing the 3.

$$\frac{3x-15}{4} = 10$$

Multiply both sides by 4.

$$3x - 15 = 40$$

Add 15 to both sides.

$$3x = 55$$

Dividing both sides by 3 yields

$$x = \frac{55}{3} = 18.\overline{3}.$$

The commutative and associative properties are useful to understand for conceptual reasons.

The commutative property says that, when adding and multiplying, the order of the numbers can be switched.

The formal definition of the **commutative property of addition** states that $a + b = b + a$.

For example, $2 + 3 = 3 + 2$.

The **commutative property of multiplication** states that $a \times b = b \times a$.

For example, $2 \times 3 = 3 \times 2$.

Notice, this idea of switching the order does not work for subtraction. For example, $10 - 5 \neq 5 - 10$. This idea of switching does not work for division either because $\frac{10}{5} \neq \frac{5}{10}$.

The associative property says that when adding and multiplying, we can move the parentheses.

The formal definition of the **associative property of addition** states that $(a + b) + c = a + (b + c)$.

For example, $(2 + 3) + 4 = 2 + (3 + 4)$.

The **associative property of multiplication** states that $(a \times b) \times c = a \times (b \times c)$.

For example, $(2 \times 3) \times 4 = 2 \times (3 \times 4)$.

Again, this idea of moving parentheses does not work for subtraction or division.

Simultaneous Equations

Those involved in the sciences must often work with two different equations that are interrelated. These types of equations are often referred to as **simultaneous equations**. In such cases you can frequently use given values for one variable to find the value of another variable and then substitute that result into another equation to find the value of yet another variable. Let's illustrate with an example. Say you are given the following equations and information:

$A = rT$, where $r = 5$ and $T = 6$.

$A = kc$, where $k = 10$

The question is, what is the value of c?

To solve this begin by substituting $r = 5$ and $T = 6$ into $A = rT$.

$$A = 5 \cdot 6 = 30$$

Now substitute this value of A, along with the fact that $k = 10$, into the equation $A = kc$, yielding

$$30 = 10 \cdot c.$$

Now divide both sides by 10 and simplify.

$$\frac{30}{10} = \frac{\cancel{10} \cdot c}{\cancel{10}}$$

We find that

$$c = 3.$$

EXAMPLE 2-8: Find the value of V given the following equations and values:

$PV = cT$, where $c = 100$ and $P = 75$.

$T = 5s$, where $s = 12$

First, substitute $s = 12$ into the equation $T = 5s$ to find T.

$$T = 5 \cdot 12 = 60$$

Next, substitute $T = 60$, $c = 100$, and $P = 75$ into the first equation, $PV = cT$.

$$75V = 100 \cdot 60$$

Simplifying the right-hand side yields

$$75V = 6{,}000.$$

Dividing both sides by 75, we get

$$V = \frac{6{,}000}{75} = 80.$$

NOTE

One way to check your answer is to substitute the found values into both of the original equations, $PV = cT$ and $T = 5s$.

$$PV = cT:\ 75 \cdot 80 = 100 \cdot 60$$

Simplifying both sides we find

$$6,000 = 6,000,$$

which is certainly true. Likewise,

$$T = 5s : 60 = 5(12) = 60,$$

which is also true.

PRACTICE PROBLEMS: Section 2.1

Solve the equations and check your answers.

1. $x + 12 = 8$

2. $2x - 3 = -9$

3. $3x + 4 = 22$

4. $5 = -7 + 4x$

5. $5x - 8 = 5 + 12$

6. $4 = -5 + 3x$

7. $8 - 6x = -58$

8. $2 = 8 - x$

9. $3(x - 5) = 30$

10. $2(x + 5) = 20$

11. $2(x - 6) - 8 = 4$

12. $4(x + 7) + 2 = 0$

13. $-(x - 6) + 3 = -12$

14. $8 - 2(x - 1) = 24$

15. $-x - 4 = -6$

16. $\frac{x}{3} = 8.2$

17. $\frac{2}{x} = 4$

18. $\frac{7}{x} = 15$

19. $\frac{2x}{5} = 8$

20. $\frac{20}{3x} = -5$

21. $\frac{7}{x} = 14$

22. $3x = \frac{9}{4}$

23. $2x = \frac{1}{2}$

24. $-5x = \frac{3}{8}$

25. $\frac{5}{8} \times \frac{1}{x} = 1,000$

26. $\frac{\frac{4}{x}}{5} = 12$

27. $5.2 \times \frac{x}{7} = \frac{4}{5}$

28. $\frac{x}{1.8} + 4.1 = 9.7$

29. $5 \times \frac{x}{3} = 10$

30. $\frac{\frac{1}{x}}{2} = 4$

31. $\frac{x}{15} = 3$

32. $\frac{2}{3}x = 8$

33. $\frac{x}{6} = 4$

34. $\frac{3}{4}x = 9$

35. $\frac{1}{4}x = 25$

36. $\frac{x}{6} = 0$

37. $\frac{4}{5}x = 12$

38. $\frac{\frac{1}{5}}{x} = \frac{2}{3}$

39. $\dfrac{5}{x} \times \dfrac{5}{6} = 1{,}200$

40. $\dfrac{x}{12.7} = 2.1$

Solve the following simultaneous equations and check your answers.

41. Find the value of x given that $a = 5$: $y = 3a$
$x = 4y$

42. Find the value of r given that $s = 3$: $t = 4s - 5$
$r = 2s + t$

43. Find the value of y given that $z = 6$ and $v = 8$: $x = \dfrac{3v}{z}$
$y = \dfrac{4x}{2}$

44. Find the value of z given that $w = 2.5$: $t = 3.5w$
$z = 4.8t - 1.9$

45. Find the value of A given that $t = 4$: $r = 1.5t$
$A = 3.14\,r^2$

46. Find the value of x given that $y = -2$: $t = 4y$
$x = -6t$

2.2 – FORMULAS

Often we work with formulas that do not have many numbers. Our approach to solving these formulas is the same as our approach to solving equations. For example, say we want to solve the equation $A = \epsilon c l$ for ϵ. (This equation is Beer's Law, where A is the absorbance, c is the concentration, l is the path length, and ϵ is some constant.) First, remember that our goal is to get ϵ by itself. So we want to get rid of c and l. How do we do this? Notice that ϵ is multiplied by both c and l. Therefore, to get rid of c and l, divide both sides by cl.

$$\frac{A}{cl} = \frac{\epsilon c l}{cl}$$

The c's and l's on the right side reduce to 1 and we get

$$\frac{A}{cl} = \frac{\epsilon\, \cancel{cl}}{\cancel{cl}}, \text{ which simplifies to } \frac{A}{cl} = \epsilon$$

or equivalently

$$\epsilon = \frac{A}{cl}.$$

Now let's say we want to solve the equation $A = kc$ for c. We want c by itself, so we must get rid of k. Because c is multiplied by k, divide both sides by k to get c by itself.

$$\frac{A}{k} = \frac{kc}{k}$$

Now the k's on the right side reduce and we get

$$\frac{A}{k} = \frac{\cancel{k}c}{\cancel{k}} \text{, which simplifies to } c = \frac{A}{k}.$$

EXAMPLE 2-9: Solve for r: $Ar = st$

Our goal is to get r by itself. Thus, we need to get rid of the A. Because A and r are multiplied, to get r by itself we must divide both sides by A.

$$\frac{\cancel{A}r}{\cancel{A}} = \frac{st}{A} \text{, which simplifies to } r = \frac{st}{A}$$

EXAMPLE 2-10: Solve for m: $y = mx + b$

First, subtract b from both sides, yielding

$$y - b = mx.$$

To get m by itself, divide both sides by x.

$$\frac{y-b}{x} = \frac{m\cancel{x}}{\cancel{x}} \text{ and simplifying we get } \frac{y-b}{x} = m$$

EXAMPLE 2-11: Solve the following equation for t. (This equation is distance equals rate times time.)

$$D = rt$$

To isolate t, get rid of r. Because r is multiplied, divide both sides by r.

$$\frac{D}{r} = \frac{rt}{r}$$

The r's reduce on the right side, and we get the solution of

$$t = \frac{D}{r}.$$

PRACTICE PROBLEMS: Section 2.2

Solve the equations for the given variable.

1. $A = \epsilon c l$; c

2. $AB = CD$; C

3. $V = lwh$; w

4. $Q = \frac{3}{4}Dh$; h

5. $A = b + c + d$; c

6. $c = 2a - r$; a

7. $A = \frac{bh}{2}$; h

8. $C = 2\pi r$; r

9. $R = \frac{h}{2}(a + b)$; a

10. $S = 4lw + 2wh$; h

11. $y = 4x - 12$; x

12. $5x - 4y = 15$; y

13. $x - y = 2$; y

14. $8x + 2y = 20$; y

15. $4y - 12x + 8 = 0$; y

16. $5x - y = 1$; y

2.3 – RATIOS AND PROPORTIONS

A **ratio** is the quotient of two quantities. The ratio of 1 to 2 is usually written in one of the following three ways:

$$1 \text{ to } 2 \quad \text{or} \quad \frac{1}{2} \quad \text{or} \quad 1 : 2.$$

All of these are read as "the ratio of 1 to 2." By definition, ratios are used to compare the relationship of two quantities with the same units. If the units are different, it is called a **rate**. Therefore, ratios have no units associated with them because the units cancel. For example, the ratio of 3 feet to 8 feet is $\frac{3 \cancel{ft}}{8 \cancel{ft}} = \frac{3}{8}$. Often we want to write the result in reduced form. For example, write the ratio of $15 to $10 in reduced form. The solution is $\frac{\$15}{\$10} = \frac{\cancel{\$}3 \cdot \cancel{5}}{\cancel{\$}2 \cdot \cancel{5}} = \frac{3}{2}$.

Two ratios are said to be in **proportion** with each other if they are equivalent. For example, $\frac{2}{3}$ is in proportion with $\frac{6}{9}$ because $\frac{2}{3} = \frac{6}{9}$. If two ratios are in proportion, their **cross products** must be equal. Using this fact we show that $\frac{2}{3}$ is in proportion with $\frac{6}{9}$ by demonstrating that their cross products are equal:

$$\frac{2}{3} \bowtie \frac{6}{9}$$

Cross product says that $3 \times 6 = 2 \times 9$ or $18 = 18$.

This fact that cross products of proportions are equal is the underlying concept of how we solve problems involving proportions. In the laboratory and health professions, many problems are solved using proportions. For example, if the concentration of a mixture is to be 5 parts serum per 2 parts H_2O, then how many parts of serum should be used to make a solution having 7 parts H_2O? Because the two mixtures have the same concentration, they are in proportion with each other. That is

$$\frac{\text{Parts serum}}{\text{Parts } H_2O} = \frac{\text{Parts serum}}{\text{Parts } H_2O} \cdot$$

In this example we have

$$\frac{5 \text{ parts serum}}{2 \text{ parts water}} = \frac{x \text{ parts serum}}{7 \text{ parts water}} \cdot$$

To solve this, cross multiply.

$$\frac{5 \text{ parts serum}}{2 \text{ parts water}} \diagdown\!\!\!\!\diagup \frac{x \text{ parts serum}}{7 \text{ parts water}}$$

After cross multiplication the resulting equation is

$$2x = 5 \times 7$$

or

$$2x = 35 \, .$$

Dividing by 2 we get

$$x = 17.5 \, .$$

Therefore, to make a 7 parts H_2O solution with the desired concentration of 5 parts serum to every 2 parts water, you would have to mix 17.5 parts of serum with the 7 parts of water.

EXAMPLE 2-12: Fifty units of glucose are needed for every 2,400 units of saline. How many units of glucose do we need if we have 15,360 units of saline and wish to keep the same concentration?

$$\frac{50 \text{ units glucose}}{2,400 \text{ units saline}} = \frac{x \text{ units glucose}}{15,360 \text{ units saline}}$$

Cross multiplying we get

$$2,400x = 50 \times 15,360$$

$$2,400x = 768,000 \, .$$

Dividing by 2,400 we get

$$x = \frac{768,000}{2,400} \cdot$$

Simplifying we find

$$x = 320 \text{ units of glucose.}$$

> When you solve proportions, the units on the left-hand side of the equation must be set up exactly as the units on the right-hand side.

In Example 2-12 we had glucose over saline on the left-hand side and glucose over saline on the right-hand side. If glucose over saline had been on the left and saline over glucose on the right, the problem would *not* have worked out. This is the primary focus when solving proportion problems—the units must be consistent on both sides.

EXAMPLE 2-13: A solution must be made such that for every 1 part serum there is a total of 4 parts solution. If the total volume is to be 100 units, how much serum is needed?

We are given 1 part serum in a total of 4 parts solution. Setting this up and keeping our units consistent on both sides we get

$$\frac{1 \text{ serum}}{4 \text{ total}} = \frac{x \text{ serum}}{100 \text{ total}}.$$

Cross multiplying we get

$$4x = 100.$$

Dividing by 4 we get

$$x = 25.$$

Therefore, we need 25 parts of serum. Note: To actually make this 100-part solution we would take 25 parts of serum and add it to 75 parts of diluent to get our desired total of 100.

EXAMPLE 2-14: A solution is to be made that has 1 part of reagent for every 9 parts of water. If a lab technician must make a total of 500 parts of this solution, how much reagent should be used and how much water should be used?

First notice that 1 part of reagent plus 9 parts water gives a solution whose total volume is 10. Therefore, our proportion is

$$\frac{1 \text{ reagent}}{10 \text{ parts total solution}} = \frac{x \text{ reagent}}{500 \text{ parts total solution}}.$$

Cross multiplying we get

$$10x = 500.$$

Dividing by 10 we find

$$x = 50.$$

Therefore, to make this solution, we must have 50 parts of reagent. Keep in mind that to make the solution we add the reagent to the water to get the total solution. If we let y equal the amount of water needed for our 500 parts of solution, then our equation would be

$$y + 50 = 500.$$

Subtracting 50 from both sides we find

$$y = 450.$$

Therefore, to make the 500 parts solution, we need 50 parts of reagent and 450 parts of water.

PRACTICE PROBLEMS: Section 2.3

Solve for x.

1. $\dfrac{5}{x} = \dfrac{11}{17}$

2. $\dfrac{x}{110} = \dfrac{200}{160}$

3. $\dfrac{x}{50} = \dfrac{1,200}{45}$

4. $\dfrac{1,500}{x} = \dfrac{2,000}{3,000}$

5. $\dfrac{1}{3} = \dfrac{5}{x}$

6. $\dfrac{3}{5} = \dfrac{12}{x}$

7. $\dfrac{15}{50} = \dfrac{x}{200}$

8. $0 = \dfrac{x}{5}$

9. $\dfrac{2}{x} = 8$

10. $\dfrac{6}{x} = \dfrac{48}{80}$

11. $\dfrac{x}{4} = \dfrac{25}{16}$

12. $\dfrac{3}{8} = \dfrac{9}{x}$

Solve the following proportion problems.

13. For every 1,800 mL of saline, 40 mL of serum is needed. How many grams of serum do we need if we have 9,450 mL of saline and wish to keep the same concentration?

14. For every 400 mL of saline, 28 mL of serum is needed. How many grams of serum do we need if we have 1,300 mL of saline and wish to keep the same concentration?

15. A solution must be made such that for every 1 part serum we have a total volume of 5 parts solution. If the total volume is to be 100 mL, how much serum do we need?

16. A solution must be made such that for every 2 parts serum we have a total volume of 5 parts solution. If the total volume is to be 400 mL, how much serum do we need?

17. A solution must be made such that for every 3 parts serum we have a total volume of 10 parts solution. If the total volume is to be 500 mL, how much serum do we need?

18. A urine sample has a total volume of 1,900 mL and a total of 800 mg of protein. Find the amount of protein in 380 mL of this same urine sample.

19. A urine sample has a total volume of 1,300 mL and a total of 700 mg of protein. Find the amount of protein in 650 mL of this same urine sample.

20. For every 1.5 L total volume, there must be 0.2 L of saline. How many liters of saline are needed if there is a total volume of 10.8 L?

21. A large 5-foot-tall plastic cylindrical barrel holds 1,500 L of saline when completely filled. How many liters of saline are in the barrel if the height of the saline is 3 feet?

22. For every 2.5 L total volume there must be 0.3 L of saline. How many liters of saline are needed if there is a total volume of 12 L?

23. For every 3 mg of drug, 20 mL of saline is needed. How many milliliters of saline are required for 170 mg of drug?

24. For every 1.8 mg of drug, 5 mL of saline is needed. How many milliliters of saline are required for 45 mg of drug?

25. A bag is being filled with saline at the rate of 50 mL per minute. How long will it take to fill a 1,000 mL bag?

26. A bag is being filled with saline at the rate of 125 mL per minute. How long will it take to fill a 1,000 mL bag?

27. A bag is being drained at the rate of 150 mL per hour. How long will it take to drain a 1,000 mL bag?

28. A bag is being drained at the rate of 400 mL per hour. How long will it take to drain a 1,000 mL bag?

29. One kilogram equals 2.2 lb. How many kilograms are in 110 pounds?

30. One kilogram equals 2.2 lb. How many kilograms are in 44 pounds?

31. Every 5 mL of solution contains 8 mg of drug. How many milligrams of drug are in 38 mL of solution?

32. Every 6 mL of solution contains 10 mg of drug. How many milligrams of drug are in 20 mL of solution?

33. Every 5 mL of solution contains 4 mg of drug. If a patient needs 30 mg of drug, how many milliliters of solution should the patient receive?

34. Every 4 mL of solution contains 12 mg of drug. If a patient needs 40 mg of drug, how many milliliters of solution should the patient receive?

2.4 – SOLVING PERCENT PROBLEMS

Normally, when we work problems involving percents, we must write the percent as a decimal. For example, how do we find 25% of a number? The answer is multiply the number by 0.25. To find 25% of 200, multiply 200 by 0.25 or

$$200 \times 0.25 = 50.$$

This makes sense because 50 is $\frac{1}{4}$ (or 0.25) of 200.

However, what if the problem reads "35% of what number is 21"? These types of problems can be solved in two different ways, namely by translating the phrase into an equation and by using proportions. The unknown will be represented by x.

$$\underline{35\%} \text{ of } \underbrace{\text{what number}} \text{ is } 21$$

Corresponding equation → $0.35 \times \quad x \quad = 21$

or

$$0.35x = 21$$

To solve this equation, divide both sides by 0.35, yielding

$$x = \frac{21}{0.35}.$$

Plugging $\frac{21}{0.35}$ into the calculator, we get

$$x = 60.$$

Therefore 35% of 60 is 21. We can check that this is true because 0.35×60 does equal 21.

Another common method utilized to solve percent problems is to use proportions. The basic formula used when solving percent problems using proportions is

$$\frac{\text{Part}}{\text{Whole}} = \frac{\text{Percent}}{100}$$

NOTE

When using the proportion method, we do not use the decimal form of the percent.

Let's now solve the problem "35% of what number is 21" using proportions. First, because we are finding 35% of some number, this unknown number is the whole portion, 21 is part of the whole portion, and 35 is the percent. Substituting these values into the preceding formula, we get

$$\frac{21}{x} = \frac{35}{100}.$$

Cross multiplying we get

$$35x = 2,100.$$

Dividing both sides by 35 we find

$$x = \frac{2,100}{35} = 60.$$

EXAMPLE 2-15: What number is 38% of 250?

a) Solving by translation:

First, we translate into an equation as follows:

$$\underbrace{\text{What number}}_{x} \text{ is } \underbrace{38\%}_{= 0.38} \text{ of } 250$$
$$\times 250$$

or

$$x = 0.38(250)$$

Next, solve this equation. In this case simply multiply the right-hand side to find

$$x = 95.$$

b) Solving the same problem by using proportions:

First, the percent is 38 and the whole portion is 250 since we are asked to find the part that is 38% of 250. Substituting these into the formula

$$\frac{\text{Part}}{\text{Whole}} = \frac{\text{Percent}}{100}$$

we obtain

$$\frac{x}{250} = \frac{38}{100}.$$

Cross multiplying we get

$$100x = (38)(250).$$

Simplify the right-hand side.

$$100x = 9,500$$

Dividing both sides by 100, we find

$$x = \frac{9,500}{100} = 95 \,.$$

EXAMPLE 2-16: 25 is what percent of 200?

a)   Solving by translation:

First, write as an equation: $25 = x \cdot 200$. To solve this divide both sides by 200, yielding

$$\frac{25}{200} = x \,.$$

Writing as a decimal, we find

$$x = \frac{25}{200} = 0.125 = 12.5\%.$$

b)   Solving by proportion:

First, we see that 25 is the part, 200 is the whole, and the percent is the unknown. Substituting these into the proportion formula, we obtain

$$\frac{25}{200} = \frac{x}{100} \,.$$

Cross multiplying we get

$$200x = 2,500 \,.$$

Dividing both sides by 200, we find

$$x = \frac{2,500}{200} = 12.5\%.$$

EXAMPLE 2-17: A test is run in the laboratory. If 825 of the test results were positive out of a total of 1,100 test results, what percent of the test results were positive? What percent of the results were negative?

Because a percent is $\dfrac{\text{Part}}{\text{Whole}}$, the percent of positive results would be $\dfrac{825}{1,100} = 0.75 = 75\%$.

To find the number of negative results, keep in mind that all the positive results plus all the negative results must total all of the results or 100% of the results. Therefore, the percent of results that are negative would be $100\% - 75\% = 25\%$.

EXAMPLE 2-18: If a technician makes a mistake on 0.7% of all his measurements performed in the laboratory, how many mistakes will be made by this technician if he performs 286 measurements?

The question really is "What is 0.7% of 286?" The answer is

$$0.7\% \times 286 = 0.007 \times 286 = 2.002 \approx 2.$$

Therefore, this technician will make a mistake in about 2 out of every 286 measurements, which is $\dfrac{2 \text{ errors}}{286 \text{ measurements}} = \dfrac{1 \text{ error}}{143 \text{ measurements}}$. Thus, we could say the technician will make an error once in every 143 measurements.

PRACTICE PROBLEMS: Section 2.4

Solve the following percent problems.

1. 16 is what percent of 100?
2. 16 is what percent of 200?
3. 16 is what percent of 400?
4. 12 is what percent of 140?
5. 50 is what percent of 200?
6. 20 is what percent of 80?
7. 25 is 50% of what number?
8. 58 is 30% of what number?
9. 121 is 20% of what number?
10. 90 is 40% of what number?

11. 10 is 25% of what number?
12. 8 is 2% of what number?
13. What number is 30% of 250?
14. What number is 7% of 60?
15. What number is $2\frac{1}{2}\%$ of 160?
16. What number is 4% of 200?
17. What number is 20% of 300?
18. What is 15% of 90?

Solve the percent problems.

19. If 100 fluid ounces of a solution contains 20 fluid ounces of a chemical, what percent of the solution is chemical?
20. If 200 fluid ounces of a solution contains 20 fluid ounces of a reagent, what percent of the solution is reagent?
21. A solution contains water and a liquid chemical. How much liquid chemical is in 150 fluid ounces of this solution if 12% of the solution is liquid chemical?

Continues

PRACTICE PROBLEMS: Section 2.4 *(continued)*

22. If 200 fluid ounces of solution contains 12 fluid ounces of some chemical, what percent of the solution is not chemical?

23. If 300 fluid ounces of solution contains 18 fluid ounces of some reagent, what percent of the solution is not reagent?

24. Two out of 30 days there is at least one laboratory technician who is unable to make it to work. What percent of the days is there at least one technician unable to make it to work? What percent of the days do all the technicians make it to work?

25. If 1.2% of all shipped volumetric flasks are damaged upon arrival, approximately how many will arrive damaged if a laboratory receives a shipment of 1,200 flasks?

26. A test is run in the laboratory. If 625 of the test results were positive out of a total of 950 test results, what percent of the test results were positive? What percent of the results were negative?

27. A test is run in the laboratory. If 312 of the test results were negative out of a total of 500 test results, what percent of the test results were positive?

28. The cholesterol count in a blood sample was 198. A few months later the count was 178. What was the percent decrease in the cholesterol count?

29. If 70 out of every 80 patients thought to have a disease tested positive, what percent tested positive?

30. If 6 out of every 120 patients thought to have a disease tested negative, what percent tested negative?

2.5 – PROPERTIES OF EXPONENTS

Let's begin by noting that exponentials are used to represent repeated multiplication, as shown in the following example:

$$3^4 = 3 \times 3 \times 3 \times 3 = 81.$$

Remember also that the 3 in the above equation is called the **base** and the 4 is called the **exponent**. The question is, what is the rule when multiplying two exponentials with the same base? The answer is that we add the exponents, but why? To answer this let's look at the following situation.

$$2^3 \cdot 2^4$$

By our rule we add the exponents to get the answer of $2^{3+4} = 2^7$. The reasoning is as follows:

$$2^3 \cdot 2^4 = \underbrace{2 \times 2 \times 2}_{2^3} \cdot \underbrace{2 \times 2 \times 2 \times 2}_{2^4} = 2^7 \text{ because there are a total of seven 2s.}$$

In general the rule is: $x^A \cdot x^B = x^{A+B}$. We refer to this rule as the **product rule**.

EXAMPLE 2-19: Simplify: $4^5 \cdot 4^6$

Adding the exponents we get $4^{5+6} = 4^{11}$.

Our next situation is the division of two exponentials with the same base. Let's simplify the following expression and then figure out what the rule is.

$$\frac{4^5}{4^3} = \frac{4 \times 4 \times 4 \times 4 \times 4}{4 \times 4 \times 4} = \frac{\cancel{4} \times \cancel{4} \times \cancel{4} \times 4 \times 4}{\cancel{4} \times \cancel{4} \times \cancel{4}} = 4 \times 4 = 4^2$$

When we reduced the 4s, we essentially subtracted. Thus, $\frac{4^5}{4^3} = 4^{5-3} = 4^2$. Therefore, our rule when dividing exponentials with the same base is to subtract the exponents. In general the rule is

$$\frac{x^A}{x^B} = x^{A-B}.$$

We refer to this rule as the **quotient rule**.

EXAMPLE 2-20: Simplify: $\dfrac{8^{10}}{8^4}$

Subtracting the exponents we get $8^{10-4} = 8^6$.

Next, we discuss what to do when an exponential is raised to an exponent such as $\left(2^3\right)^4$. We will simplify this expression and logically deduce what the formula is.

By the definition of exponents,

$$\left(2^3\right)^4 = 2^3 \times 2^3 \times 2^3 \times 2^3.$$

But from the product rule, we know to add the exponents:

$$\left(2^3\right)^4 = 2^3 \times 2^3 \times 2^3 \times 2^3 = 2^{3+3+3+3} = 2^{12}.$$

In Chapter 1 we discussed that repeated addition (i.e., $3 + 3 + 3 + 3$) is nothing more than multiplication. Therefore, all we have to do is multiply the exponents. That is

$$\left(2^3\right)^4 = 2^{3 \times 4} = 2^{12}.$$

In general our rule is $\left(x^A\right)^B = x^{A \times B}$. We refer to this rule as the **power rule**.

EXAMPLE 2-21: Simplify: $\left(3^5\right)^4$

Multiplying the exponents we get $3^{5\times4} = 3^{20}$.

Our next question is, when applying the quotient rule, what if the value of the exponent in the numerator is smaller than the exponent in the denominator? When we subtract, the exponent will be negative. To investigate further we inspect the following concrete example:

$$\frac{4^3}{4^5} = 4^{3-5} = 4^{-2}.$$

We could also have simplified this by reducing as follows:

$$\frac{4^3}{4^5} = \frac{\cancel{4}\times\cancel{4}\times\cancel{4}}{\cancel{4}\times\cancel{4}\times\cancel{4}\times4\times4} = \frac{1}{4^2}.$$

From the previous two facts, we can conclude that $4^{-2} = \frac{1}{4^2}$. In general our rule is $x^{-A} = \frac{1}{x^A}$. We refer to this rule as the **negative exponent rule**.

EXAMPLE 2-22: Simplify: $\frac{10^5}{10^8}$

Subtracting the exponents we get $10^{5-8} = 10^{-3} = \frac{1}{10^3} = \frac{1}{1,000}$.

Following is a summary of the exponent rules:

EXPONENT RULES

Product rule: $x^A \cdot x^B = x^{A+B}$

Quotient rule: $\frac{x^A}{x^B} = x^{A-B}$

Power rule: $\left(x^A\right)^B = x^{A\times B}$

Negative exponent rule: $x^{-A} = \frac{1}{x^A}$

Let's continue with a few examples.

EXAMPLE 2-23: Simplify the following.

a) $10^8 \times 10^{-5}$

Adding the exponents, $10^{8+(-5)} = 10^3$.

b) $\left(4^3\right)^{-2}$

Multiplying the exponents, $4^{3\times(-2)} = 4^{-6} = \frac{1}{4^6} = \frac{1}{4,096}$.

c) $\dfrac{3^4}{3^{-2}}$

Subtracting the exponents, $3^{4-(-2)} = 3^{4+2} = 3^6$.

Remember, these rules apply only when the bases are the same. If the bases are different, the rules do not apply. For example,

$$2^3 \times 4^2 \neq 8^5.$$

To evaluate this we must evaluate each piece and then multiply.

$$2^3 \times 4^2 = 8 \times 16 = 128$$

We must also be careful when adding. For example,

$$3^2 + 3^2 = 9 + 9 = 18.$$

There is no exponent rule for adding. Remember, exponentials mean multiply. Therefore, to add $10^{-2} + 10^{-3}$ we cannot apply any of our exponent rules because none of the rules apply for addition. To add these, first apply the negative exponent rule:

$$\frac{1}{10^2} + \frac{1}{10^3}.$$

At this point we are back to the basics of adding fractions. Remember, we need a common denominator. In this case the LCD would be 10^3. Therefore, multiply the first fraction by $\dfrac{10}{10}$ to get a common denominator so we can add:

$$\frac{10}{10} \cdot \frac{1}{10^2} + \frac{1}{10^3} = \frac{10}{10^3} + \frac{1}{10^3} = \frac{10+1}{10^3} = \frac{11}{10^3} = \frac{11}{1{,}000}.$$

EXAMPLE 2-24: Add $10^5 + 10^{-4}$.

First, rewrite 10^{-4} as a fraction: $10^5 + \dfrac{1}{10^4}$. Now we are right back to adding fractions; thus, we need a common denominator. In this case that would be 10^4. Now manipulate the problem so each fraction has a denominator of 10^4 as follows:

$$\frac{10^4}{10^4} \cdot \frac{10^5}{1} + \frac{1}{10^4} = \frac{10^9}{10^4} + \frac{1}{10^4} = \frac{10^9+1}{10^4}.$$

PRACTICE PROBLEMS: Section 2.5

Simplify and express your answers with positive exponents.

1. $3^4 \cdot 3^7$
2. $10^{-3} \cdot 10^2$
3. $10^3 \cdot 10^3$
4. $2^0 \cdot 2^4$
5. $5^3 \cdot 4^6$
6. $2^2 \cdot 3^2$
7. $x^5 \cdot x^{-2}$
8. $x^3 \cdot x^8$
9. $y^{-5} \cdot y^{-4}$
10. $a^{-6} \cdot a^3$
11. $x^{-1} \cdot x^{-7}$
12. $x^4 \cdot x^0$
13. $\left(x^3\right)^4$
14. $\left(x^2\right)^7$
15. $\left(x^5\right)^{-2}$
16. $\left(c^{-5}\right)^{-6}$

17. $\left(x^{-2}\right)^9$
18. $\left(x^{-4}\right)^{-8}$
19. $\dfrac{x^8}{x^5}$
20. $\dfrac{y^4}{y^{-3}}$
21. $\dfrac{x^3}{x^9}$
22. $\dfrac{x^4}{x^{-2}}$
23. $\dfrac{y^{-7}}{y^{-3}}$
24. $\dfrac{a^{-2}}{a^5}$
25. $\left(10^{-3}\right)^2$
26. $\dfrac{10^{-6}}{10^{-2}}$
27. $\dfrac{10^{-8}}{10^3}$

28. $\left(10^4\right)^{-3}$
29. $\dfrac{10^{-1}}{10^{-2}}$
30. $\dfrac{10^{-9}}{10^{-3}}$
31. $10^{-12} \times 10^8$
32. $\dfrac{10^7 \times 10^{-10}}{10^{-5}}$
33. $10^{-5} \times 10^{-1}$
34. $10^{-10} \times 10$
35. $\dfrac{10^{-5} \times 10^{-2}}{10^{-3}}$
36. $\dfrac{10^3 \times 10^5 \times 10^{-2}}{10^{-6}}$
37. $\dfrac{10 \times 10^3}{10^{-3}}$
38. $\dfrac{10^{-2} \times 10^{10}}{10^8}$

Evaluate the following, leaving your answer in exponential form.

39. $10^2 + 10^5$
40. $10^4 + 10^{-2}$
41. $10^{-1} + 10^{-2}$
42. $5^{-2} + 5^{-3}$
43. $10 + 10^{-1}$
44. $10^{-1} + 10^{-1}$

2.6 – ORDER OF OPERATIONS

The order of operations is a systematic way of calculating the value of a mathematical expression such as

$$(3+3)^2 \div 4 + 5.$$

It is important to understand order of operations because calculators and computers are programmed to use this same procedure when they calculate the value of a mathematical expression. You must keep this in mind whenever you are typing a problem into a calculator (or computer). It must be typed in correctly by taking into consideration the order of operations! Next is a step-by-step process for following the order of operations.

THE ORDER OF OPERATIONS

1) Simplify parentheses and brackets (in general grouping symbols).
2) Evaluate exponents.
3) Multiply and divide as operations occur from left to right.
4) Add and subtract (as these operations occur from left to right).

One way to remember the order of operations is to think of the acronym **PEMDAS**. The P stands for parentheses, E for exponents, M for multiplication, D for division, A for addition, and S for subtraction.

EXAMPLE 2-25:

a) Evaluate: $3 \times 4 + 6 \div 2 + 4 \times 3$

First, we see there are no grouping symbols. Therefore, we move to step 2. There are no exponents either, so we move to step 3, which instructs us to do all multiplications and divisions from left to right. Doing this we end up with

$$12 + 3 + 12 \,.$$

Last, we add, giving us the end result of 27.

b) Evaluate: $(2 + 4)^2 \div 4 \times 2$

Simplifying the parentheses we get $(6)^2 \div 4 \times 2$.

After step 2 (evaluate exponents), we get $36 \div 4 \times 2$.

For step 3 remember to multiply and divide *from left to right*.

$$\underset{9}{\underline{36 \div 4}} \times 2 \text{ gives us } 9 \times 2 = 18$$

Therefore, our answer is 18.

c) Evaluate: $(5 + 4 + 6) \div (2 + 3) - 1$

Simplifying parentheses: $15 \div 5 - 1$.

There are no exponents, so we move to step 3. After we do the division, we get $3 - 1$.

The last step is subtract and thus the answer is 2.

d) Compare the result of $4 \times 4 \div 4 \times 4$ with $4 \times 4 \div (4 \times 4)$.

To evaluate $4 \times 4 \div 4 \times 4$, multiply and divide as these operations occur from left to right.

$$4 \times 4 \div 4 \times 4 = \underset{16}{\underline{4 \times 4}} \div 4 \times 4 = \underset{4}{\underline{16 \div 4}} \times 4 = 4 \times 4 = 16$$

To evaluate $4 \times 4 \div (4 \times 4)$, first simplify the parentheses and then multiply and divide from left to right.

$$4 \times 4 \div (4 \times 4) = 4 \times 4 \div 16 = 16 \div 16 = 1$$

NOTE

There is a significant difference in the end results with and without the parentheses. Understanding the use of parentheses, or the lack thereof, is very important when using the calculator to evaluate mathematical expressions. We discuss this further in Section 2.10.

PRACTICE PROBLEMS: Section 2.6

Evaluate by using the order of operations.

1. $4^2 - (-3)^2$

2. $\dfrac{-8 - 4^2}{2^3 - 2}$

3. $\left((5 - 3)^2 \right)^2$

4. $\dfrac{(3 - 5)^2 \div 2 + 4}{2^4 - 13}$

5. $\dfrac{3}{4} \times 16 \div 2 + 2$

6. $5 - 4 \times \dfrac{1}{2} \div 4 + \dfrac{1}{2}$

7. $\dfrac{(-2)^3 \cdot [4^2 - 12]}{3^2 \div 3 - 1}$

8. $3 + 2(4 - 1)$

9. $8 - 4(3^2 - 7)$

10. $4 \times 6 \div 4 + 4$

11. $(2^2 + 8) \div 4 - 2$

12. $\dfrac{10 + 2}{8 - 6}$

13. $7 + 3 \cdot 2$

14. $\dfrac{6^2 + 2(4 + 2)}{2 \cdot 4}$

2.7 – SIGNIFICANT DIGITS AND ROUNDING

When rounding decimal numbers to the nearest tenths, hundredths, thousandths, and so on, look to the immediate right of the digit located in the position to be rounded. If the number to the direct right is 5 or larger, round the position being rounded up one number and drop everything that follows. If the number to the direct right is 4 or smaller, leave the position being rounded as is and drop everything that follows. Following are some examples.

EXAMPLE 2-26:

a) Round 12.486 to the tenths position.

First, identify the tenths position. Clearly the 4 is in the tenths position. The number directly to the right of 4 is 8, which is 5 or larger; therefore, increase 4 by one and drop the remaining portion, giving the end result of 12.5.

b) Round 36.1529 to the nearest hundredths position.

First, identify the hundredths position. Clearly the 5 is in the hundredths position. The number directly to the right of 5 is 2, which is 4 or less; therefore, leave the 5 as is and drop the remaining portion, giving the end result of 36.15.

c) Round 1.49548 to the nearest thousandth.

First, identify the thousandths position. Clearly the 5 is in the thousandths position. The number directly to the right of 5 is 4, which is 4 or less; therefore, leave the 5 as is and drop the remaining portion, giving the end result of 1.495.

Significant Digits

When using an instrument to measure quantities in the laboratory, the results will not be exact. As a consequence there is always some amount of uncertainty. For example, if we are measuring the volume of a solution, maybe we can measure "correctly" only to the nearest tenths position. Therefore, the answer would most likely contain two decimal places. This is because the last significant digit is the first estimated position. So, the number of digits contained in our answer tells us about how uncertain (or certain) our measurement is. The **significant digits** in a number tell us about the accuracy of a measurement. To determine how many significant digits are contained in a given number, use the following rules:

RULE 1: DETERMINING WHETHER A DIGIT IS SIGNIFICANT

a) All nonzero digits are significant.
b) Zeros are significant if they are on the right side of a *decimal* number.
c) Zeros are significant if they are between two significant digits.

RULE 2: DETERMINING WHETHER A ZERO IS NOT SIGNIFICANT

a) A zero is not significant if it is on the right side of a *whole* number.
b) A zero is not significant if it is on the left side of a *decimal* number.

EXAMPLE 2-27: Determine the number of significant digits in the following numbers:

a) 5.07

There are three significant digits by rule 1, part c.

b) 45,000

There are two significant digits by rule 2, part a.

c) 12.430

There are five significant digits by rule 1, part b.

d) 0.0037

There are two significant digits by rule 2, part b.

e) 400.0

There are four significant digits by rule 1, part c.

Let's continue with a couple of definitions before we discuss adding and subtracting significant digits.

The **precision** of a number is determined by the place value (tenths, hundredths, thousandths, and so on) of the last significant digit.

The **accuracy** of a number tells us about the quantity of significant digits in the number. In general, the more significant digits a number has, the more accurate the measurement.

When two numbers are added or subtracted, the result should not have more decimal places than the least precise number. In other words, the answer must be rounded to the place value that the least precise number contains. For example, if we are adding $4.332 + 3.51$, the number 3.51 is less precise (precise to the hundredths position) than 4.332 (precise to the thousandths position); therefore, we want the answer to stop at the hundredths position and thus the answer would be 7.84. Following is another example:

$$2.12 + 3.118 + 1.3 = 6.538.$$

However, our answer must stop at the tenths position because 1.3 is the least precise number. Therefore, the answer is 6.5 and not 6.538.

When multiplying or dividing, perform the operation and the answer should be as *accurate* as the least accurate number. In other words, look at the number of significant digits, not the number of decimal places.

PRACTICE PROBLEMS: Section 2.7

Determine the number of significant digits.

1. 0.0018
2. 5,000
3. 90.020
4. 31.0
5. 10
6. 1.320

7. 0.0001
8. 200
9. 9,004
10. 8,020
11. 9
12. 57.006

13. 6,001
14. 12.7070
15. 0.00502
16. 12.0
17. 5.002

Round to the nearest tenth.

18. 15.952
19. 1.05
20. 5.348
21. 0.999

22. 6.929
23. 8.255
24. 5.555

25. 0.1392
26. 0.0115
27. 99.91

Round to the nearest hundredth.

28. 12.5455
29. 334.0946
30. 1.5555
31. 87.293

32. 90.95482
33. 1,500.0080
34. 0.00513

35. 0.90909
36. 0.11650
37. 287.499

Add the following.

38. 5.92 + 4.853
39. 4.1 + 5.542

40. 0.052 + 0.19
41. 3.12 + 5.8

42. 5.321 + 2.53 + 6.812
43. 9.93 + 8.60 + 7.1

2.8 – SCIENTIFIC NOTATION

Scientific notation is used when dealing with very large or very small numbers. In science we often deal with such numbers, hence the name **scientific notation**. A number written in scientific notation has the following form:

$$A \times 10^{n}, \text{ where } 1 \leq A < 10 \text{ and } n \text{ is an integer}$$

Following are two examples of numbers written in scientific notation:

$$1.8 \times 10^9 \text{ and } 4.62 \times 10^{-7}.$$

Notice the first involves a positive exponent (i.e., 9) and the second involves a negative exponent (i.e., -7). Whenever a number in scientific notation has a positive exponent, it is representing a large number; if the exponent is negative, it is representing a small number. This is because of the nature of exponents: $10^9 = 1,000,000,000$ and if we multiply a number such as 1.8 by this, we will certainly get a very large number; on the other hand, remember that $10^{-7} = \dfrac{1}{10^7} = \dfrac{1}{10,000,000}$ and in this case if we multiply a number such as 4.62 by this fraction, we get $4.62 \times \dfrac{1}{10,000,000} = \dfrac{4.62}{10,000,000}$ and when we divide by such a big number the end result is a very small number. Recalling our arithmetic rules, when we multiply any number by 10, it moves the decimal to the *right* one place. If we multiply by 100, it moves the decimal to the right two places and so forth. In general, for every factor of 10 that we multiply by, the decimal moves to the right one place. On the other hand, if we divide a number by 10, it moves the decimal to the *left* one place. If we divide by 100, it moves the decimal to the left two places and so on. In general, for every factor of 10 that we divide by, we move the decimal to the left one place. This is why numbers in scientific notation with positive exponents are large and numbers with negative exponents are small. Keeping this in mind, following are two examples of rewriting a number in scientific notation into fixed-point notation.

1) 3.2×10^4

   We first note that the exponent is positive and there are four factors of 10. Therefore, we move the decimal to the right four places. Thus,

$$3.2 \times 10^4 = 3.\underbrace{2000}_{4 \text{ places}} = 32,000.$$

2) 6.7×10^{-5}

   We first note that the exponent is negative and there are five factors of 10. Therefore, we move the decimal to the left five places. Thus,

$$6.7 \times 10^{-5} = \underbrace{00006}_{5 \text{ places}}.7 = 0.000067.$$

We will now do two examples of converting a number in fixed-point form into scientific notation.

1)   5,100,000,000

   We first note this is a large number. Therefore, the exponent will be positive. Now all we must do is count the number of decimal places and place that number as a positive exponent with the 10. Note that we move the decimal until it is placed in a position such that the resulting *nonzero* digit is between 1 and 10. In this case that would be 5.1.

$$5,\underbrace{100,000,000}_{9 \text{ places}} = 5.1 \times 10^9$$

2) 0.00000000000673

We first note this is a small number. Therefore, the exponent will be negative. Now all we must do is count the number of decimal places and place that number as a negative exponent with the 10. Again, note that we move the decimal until it is placed in a position such that the resulting *nonzero* digit is between 1 and 10. In this case that would be 6.73.

$$0.\underbrace{00000000000}_{12 \text{ places}}673 = 6.73 \times 10^{-12}$$

EXAMPLE 2-28: The following examples involve mathematical manipulations found in many calculations in clinical laboratory courses.

Simplify the following:

a) $\dfrac{0.03 \times 10^{12}}{6 \times 10^{-2}}$

$$= \frac{0.03}{6} \times \frac{10^{12}}{10^{-2}} = 0.005 \times 10^{14} = (5 \times 10^{-3}) \times 10^{14} = 5 \times 10^{11}$$

b) $\dfrac{(4 \times 10^{-9})(8 \times 10^{2})}{2 \times 10^{-3}}$

$$= \frac{32 \times 10^{-7}}{2 \times 10^{-3}} = \frac{32}{2} \times 10^{-4} = 16 \times 10^{-4} = (1.6 \times 10^{1}) \times 10^{-4} = 1.6 \times 10^{-3}$$

c) $\dfrac{0.186}{3.0 \times 10^{3}}$

$$= \frac{0.186}{3.0} \times \frac{1}{10^{3}} = 0.062 \times 10^{-3} = (6.2 \times 10^{-2}) \times 10^{-3} = 6.2 \times 10^{-5}$$

d) $\dfrac{(2 \times 10^{-1})(8 \times 10^{-3})}{(5 \times 10^{-5})(4 \times 10^{3})}$

$$= \frac{16 \times 10^{-4}}{20 \times 10^{-2}} = \frac{16}{20} \times \frac{10^{-4}}{10^{-2}} = 0.8 \times 10^{-2} = (8 \times 10^{-1}) \times 10^{-2} = 8 \times 10^{-3}$$

PRACTICE PROBLEMS: Section 2.8

Write in scientific notation.

1. 0.00002

2. 0.0008976

3. 0.28

4. 93,000,000

5. 123,000,000,000

6. 9,050

7. 17

8. 0.00000085

9. 0.000092

10. 0.0621

11. 435,000

Write in fixed-point notation.

12. 5.21×10^4

13. 6.502×10^5

14. 4.8×10^1

15. 9.92×10^3

16. 8×10^7

17. 9.0×10^5

18. 6.2×10^{-1}

19. 5.5×10^{-4}

20. 2.15×10^{-6}

21. 8.7×10^{-2}

22. 2×10^{-3}

23. 7.0×10^{-6}

Simplify the following and give your answer in scientific notation.

24. $(6 \times 10^3)(5 \times 10^5)$

25. $(12.4 \times 10^{-8})(6.1 \times 10^{-2})$

26. $(0.23 \times 10^{-7})(0.08 \times 10^{-1})$

27. $\dfrac{3.0 \times 10^{16}}{15.0 \times 10^{-2}}$

28. $\dfrac{6.3 \times 10^{-9}}{9.0 \times 10^4}$

29. $\dfrac{(20 \times 10^{-2})(6 \times 10^3)}{(1.5 \times 10^{-5})(2 \times 10^9)}$

30. $\dfrac{0.0325}{5 \times 10^8}$

31. $\dfrac{2 \times 10^{-19}}{5 \times 10^{-12}}$

32. $\dfrac{3.0 \times 10^{12}}{(2.0 \times 10^{-3})(6.0 \times 10^{-2})}$

33. $(2 \times 10^{-5})(5 \times 10^4)$

34. $\dfrac{4 \times 10^{-2}}{8 \times 10^{-1}}$

35. $\dfrac{9 \times 10^6}{3 \times 10^{-4}}$

36. $\dfrac{5 \times 10^{-12}}{10^3}$

37. $\dfrac{10^9}{2 \times 10^{-6}}$

38. $\dfrac{6 \times 10^{16}}{(6 \times 10^{12})(2 \times 10^{-4})}$

39. $\dfrac{(8 \times 10^3)(10^4)}{(5 \times 10^{-1})(1 \times 10^{-2})}$

2.9 – AREA VERSUS VOLUME AND UNITS

Area is defined as the amount of surface within a given boundary. Most of us remember that the area of a rectangle is length times width. For example, in the following diagram we know the area is 3 in $\times$ 2 in = 6 in^2 = 6 sq in. (Remember, just as $3 \times 3 = 3^2$, units work the same so that in $\times$ in = in^2.)

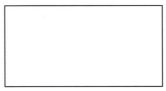

2 in

3 in

But what does this mean? To answer this let's take a closer look. Because the length is 3 inches and the width is 2 inches, we can partition the rectangle into a length with three 1-inch pieces and the width into two 1-inch pieces as follows:

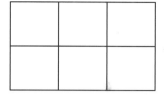

Notice this rectangle now has six squares, each square having a dimension of 1 inch by 1 inch. There is a total of 6 square inches, notated as 6 in². This is why area has units of "square" units. However, keep in mind that if we wanted to find the perimeter (distance around the outside) of this rectangle, the answer would have units of inches because this is a *distance* not an area.

On the other hand, **volume is the amount of space a three-dimensional object encloses.** The volume of a rectangular prism is length × width × height or $V = L \times W \times H$. For example,

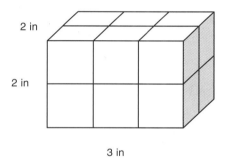

This rectangular prism has a volume of

$$V = 3 \, \text{in} \times 2 \, \text{in} \times 2 \, \text{in} = 12 \, \text{in}^3 = 12 \, \text{cubic inches}.$$

The reason the units are cubic inches is because this rectangular prism can hold 12 smaller cubes, each having a size of 1 in × 1 in × 1 in. There is a total of 12 cubes, with each cube being 1 cubic inch. This is illustrated in the diagram that follows.

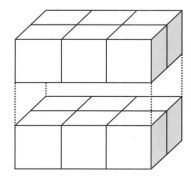

EXAMPLE 2-29: How many square inches are in the following diagram?

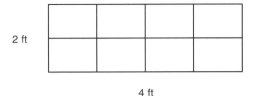

First, we must note that the diagram has an area of 8 square feet. However, the question is how many square inches are in the diagram (not square feet). Thus, to answer the question, we need to find how many square inches are in 1 square foot. Then we multiply our answer by 8 because this diagram has 8 sq ft. We know 1 square foot has 144 square inches because 1 square foot is a 12×12-inch square, which has 144 square inches. Therefore, this diagram has $8 \times 144 = 1,152$ sq in.

EXAMPLE 2-30: For each situation that follows, determine which unit—inches, square inches, or cubic inches—would be suitable.

a)   Amount of air a box can hold

This would be *cubic inches* because we are talking about volume.

b)   Length around a rectangle

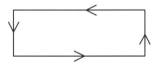

This would be *inches* because we are talking about distance.

c)   Amount of space on one wall of a home

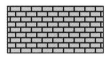

This would be *square inches* because we are talking about the amount of surface, which is measured in square units.

As we have just seen, when multiplying with units, the same exponent rules of algebra apply. Also note that if the same units are involved within a fraction, they cancel. We will illustrate with some examples. Metric units are discussed more thoroughly in Chapter 3, so only a brief summary of some basic metric notation is given here.

Basic Metric Units

- m is the metric symbol for meter

- g is the metric symbol for gram

- L is the metric symbol for liter

- mL is the metric symbol for milliliter

- kg is the metric symbol for kilogram

- mg is the metric symbol for milligram

- mm is the metric symbol for millimeter

EXAMPLE 2-31: Simplify: $L^{-1} \cdot g$

Applying the rules of exponents, $L^{-1} \cdot g = \frac{g}{L}$. Notice that these units are saying "grams per liter."

EXAMPLE 2-32: Simplify: $6 \, kg \cdot day^{-1}$

$6 \, kg \cdot day^{-1} = \frac{6 \, kg}{day}$, which is saying "6 kilograms per day"

EXAMPLE 2-33: Simplify: $\frac{mg \cdot hr}{mL} \cdot mL \cdot hr^{-1}$ (where hr represents hours)

First, note that the mL's cancel.

$$\frac{mg \cdot hr}{\cancel{mL}} \cdot \cancel{mL} \cdot hr^{-1} = mg \cdot hr \cdot hr^{-1}$$

Using the properties of negative exponents, this can be rewritten as

$$\frac{mg \cdot hr}{hr} \ .$$

Canceling the hr's we get

$$\frac{mg \cdot \cancel{hr}}{\cancel{hr}} = mg \ .$$

Next we present some basic ideas behind area and volume, ideas that arise in the study of hematology. Note that the volume of a cube is $V = L \times W \times H$. We could, however, express this as

$$V = (L \times W) \times H .$$

Remember, the area of a rectangle is $L \times W$ and if we think of the height, H, as depth, then this equation becomes

$$V = \text{Area} \times \text{Depth} .$$

The concept of Volume = Area × Depth arises in counting cells in hematology. We go further in depth when we study hematology in Chapter 7. For now we will do some basic examples involving the calculation of the volume of a sample of blood.

EXAMPLE 2-34: A blood sample is placed on a 20×20 mm slide in order to count the number of white blood cells. The thickness, or depth, of the blood sample between the slide and the cover slip is 0.1 mm. What is the volume of blood in this sample?

Volume is length × width × height, or $V = (L \times W) \times H$, thus the volume is

$$V = (20 \text{ mm} \times 20 \text{ mm}) \times \frac{1}{10} \text{ mm} = \frac{400}{10} \text{ mm}^3 = 40 \text{ mm}^3.$$

EXAMPLE 2-35: A blood sample is placed on a 24×40 mm slide and the depth of the sample between the slide and the cover slip is 0.1 mm. What is the volume of this blood sample?

$$V = (L \times W) \times H = (24 \text{ mm} \times 40 \text{ mm}) \times \frac{1}{10} \text{ mm} = \frac{960}{10} \text{ mm}^3 = 96 \text{ cubic millimeters}$$

PRACTICE PROBLEMS: Section 2.9

For each of the following situations, determine which unit—ft, ft², or ft³—would be suitable.

1. Width of a rectangle
2. Perimeter of a triangle
3. Surface of a circle
4. Amount of fluid a test tube holds
5. Length around a circle.
6. Amount of storage inside a box

7. Distance around the top of a desk
8. How far an elevator moves
9. Amount of space in a refrigerator
10. Wall space covered by a picture
11. Size of the inside of a filing cabinet

Simplify the units and then write your answer in words.

12. $mg \, L^{-1}$

13. $6 \, g \, hr^{-1}$

14. $mL \cdot day^{-1} \cdot \dfrac{7 \text{ day}}{\text{week}}$

15. $\dfrac{\frac{mg}{L} \cdot \frac{mL}{min}}{\frac{mg}{L}}$

16. $\dfrac{mL}{M^{-1} \, cm^{-1}} \cdot \dfrac{M^{-1}}{cm}$

17. $g \, cm^{-1} \, cm$

18. $\dfrac{\frac{g}{g}}{dL}$

19. $\dfrac{\frac{g}{\frac{g}{mole}}}{L}$

20. A blood sample is placed on an 18 × 18 mm slide in order to count the number of red blood cells. The thickness, or depth, of the blood sample is $\frac{1}{10}$ mm. What is the volume of blood in this sample?

21. A blood sample is placed on a 24 × 24 mm slide in order to examine the platelets. The thickness, or depth, of the blood sample is $\frac{1}{10}$ mm. What is the volume of blood in this sample?

22. An instrument measured an anemic blood sample and found it to have $\frac{7{,}800 \text{ white blood cells}}{\text{mm}^3}$. How many white blood cells should a $2 \times 2 \times \frac{3}{10}$ mm sample of this blood contain?

2.10 – USING THE CALCULATOR

If calculators are allowed in your program of study, the type allowed will most likely be a scientific calculator rather than a graphing calculator. Therefore, this section concentrates on how to use a scientific calculator.

When you use a scientific calculator, one concept to keep in mind when entering problems is the order of operations. Remember, parentheses first, then exponents, then multiplication and division (as they occur from left to right), and addition and subtraction last. It is especially important to become familiar with the use of parentheses—when to use them and when not to.

Before moving on to some examples, let's first discuss some of the more relevant keys on the scientific calculator and keys that often create confusion.

- The $\boxed{y^x}$ key is used to enter expressions containing exponents. For example, to enter 6^3, first enter 6, then press the $\boxed{y^x}$ key, and then enter 3. The answer should be 216. Scientific calculators also have a key with $\boxed{\text{EE}}$ on it. Be careful when using this key! For example, to enter 10^3 using the $\boxed{\text{EE}}$ key, you first need to think of this as 1×10^3. Now enter 1, press the $\boxed{\text{EE}}$ key, and then enter 3. This is because the $\boxed{\text{EE}}$ key already has the 10 programmed into it. Thus the $\boxed{\text{EE}}$ key is used only when we have 10 raised to a power.

- To enter a negative number, enter the number first and then enter the $\boxed{+/-}$ key. Therefore, to enter −5, first enter 5 and then press $\boxed{+/-}$. To enter −5 − 2, first enter 5, press the $\boxed{+/-}$ key, press the subtraction key, enter 2, and then press the $\boxed{=}$ key. Try it.

EXAMPLE 2-36: Evaluate $(3.8 \times 10^4)(2.6 \times 10^{-2})$ by using your calculator.

When entering a problem into the calculator, first rewrite the expression, including any mathematical symbols that do not physically show up (such as multiplication, division, or parentheses). In this example the parentheses imply multiplication, but the × symbol is clearly missing. Rewriting, we have the equivalent expression $(3.8 \times 10^4) \times (2.6 \times 10^{-2})$. Enter this into the calculator just as you read it from left to right. Following are the keystrokes for this particular problem.

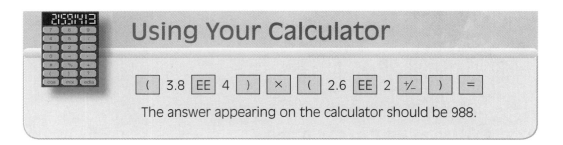

Using Your Calculator

(3.8 EE 4) × (2.6 EE 2 +/−) =

The answer appearing on the calculator should be 988.

NOTE

We could have done this problem without using any parentheses. This is because everything is being multiplied (keep in mind the order of operations). If we do this computation using no parentheses, we would enter it as

3.8   EE   4   ×   2.6   EE   2   +/−   =

Enter 3.8

Press the EE key

Enter 4

Press the multiplication key ×

Enter 2.6

Press the EE key

Enter 2

Press the +/− key

Press the equal key =

EXAMPLE 2-37: Evaluate $\dfrac{8.4 \times 10^5}{2.4 \times 10^{-3}}$ by using your calculator.

First, notice this problem can be rewritten as $(8.4 \times 10^5) \div (2.4 \times 10^{-3})$.

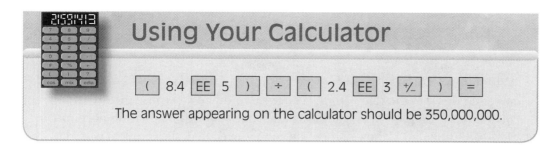

Using Your Calculator

(8.4 EE 5) ÷ (2.4 EE 3 +/-) =

The answer appearing on the calculator should be 350,000,000.

Press the (key

Enter 8.4

Press the EE key

Enter 5

Press the division key ÷

Press the) key

Press the (key

Enter 2.4

Press the EE key

Enter 2

Press the +/- key

Press the) key

Press the equal key =

EXAMPLE 2-38: Evaluate $\frac{8+12}{6-2}$ by using your calculator.

This problem can be rewritten as $(8 + 12) \div (6 - 2)$. It is important to realize when working with fractions that the entire numerator is being divided by the entire denominator. Therefore, when you enter the example problem into the calculator, you must remember to use parentheses around the entire numerator and parentheses around the entire denominator.

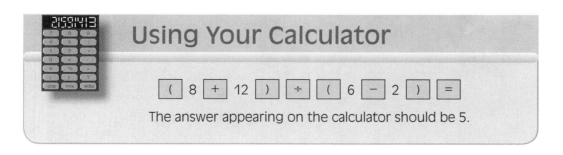

Using Your Calculator

(8 + 12) ÷ (6 - 2) =

The answer appearing on the calculator should be 5.

NOTE

Without parentheses our problem would have appeared as $8 + 12 \div 6 - 2$. If we enter this into the calculator, the answer would be 8 because the order of operations is division before addition and subtraction. The division portion, $12 \div 6$, is equal to 2, thus after the division is executed, the problem would appear as $8 + 2 - 2$, and this is equal to 8. Enter this problem into your calculator, without parentheses, to see that the answer is 8. The point here is that the calculator follows the order of operations. This is one of the primary reasons it is so important to understand the order of operations.

EXAMPLE 2-39: Evaluate $\frac{(2+4)^2}{6+3}$ by using your calculator.

This can be rewritten as $(2 + 4)^2 \div (6 + 3)$. Enter this into the calculator just as you read it from left to right, keeping in mind the order of operations and how the proper use of parentheses is very important.

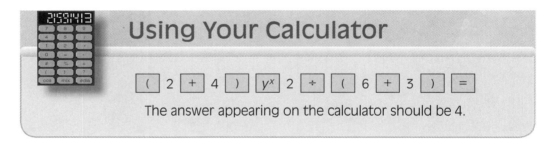

Using Your Calculator

(2 + 4) y^x 2 ÷ (6 + 3) =

The answer appearing on the calculator should be 4.

EXAMPLE 2-40: Evaluate $\frac{4.8 \times 10^{-2}}{(1.5 \times 10^{-1})(3.2 \times 10^5)}$ by using your calculator.

First, we can write this problem as $(4.8 \times 10^{-2}) \div (1.5 \times 10^{-1} \times 3.2 \times 10^5)$. Again, the correct use of parentheses is very important.

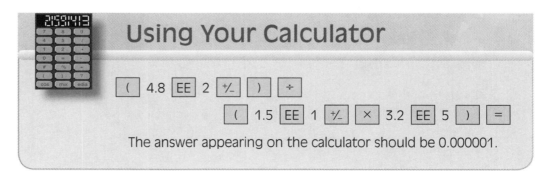

Using Your Calculator

(4.8 EE 2 +/-) ÷

(1.5 EE 1 +/- × 3.2 EE 5) =

The answer appearing on the calculator should be 0.000001.

If we enter the problem from example 2-40 without using parentheses, it would appear as

$$4.8 \times 10^{-2} \div 1.5 \times 10^{-1} \times 3.2 \times 10^5$$

and our answer would be 1,024. The point again is how important the correct use of parentheses is. Remember, multiplication and division are executed *as they occur from left to right*.

EXAMPLE 2-41: Evaluate $10^{-5} \times 10^3$ by using your calculator.

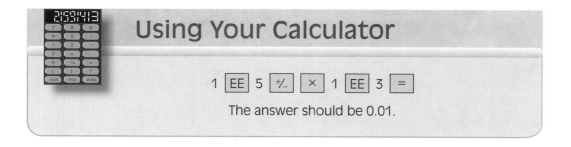

Using Your Calculator

1 EE 5 +/- × 1 EE 3 =

The answer should be 0.01.

EXAMPLE 2-42: Evaluate $3\frac{2}{5} + 4\frac{1}{2}$ by using your calculator.

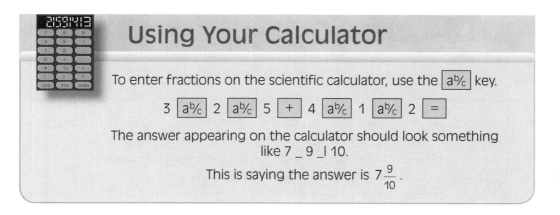

Using Your Calculator

To enter fractions on the scientific calculator, use the a b/c key.

3 a b/c 2 a b/c 5 + 4 a b/c 1 a b/c 2 =

The answer appearing on the calculator should look something like 7 _ 9 _| 10.

This is saying the answer is $7\frac{9}{10}$.

EXAMPLE 2-43: Try to work the following problems using your scientific calculator. The correct answers are given to check your work.

a) $\dfrac{0.050}{0.125} \times 10^5 \times \dfrac{1}{4}$

Answer: 10,000

b) $\dfrac{3 \times 10^4}{10^{-2}}$

Answer: 3,000,000

c) $\dfrac{1}{2+3} + 2 \times 3$

Answer: 6.2

d) $\dfrac{3 \times 10^{-2}}{2+4} + 0.1$

Answer: 0.105

PRACTICE PROBLEMS: Section 2.10

Use a scientific calculator to find the value of the following expressions.

1. $10^{-2} \times 10^{10}$

2. $\dfrac{4}{5} \times 10^3 \times 10^4$

3. $5 \times 10^6 \times 10^{12}$

4. $(2.45 \times 10^{-7})(5.42 \times 10^{-3})$

5. $\dfrac{5.00\% \times \dfrac{1}{2}}{2.5}$

6. $\dfrac{4 \times 10^2 \times \dfrac{3}{4}}{3.2 - 2.8}$

7. $\dfrac{4 \times 10^5}{3.2(7.8 \times 10^{-2})}$

8. $(5 \times 10^{-2})(10^3)$

9. $10^8 \times 10^{-10}$

10. $\dfrac{6 \times 10^2}{3 \times 10^{-1}}$

11. $\dfrac{(2 \times 10^{-6})(5 \times 10^2)}{4 \times 10^{-3}}$

12. $(4.1 \times 10^{-2})(8.6 \times 10^{-5})$

13. $\dfrac{80}{2.0 \times 10^{-4}}$

CHAPTER SUMMARY

- If the product of two numbers is 1, then the two numbers are said be *reciprocals* of each other.
- When solving an equation, the goal is to get the variable (x) by itself. To accomplish this, remember that whatever operation is performed on one side of the equation must also be performed on the other side.
- When setting up proportions to solve a problem, the units on both sides of the equal sign must be set up in exactly the same order.
- Percent problems can be solved by setting up an equation or by using a proportion.
- Following are the four main rules for exponents:
  - Product rule: $x^A \cdot x^B = x^{A+B}$
  - Quotient rule: $\dfrac{x^A}{x^B} = x^{A-B}$
  - Power rule: $(x^A)^B = x^{A \times B}$
  - Negative exponent rule: $x^{-A} = \dfrac{1}{x^A}$

■ The order of operations is as follows:
  1) Simplify parentheses and brackets (in general grouping symbols).
  2) Evaluate exponents.
  3) Multiply and divide as the operations occur from left to right.
  4) Add and subtract (from left to right).
■ Rules to determine the number of significant digits
  Rule 1: Determining whether a digit is significant:
  • All nonzero digits are significant.
  • Zeros are significant if they are on the right side of a *decimal number*.
  • Zeros are significant if they are between two significant digits.
  • Zeros are significant if they are marked with an over bar, $\bar{0}$.
  Rule 2: Determining whether a zero is not significant:
  • A zero is not significant if it is on the right side of a *whole number*.
  • A zero is not significant if it is on the left side of a *number*.
■ A number less than zero expressed in scientific notation will have a negative exponent. A number greater than 10 expressed in scientific notation will have a positive exponent.
■ Area deals with the amount of surface on a flat or two-dimensional object. Volume deals with the amount of space inside a three-dimensional object. Perimeter is the distance around an object.

CHAPTER TEST

1. Solve: $2(x - 8) = 20$

2. Solve: $\frac{2}{3}x - 1 = 5$

3. Solve: $\frac{3x-6}{4} = 12$

4. Solve: $\frac{x}{8} = \frac{5}{6}$

5. Solve: $\frac{3x}{2} = 9$

6. Solve: $\frac{\frac{2}{x}}{3} = 8$

7. Solve for a: $r = \frac{a+b}{3}$

8. Find the value of y given that $z = 6$: $x = \frac{2z+8}{5}$
$$y = -3x + 4$$

9. A solution must be made such that for every 2 parts serum we have a total of 8 parts solution. If the total volume is to be 300 mL, how much serum do we need?

10. Every 5 mL of a solution contains 12 mg of chemical. How many milligrams of chemical are in 24 mL of solution?

11. What percent of 250 is 16?

12. What is 12% of 80?

13. Twenty-five is 20% of what number?

14. If 500 fluid ounces of a solution contains 40 fluid ounces of a liquid chemical, what percent of the solution is liquid chemical?

15. If 6 out of every 400 patients test positive for a disease, what percent test positive?

16. Simplify: $\dfrac{10^{-5} \times 10^{2}}{10^{-4}}$

17. Simplify: $\dfrac{x^{15}}{x^{-4}}$

18. Simplify: $x^{-7} \cdot x^{-2}$

19. Simplify: $(x^{-5})^{6}$

20. Round 291.1945 to the nearest hundredth.

21. Round 3.0496 to the nearest tenth.

22. Write 0.00000215 in scientific notation.

23. Simplify $2 + 3(5 - 3)^{2} \div 6$ by using the order of operations.

24. How many significant digits are in the number 0.0320?

25. How many significant digits are in the number 5.052?

26. Simplify: $\dfrac{(9 \times 10^{-2})(8 \times 10^{-3})}{2 \times 10^{-1}}$

27. Write $g \cdot L^{-1}$ in words.

28. Explain what perimeter, area, and volume mean and give an example of a unit associated with each.

29. Evaluate $2 \times 10^{2} \times 10^{-4}$ by using your calculator.

Measurement Systems and Conversion Procedures

$$y = -\frac{2}{5}x + 8$$

INTRODUCTION

This chapter focuses on conversions. We begin with conversions within the metric system and move to conversions between metric and nonmetric. A few different approaches to performing conversions are discussed. Understanding every approach will help to alleviate difficulty and confusion in subsequent courses. The last topic in this chapter is temperature conversions.

The U.S. Customary System

In the United States, the type of measurement typically used is called the United States Customary System of Measurement. Following are some of the standard units and their relationships involving distance:

> 1 ft = 12 in
> 1 yd = 3 ft
> 1 mi = 5,280 ft

Following are some of the standard units that involve **volume**:

> 8 fl oz = 1 cup
> 1 pt = 2 cups
> 1 qt = 2 pt
> 4 qt = 1 gal

Following are some of the standard units that involve weight:

$$16\,\text{oz} = 1\,\text{lb} \qquad\qquad\qquad 2{,}000\,\text{lb} = 1\,\text{short ton}$$

These are a part of what is called the avoirdupois system.

The Metric System

Notice the units for distance. In just those three relationships, there are inches, feet, yards, and miles. The nice part about the metric system is that there is one basic unit for distance, one basic unit for volume, and one basic unit for weight, and those basic units are as follows:

$$\begin{array}{ccc}
\text{m} & \to \text{meter} & \to \text{Length} \\
\text{l or L} & \to \text{liter} & \to \text{Volume} \\
\text{g} & \to \text{gram} & \to \text{Weight}
\end{array}$$

A meter is slightly longer than a yard, a liter is slightly more than a quart, and a penny typically weighs around $1\frac{1}{2}$ grams. Following are the equations that relate these units:

$$0.91\,\text{m} = 1\,\text{yd}$$
$$3.79\,\text{L} = 1\,\text{gal}$$
$$28.3\,\text{g} = 1\,\text{oz}$$

Metric System Prefixes

As just noted, the three basic units in the metric system are meter, liter, and gram. In the metric system, prefixes are used to inform the reader how many basic units are involved. For example, a microgram is notated as μg, where μ is the prefix and g is the basic unit. Micro implies 10^{-6} or $1/1{,}000{,}000$; therefore, μg means $1/1{,}000{,}000$ of a gram. On the other hand, μm means $1/1{,}000{,}000$ of a meter. Likewise, μL means $1/1{,}000{,}000$ of a liter. Table 3–1 gives the prefixes used in the metric system along with their abbreviated symbol and corresponding values. The corresponding value is the number of basic units the prefix represents. That is to say, cg is centigram, and we see from Table 3–1 that c (or centi) corresponds to 10^{-2}, which we know is the same as $\frac{1}{10^2}$, which is equivalent to $\frac{1}{100}$. Thus, cg means one one-hundredth of a gram. We can also think of this as 100 cg equals 1 gram. It is very helpful to think of metric units in both of these ways. By the nature of negative exponents, a topic covered in Section 2.5, prefixes with negative exponents represent a fractional (or small) amount, and prefixes with positive exponents represent a large amount.

The International System of Units

The International System of Units, often referred to as the SI system, has become the prevailing scientific language used for trade and commerce. The SI system consists of seven basic units:

1) meter (length)

2) kilogram (mass)

3) mole (amount of substance)

4) second (time)

5) kelvin (temperature)

6) ampere (current—electricity)

7) candela (luminous intensity—light)

TABLE 3–1 Metric System Prefixes, Abbreviations, and Basic Units

PREFIX	ABBREVIATION	NUMBER OF BASIC UNITS
peta	P	10^{15}
tera	T	10^{12}
giga	G	10^{9}
mega	M	10^{6}
kilo	k	10^{3}
hecto	h	10^{2}
deka	da	10^{1}
Basic Unit	g, m, or L	10^{0}
deci	d	10^{-1}
centi	c	10^{-2}
milli	m	10^{-3}
micro	μ	10^{-6}
nano	n	10^{-9}
pico	p	10^{-12}
femto	f	10^{-15}

Table 3–1 can be expressed in a horizontal format as well.

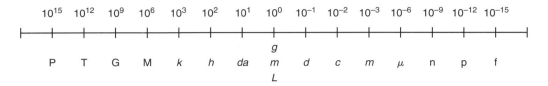

Understanding Metric Conversions

The horizontal format can be used for simple conversions. However, we need to thoroughly understand Table 3–1 to perform more involved conversions. To begin, look at the prefixes *centi*, *milli*, and *micro* together with the basic unit of gram.

Referring to Table 3–1, note that 1 centigram equals 10^{-2} grams or, in other words, 1 cg equals $\frac{1}{100}$ of a gram. As an equation we can write this as

$$1 \text{ cg} = 10^{-2} \text{ g.*}$$

If we multiply both sides of this equation by 10^2, we get

$$10^2 \cdot 1 \text{ cg} = 10^2 \cdot 10^{-2} \text{ g.}$$

Simplifying both sides we obtain

$$10^2 \text{ cg} = 1 \text{ g.**}$$

Therefore, it takes 10^2 (or 100) centigrams to make 1 gram; this is another way of interpreting *centigram*.

The importance of understanding that the two equations labeled * and ** are equivalent becomes very pertinent when doing conversions. This same concept applies to all of the prefixes in Table 3–1. For example, we see from Table 3–1 that 1 milligram equals $\frac{1}{1,000}$ of a gram. We can also think of this as 1 gram equals 1,000 milligrams. Likewise, from Table 3–1 we see that 1 μg equals 1/1,000,000 of a gram. We can also look at this as 1 gram equals 1,000,000 μg.

In conversions, if we place the 1 with the basic unit (g, L, or m), the exponent with the 10 will be the opposite of what is given in Table 3–1. However, when the 1 is placed with the two-lettered unit (i.e., μg, cg, or mg), the exponent with the 10 is exactly the same as given in Table 3–1.

3.1 – CONVERSIONS WITHIN THE METRIC SYSTEM

In the sciences (and the laboratory sciences are no exception), it is often necessary to convert a given measurement in metric to another equivalent measurement in metric. For example, we may need to know how many microliters are in a milliliter. To complete this type of conversion, we can perform a manipulation called **dimensional analysis**. We can also use the horizontal format. However, the horizontal format works only when we are converting *within* the metric system.

Using the Horizontal Format

The horizontal format is arguably the easiest method to use when converting within the metric system. However, when we do metric to nonmetric, this method breaks down. Following is a procedure for using the horizontal format:

1) Identify where the decimal is located in the numerical portion of the quantity being converted.

2) Identify the location of each *prefix* on the horizontal diagram.

3) Find the difference between the two exponents associated with each prefix.

4) If the conversion is moving to the *right* on the horizontal diagram, move the decimal to the *right* by the amount calculated in step 3.

5) If the conversion is moving to the *left* on the horizontal diagram, move the decimal to the *left* by the amount calculated in step 3.

EXAMPLE 3-1: Convert 12 mL to μL using the horizontal format.

1) Identify the decimal location: 12 can be thought of as 12.0.

2) Identify where the two prefixes are located on the horizontal diagram. In this example the first prefix is m and the second is μ. Their locations are as follows:

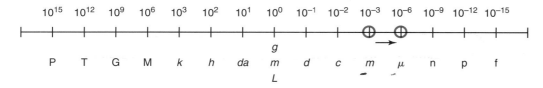

3) The difference between the exponents is $-3 - (-6) = 3$.

4) We are converting from m to μ, so we are moving to the right. Because we are moving to the right, we must move the decimal place to the right by three places as follows:

$$12\,0\,0\,0.$$

This is equivalent to 12000 or 12,000. Therefore, 12 mL = 12,000 μL.

EXAMPLE 3-2: Convert 8 ng to mg using the horizontal format.

1) Identify the decimal location: 8 can be thought of as 8.0.

2) Identify where the two prefixes are located on the horizontal diagram. In this example the first prefix is n and the second is m. Their locations are as follows:

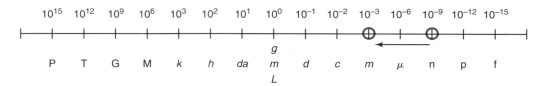

3) The difference between the exponents is $-3 - (-9) = 6$.

4) We are converting from n to m, so we are moving to the left. Because we are moving to the left, we must move the decimal place to the left by six places as follows:

$$.0\,0\,0\,0\,0\,8$$

This is equivalent to .000008 or 0.000008; therefore, 8 ng = 0.000008 mg.

Applying Dimensional Analysis

In the application of dimensional analysis, the main concern is where the 1 is placed. When we place the 1 with the two-lettered unit and not with the basic unit, we just read the values from Table 3–1 and place them in the problem. However, when we place the 1 with the basic unit, we must use the opposite sign associated with the exponent of 10.

Some of the conversions in the following examples are not typically done in a laboratory science setting; however, these examples are to illustrate the concept of how to perform conversions, and all conversions are done using the same concept.

EXAMPLE 3-3: Convert 15 μg to ng. First, place the 1 with the basic unit. Remember, doing it this way requires use of an exponent that is opposite of the one given in Table 3–1.

In this example we will place the 1 with the basic unit.

First, convert to the basic unit, which in this case is grams. Note that μg must be placed in the denominator so the μg's cancel and we are left with grams.

$$15\,\mu g\left(\frac{1\,g}{10^6\,\mu g}\right)$$

Next, we complete the conversion by going to ng. Again note that g must be in the denominator so the g's cancel.

$$15 \, \mu\text{g} \left(\frac{1 \text{g}}{10^6 \, \mu\text{g}} \right) \left(\frac{10^9 \, \text{ng}}{1 \text{g}} \right)$$

Last, we simplify.

$$15 \, \mu\text{g} \left(\frac{1 \text{g}}{10^6 \, \mu\text{g}} \right) \left(\frac{10^9 \, \text{ng}}{1 \text{g}} \right) = 15 \times \frac{10^9}{10^6} \text{ng} = 15 \times 10^3 \, \text{ng} = \underbrace{1.5 \times 10^1}_{\text{Equivalent to 15}} \times 10^3 \, \text{ng} = 1.5 \times 10^4 \, \text{ng}$$

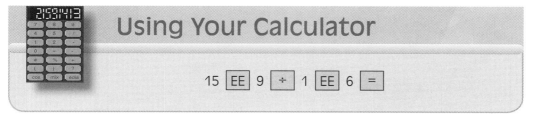

Using Your Calculator

15 [EE] 9 [÷] 1 [EE] 6 [=]

Let's do the same problem now by placing the 1 with the two-lettered unit instead of placing the 1 with the basic unit. Remember, when doing it this way, just read the values directly off of Table 3–1.

First, convert to the basic unit, which in this case is grams. Note that μg must be placed in the denominator so the μg's cancel.

$$15 \, \mu\text{g} \left(\frac{10^{-6} \, \text{g}}{1 \, \mu\text{g}} \right)$$

Second, complete the conversion by going to ng. Again note that g must be in the denominator so the g's cancel.

$$15 \, \mu\text{g} \left(\frac{10^{-6} \, \text{g}}{1 \, \mu\text{g}} \right) \left(\frac{1 \, \text{ng}}{10^{-9} \, \text{g}} \right)$$

Last, simplify.

$$15 \, \mu\text{g} \left(\frac{10^{-6} \, \text{g}}{1 \, \mu\text{g}} \right) \left(\frac{1 \, \text{ng}}{10^{-9} \, \text{g}} \right) = 15 \times \frac{10^{-6}}{10^{-9}} \text{ng} = 15 \times 10^3 \, \text{ng} = \underbrace{1.5 \times 10^1}_{\text{Equivalent to 15}} \times 10^3 \, \text{ng} = 1.5 \times 10^4 \, \text{ng}$$

↑
Subtract exponents $[-6 - (-9) = 3]$

Notice that the choice of method made no difference; the answer is the same.

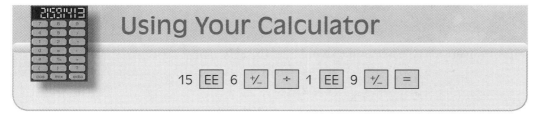

Using Your Calculator

15 [EE] 6 [+/−] [÷] 1 [EE] 9 [+/−] [=]

EXAMPLE 3-4: Convert 12 μL to mL.

Place the 1 with the two-lettered unit. First convert to the basic unit L. Note how the μL's cancel.

$$12\,\mu\mathrm{L}\left(\frac{10^{-6}\,\mathrm{L}}{1\,\mu\mathrm{L}}\right)$$

Then convert to mL. Note that L is in the denominator in the second set of parentheses so the L's cancel.

$$12\,\mu\mathrm{L}\left(\frac{10^{-6}\,\mathrm{L}}{1\,\mu\mathrm{L}}\right)\left(\frac{1\,\mathrm{mL}}{10^{-3}\,\mathrm{L}}\right)=12\times\frac{10^{-6}}{10^{-3}}\,\mathrm{mL}=12\times10^{-3}\,\mathrm{mL}=\underbrace{1.2\times10^{1}}_{\text{Equivalent to 12}}\times10^{-3}\,\mathrm{mL}=1.2\times10^{-2}\,\mathrm{mL}$$

↑

Subtract exponents $[-6-(-3)=-3]$

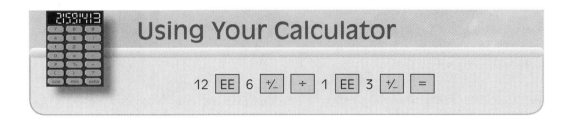

Using Your Calculator

12 [EE] 6 [+/−] [÷] 1 [EE] 3 [+/−] [=]

Now let's do the same problem by placing the 1 with the basic unit. First, convert to the basic unit L, then convert to mL.

$$12\,\mu\mathrm{L}\left(\frac{1\,\mathrm{L}}{10^{6}\,\mu\mathrm{L}}\right)\left(\frac{10^{3}\,\mathrm{mL}}{1\,\mathrm{L}}\right)=12\times\frac{10^{3}}{10^{6}}=12\times10^{-3}\,\mathrm{mL}=\underbrace{1.2\times10^{1}}_{\text{Equivalent to 12}}\times10^{-3}\,\mathrm{mL}=1.2\times10^{-2}\,\mathrm{mL}$$

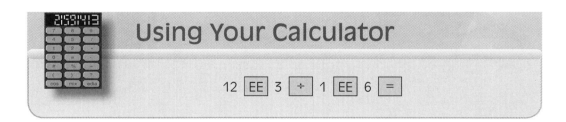

Using Your Calculator

12 [EE] 3 [÷] 1 [EE] 6 [=]

EXAMPLE 3-5: Convert by placing the 1 with the two-lettered unit:
28 cg = _____ dg.

First, convert to the basic unit g. Note how the cg's cancel.

$$28\,\mathrm{cg}\left(\frac{10^{-2}\,\mathrm{g}}{1\,\mathrm{cg}}\right)$$

Then convert to dg. Note that g is in the denominator in the second set of parentheses so the g's cancel.

$$28 \, \cancel{cg} \left(\frac{10^{-2} \, \cancel{g}}{1 \, \cancel{cg}} \right) \left(\frac{1 \, dg}{10^{-1} \, \cancel{g}} \right) = 28 \times 10^{-1} \, dg = 2.8 \times 10^{0} \, dg = 2.8 \, dg$$

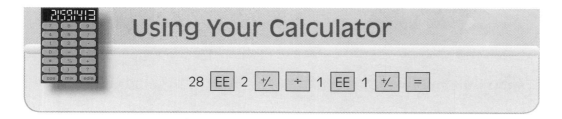

Using Your Calculator

28 [EE] 2 [+/−] [÷] 1 [EE] 1 [+/−] [=]

EXAMPLE 3-6: Convert by placing the 1 with the basic unit: 7.0 kL = _____ PL.

First, convert to the basic unit L. Note how the kL's cancel.

$$7.0 \, \cancel{kL} \left(\frac{1 \, L}{10^{-3} \, \cancel{kL}} \right)$$

Then convert to PL. Note that L is in the denominator in the second set of parentheses so the L's cancel.

$$7.0 \, \cancel{kL} \left(\frac{1 \, \cancel{L}}{10^{-3} \, \cancel{kL}} \right) \left(\frac{10^{-15} \, PL}{1 \, \cancel{L}} \right) = 7.0 \times 10^{-12} \, PL$$

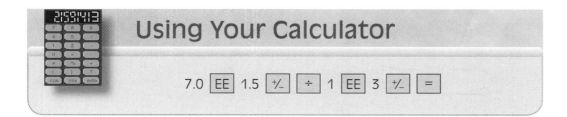

Using Your Calculator

7.0 [EE] 1.5 [+/−] [÷] 1 [EE] 3 [+/−] [=]

EXAMPLE 3-7: Convert by placing the 1 with the basic unit: 0.6 cm = _____ Tm.

First, convert to the basic unit m. Note that cm in the first set of parentheses is in the denominator so the cm's cancel. Then convert to Tm. Note that m is in the denominator in the second set of parentheses so the m's cancel.

$$0.6 \, \cancel{cm} \left(\frac{10^{-2} \, \cancel{m}}{1 \, \cancel{cm}} \right) \left(\frac{1 \, Tm}{10^{12} \, \cancel{m}} \right) = 0.6 \times 10^{-14} \, Tm = 6.0 \times 10^{-1} \times 10^{-14} \, Tm = 6.0 \times 10^{-15} \, Tm$$

EXAMPLE 3-8: Convert $20 \, \text{g/mL}$ to g/L.

We need to multiply by an appropriate factor so we end up with the units we need. In this case that would be milliliters over liters so the milliliters cancel and we are left with grams per liter. Do this by placing the 1 with the basic unit.

$$\frac{20 \, \text{g}}{\text{mL}} \left(\frac{10^3 \, \text{mL}}{1 \, \text{L}} \right) = 20 \times 10^3 \, \text{g/L} = 2.0 \times 10^4 \, \text{g/L}$$

EXAMPLE 3-9: Convert $30 \, \text{mg/dL}$ to g/L.

We first convert to grams per deciliter (this cancels the mg's) by placing the 1 with the two-lettered unit.

$$\frac{30 \, \text{mg}}{\text{dL}} \left(\frac{10^{-3} \, \text{g}}{1 \, \text{mg}} \right)$$

Next we convert to grams per liter (this cancels the dL's so we are left with grams per liter).

$$\frac{30 \, \text{mg}}{\text{dL}} \left(\frac{10^{-3} \, \text{g}}{1 \, \text{mg}} \right) \left(\frac{1 \, \text{dL}}{10^{-1} \, \text{L}} \right) = 30 \times 10^{-2} \, \text{g/L} = 3.0 \times 10^{-1} \, \text{g/L}$$

EXAMPLE 3-10: Convert $15 \, \mu\text{g/mL}$ to ng/dL.

First, convert to grams per milliliter (this cancels the μg's) by placing the 1 with the two-lettered unit.

$$\frac{15 \, \mu\text{g}}{\text{mL}} \left(\frac{10^{-6} \, \text{g}}{1 \, \mu\text{g}} \right)$$

Next, convert to nanograms per milliliter.

$$\frac{15 \, \mu\text{g}}{\text{mL}} \left(\frac{10^{-6} \, \text{g}}{1 \, \mu\text{g}} \right) \left(\frac{1 \, \text{ng}}{10^{-9} \, \text{g}} \right)$$

Next, convert to nanograms per liter.

$$\frac{15 \, \mu\text{g}}{\text{mL}} \left(\frac{10^{-6} \, \text{g}}{1 \, \mu\text{g}} \right) \left(\frac{1 \, \text{ng}}{10^{-9} \, \text{g}} \right) \left(\frac{1 \, \text{mL}}{10^{-3} \, \text{L}} \right)$$

Last, convert to nanograms per deciliter.

$$\frac{15 \, \mu\text{g}}{\text{mL}} \left(\frac{10^{-6} \, \text{g}}{1 \, \mu\text{g}} \right) \left(\frac{1 \, \text{ng}}{10^{-9} \, \text{g}} \right) \left(\frac{1 \, \text{mL}}{10^{-3} \, \text{L}} \right) \left(\frac{10^{-1} \, \text{L}}{1 \, \text{dL}} \right) = 15 \times \frac{10^{-7}}{10^{-12}} \, \text{ng/dL} = 15 \times 10^5 = 1.5 \times 10^6 \, \text{ng/dL}$$

EXAMPLE 3-11: Convert $8.2 \, {}^{mg}\!/_{\mu L}$ to ${}^{dg}\!/_{mL}$.

First, convert to grams per microliter by placing the 1 with the basic unit.

$$8.2 \frac{mg}{\mu L}\left(\frac{1 \, g}{10^3 \, mg}\right)$$

Next, convert to grams per liter.

$$8.2 \frac{mg}{\mu L}\left(\frac{1 \, g}{10^3 \, mg}\right)\left(\frac{10^6 \, \mu L}{1 \, L}\right)$$

Now we have grams per liter but need decigrams per milliliter, so we will next convert to grams per milliliter.

$$8.2 \frac{mg}{\mu L}\left(\frac{1 \, g}{10^3 \, mg}\right)\left(\frac{10^6 \, \mu L}{1 \, L}\right)\left(\frac{1 \, L}{10^3 \, mL}\right)$$

Last, convert to decigrams per milliliter.

$$8.2 \frac{mg}{\mu L}\left(\frac{1 \, g}{10^3 \, mg}\right)\left(\frac{10^6 \, \mu L}{1 \, L}\right)\left(\frac{1 \, L}{10^3 \, mL}\right)\left(\frac{10^1 \, dg}{1 \, g}\right) = 8.2 \times \frac{10^7 \, dg}{10^6 \, mL} = 8.2 \times 10^1 \, {}^{dg}\!/_{mL}$$

PRACTICE PROBLEMS: Section 3.1

Perform the metric conversions and give your answer in scientific notation.

1. 25.5 μg = _____ g
2. 10 mL = _____ L
3. 75 mm = _____ cm
4. 5.0 μm = _____ dm
5. 1.0 Mg = _____ dag
6. 15 nL = _____ mL
7. 12.5 Gm = _____ km
8. 1.07 ng = _____ dg

9. 6 dL = _____ mL
10. 9.0 mL = _____ pL
11. 100 g = _____ mg
12. 2,500 nm = _____ m
13. 15.1 mm = _____ μm
14. 3 μm = _____ km
15. 500 mg = _____ dg

16. 7 hg = _____ pg
17. 1,200 cm = _____ km
18. 12 dL = _____ cL
19. 15 daL = _____ mL
20. 3.8 nm = _____ mm
21. 9.1 mg = _____ kg
22. 3.8 kg = _____ cg

Perform the following conversions.

23. $3.0 \, {}^{mg}\!/_{mL}$ = _____ ${}^{mg}\!/_{L}$
24. $12 \, {}^{mg}\!/_{L}$ = _____ ${}^{mg}\!/_{dL}$
25. $50 \, {}^{mg}\!/_{dL}$ = _____ ${}^{g}\!/_{L}$
26. 2.5 dL = _____ ${}^{ng}\!/_{mL}$

27. $27 \, {}^{g}\!/_{L}$ = _____ ${}^{mg}\!/_{dL}$
28. $60 \, {}^{\mu g}\!/_{mL}$ = _____ ${}^{g}\!/_{dL}$
29. $42 \, {}^{g}\!/_{L}$ = _____ ${}^{mg}\!/_{mL}$
30. $15 \, {}^{ng}\!/_{dL}$ = _____ ${}^{dg}\!/_{mL}$

31. $30 \, {}^{mg}\!/_{dL}$ = _____ ${}^{mg}\!/_{mL}$
32. $5 \, {}^{mg}\!/_{dL}$ = _____ mL
33. $5.5 \, {}^{g}\!/_{dL}$ = _____ ${}^{g}\!/_{L}$
34. $8 \, {}^{g}\!/_{dL}$ = _____ ${}^{mg}\!/_{mL}$

3.2 – CONVERSIONS BETWEEN METRIC AND NONMETRIC

The idea behind converting from metric units to nonmetric units or visa versa is the same as from metric to metric—the goal is to get the units to all cancel except for the last unit (to which we are converting). Before doing some examples, let's refresh our memories with some of the primary relationships between units, as shown in Table 3–2.

TABLE 3-2 Common Unit Conversions

DISTANCE	VOLUME	WEIGHT/MASS
12 in = 1 ft	1 fl oz = 2 tbsp	16 oz = 1 lb
0.91 m = 1 yd	8 fl oz = 1 cup	28.3 g = 1 oz
1 yd = 3 ft	2 cups = 1 pt	2,000 lb = 1 short ton
1 mi = 5,280 ft	4 cups = 1 qt	2,200 lb = 1 metric ton
1.61 km = 1 mi	2 pt = 1 qt	2.2 lb = 1 kg
	4 qt = 1 gal	
	3.79 L = 1 gal	
	1 L = 1.06 qt	
	1 cm³ = 1 mL	
	128 fl oz = 1 gal	
	29.9 mL = 1 fl oz	
	1 qt = 32 fl oz	

EXAMPLE 3-12: Convert: 5 kg = _____ oz

First, convert to pounds. Second, convert pounds to ounces. Note how the units are chosen and set up so that they cancel and the only unit left is ounces. This is the main idea in these types of conversions—all the units cancel except the last unit.

$$5 \, \cancel{kg} \left(\frac{2.2 \, \cancel{lb}}{1 \, \cancel{kg}} \right) \left(\frac{16 \, oz}{1 \, \cancel{lb}} \right) = 176 \, oz$$

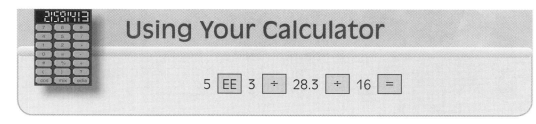

Using Your Calculator

5 [EE] 3 [÷] 28.3 [÷] 16 [=]

EXAMPLE 3-13: Convert: 50 mL = _____ cups

First, convert to ounces. Second, convert ounces to cups. Note how the units are chosen and set up so that they cancel and the only unit left is fluid cups. Again, this is the main idea in these types of conversions—all the units cancel except the last unit.

$$50 \, \text{mL} \left(\frac{1 \, \text{fl oz}}{29.9 \, \text{mL}} \right) \left(\frac{1 \, \text{cup}}{8 \, \text{fl oz}} \right) = 2.1 \times 10^{-1} \, \text{cup}$$

Using Your Calculator

50 [EE] 3 [+/−] [×] 128 [÷] 3.79 [=]

EXAMPLE 3-14: How many cubic centimeters are in 6 cups of H_2O?

First, convert to quarts. Second, convert to gallons. Third, convert to liters and fourth to milliliters. Last, convert to cubic centimeters.

$$6 \, \text{cups} \left(\frac{1 \, \text{qt}}{4 \, \text{cups}} \right) \left(\frac{1 \, \text{gal}}{4 \, \text{qt}} \right) \left(\frac{3.79 \, \text{L}}{1 \, \text{gal}} \right) \left(\frac{1 \, \text{mL}}{10^{-3} \, \text{L}} \right) \left(\frac{1 \, \text{cm}^3}{1 \, \text{mL}} \right) = 1.42 \times 10^3 \, \text{cm}^3$$

EXAMPLE 3-15: How many fluid ounces are in 25 mL?

First convert to liters, second to gallons, and last to fluid ounces.

$$25 \, \text{mL} \left(\frac{10^{-3} \, \text{L}}{1 \, \text{mL}} \right) \left(\frac{1 \, \text{gal}}{3.79 \, \text{L}} \right) \left(\frac{128 \, \text{fl oz}}{1 \, \text{gal}} \right) = 8.44 \times 10^{-1} \, \text{fl oz}$$

EXAMPLE 3-16: How many inches is 30 Gigameters?

$$30 \, \text{Gm} \left(\frac{10^9 \, \text{m}}{1 \, \text{Gm}} \right) \left(\frac{1 \, \text{yd}}{0.91 \, \text{m}} \right) \left(\frac{3 \, \text{ft}}{1 \, \text{yd}} \right) \left(\frac{12 \, \text{in}}{1 \, \text{ft}} \right) = 1.19 \times 10^{12} \, \text{in}$$

Using Your Calculator

30 [EE] 9 [×] 3 [×] 12 [÷] 0.91 [=]

EXAMPLE 3-17: How many grams are in 25 pounds?

$$25 \, \cancel{lb} \left(\frac{16 \, \cancel{oz}}{1 \, \cancel{lb}} \right) \left(\frac{28.3 \, g}{1 \, \cancel{oz}} \right) = 1.1 \times 10^4 \, g$$

EXAMPLE 3-18: A car gets 20 miles per gallon. At this rate how many liters will it take to drive 100 kilometers?

First, convert 20 miles per gallon to kilometers per liter.

$$\frac{20 \, \cancel{mi}}{\cancel{gal}} \left(\frac{1.61 \, km}{1 \, \cancel{mi}} \right) \left(\frac{1 \, \cancel{gal}}{3.79 \, L} \right) = \frac{32.20 \, km}{3.79 \, L}$$

So this car can travel 32.2 kilometers on 3.79 liters. Now we can determine how many liters it takes to drive 100 kilometers, as expressed by

$$\frac{100 \, km}{x \, L} \, ,$$

and we see the units in the first step are the same (kilometers over liters); therefore, this is nothing more than a proportion. Thus, we set up a proportion, cross multiply, and solve.

$$\frac{32.20 \, km}{3.79 \, L} = \frac{100 \, km}{x \, L}$$

Cross multiplying we get

$$32.20x = 379.$$

Dividing by 32.2 we find

$$x = 11.77.$$

Therefore, this car will need 11.77 liters of gasoline to travel 100 kilometers.

EXAMPLE 3-19: How many fluid ounces are in a 500 mL test tube? Solve using two different methods.

Solution 1: Convert 500 mL to fluid ounces.

$$500 \, \cancel{mL} \left(\frac{1 \, fl \, oz}{29.9 \, \cancel{mL}} \right) = 16.7 \, fl \, oz$$

Solution 2: We could solve this by setting up a proportion.

$$\frac{1 \, fl \, oz}{29.9 \, mL} = \frac{x \, fl \, oz}{500 \, mL}$$

Cross multiplying we get

$$29.9x = 500.$$

Dividing both sides by 29.9, we find

$$x = 16.7 \text{ fl oz.}$$

EXAMPLE 3-20: A blood sample had a glucose value of $75\ ^{mg}\!/_{dL}$. Convert this glucose value so its units are $^{g}\!/_{L}$.

First, get the milligrams to cancel. Last, get the deciliters to cancel so the only units left are grams in the numerator and liters in the denominator.

$$\frac{75\ \cancel{mg}}{1\ \cancel{dL}} \left(\frac{1\ g}{10^3\ \cancel{mg}} \right) \left(\frac{10\ \cancel{dL}}{1\ L} \right) = \frac{0.75\ g}{1\ L} = 0.75\ ^{g}\!/_{L}$$

PRACTICE PROBLEMS: Section 3.2

Perform the following conversions.

1. 5.00 oz = _____ g
2. 70 in = _____ m
3. 1.5 qt = _____ mL
4. 2.0 L = _____ gal
5. 3.9 Mg = _____ lb
6. 42.8 kg = _____ lb
7. 2.4 gal = _____ mL
8. 15 mL = _____ cups
9. 5 mi = _____ m
10. 3 yd = _____ mm
11. 28 mg = _____ lb
12. 25 ft = _____ m
13. 20 mL = _____ fl oz
14. 5 in = _____ mm
15. 18.5 lb = _____ kg
16. 98 lb = _____ kg
17. 48.3 kg = _____ lb

18. 20 kg = _____ lb
19. 0.19 lb = _____ g
20. 2 mg = _____ lb
21. A car gets 25 miles per gallon. At this rate how many liters will it take to drive 200 kilometers?
22. A car gets 18 miles per gallon. At this rate how many liters will it take to drive 250 kilometers?
23. A car gets 12 kilometers per liter. At this rate how many gallons will it take to drive 150 miles?
24. How many cubic centimeters are in 8 cups of water?
25. How many cubic centimeters are in 2 quarts of hydrochloric acid?
26. How many cubic centimeters are in 6 liters of saline?

3.3 – APOTHECARIES' AND HOUSEHOLD SYSTEMS

The apothecaries' system is sometimes used to measure drug dosages. Some of the primary units along with their relationships are given in the following list:

$$1 \text{ fluid ounce} = 8 \text{ fluid drams}$$
$$5 \text{ mL} = 1 \text{ tsp}$$
$$4 \text{ mL} = 1 \text{ fluid dram}$$
$$60 \text{ minims} = 1 \text{ fluid dram}$$
$$1 \text{ gram} = 15 \text{ grains}$$
$$1 \text{ grain} = 60 \text{ mg}$$
$$1 \text{ mL} = 16 \text{ minims}$$
$$1 \text{ pt} = 16 \text{ fl oz}$$
$$1 \text{ qt} = 2 \text{ pt}$$

In the apothecaries' system, fluid ounce and fluid dram imply liquid volume. As we see, grain is associated with gram and thus the grain is the basic unit of weight in the apothecaries' system. Also, in the apothecaries' system there are 12 ounces in a pound (not 16). It is also worth noting that the conversions used in the apothecaries' system of measure are approximations. Thus, when using this system, be careful about the answers obtained and conclusions drawn.

In the apothecaries' system, the proper notation is for the unit of measure to be written before the numerical value; if the numerical value is less than 1, fractions are used rather than decimals. The exception to this rule is the fraction $\frac{1}{2}$. To indicate one-half we use ss. Also, in the apothecaries' system, lowercase letters are used instead of uppercase for roman numerals. When roman numerals are used, a bar is often placed over the numerals to avoid errors and confusion.

EXAMPLE 3-21: How many grains is 50 mg?

$$50 \text{ mg} \left(\frac{1 \text{ grain}}{60 \text{ mg}} \right) = \text{gr} \frac{5}{6} = \text{gr } 0.83$$

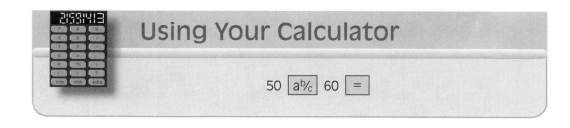

Using Your Calculator

50 [a b/c] 60 [=]

EXAMPLE 3-22: How many milliliters is 250 fluid drams?

$$250 \, \text{fl dr} \left(\frac{4 \, \text{mL}}{1 \, \text{fl dr}} \right) = 1,000 \, \text{mL}$$

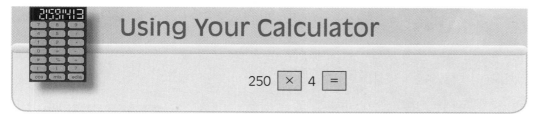

Using Your Calculator

$$250 \boxed{\times} \, 4 \, \boxed{=}$$

EXAMPLE 3-23: How many fluid drams is 4 fl oz?

$$4 \, \text{fl oz} \left(\frac{8 \, \text{fl dr}}{1 \, \text{fl oz}} \right) = \text{fl dr } 32$$

EXAMPLE 3-24: How many grains is 2 grams?

$$2 \, \text{g} \left(\frac{15 \, \text{gr}}{1 \, \text{g}} \right) = \text{gr } 30$$

EXAMPLE 3-25: How many milligrams is $\text{gr } \frac{1}{200}$?

$$\text{gr } \frac{1}{200} \left(\frac{60 \, \text{mg}}{1 \, \text{gr}} \right) = \frac{60}{200} \, \text{mg} = \frac{3}{10} \, \text{mg}$$

EXAMPLE 3-26: How many fluid drams is $\frac{1}{2}$ mL?

$$\frac{1}{2} \, \text{mL} \left(\frac{1 \, \text{fl dr}}{4 \, \text{mL}} \right) = \text{fl dr } \frac{1}{2 \times 4} = \text{fl dr } \frac{1}{8}$$

EXAMPLE 3-27: Express $5 \frac{1}{2}$ grain using roman numerals.

Since v represents 5 and ss represents $\frac{1}{2}$, $5 \frac{1}{2}$ grain would be expressed as

$$\text{gr vss or gr } \overline{\text{vss}}.$$

The Household System

The **household system** is a system used when dispensing medication in the household. The following units and their associated equivalents are used in this system. The units, such as teaspoon, tablespoon, and cup, are commonly found in most every household, hence the name *household system*.

$$60 \text{ drops} = 1 \text{ tsp}$$
$$1 \text{ fl oz} = 30 \text{ mL}$$
$$2 \text{ tbs} = 1 \text{ oz}$$
$$6 \text{ fl oz} = 1 \text{ teacup}$$
$$8 \text{ fl oz} = 1 \text{ glass}$$
$$16 \text{ oz} = 1 \text{ lb}$$
$$1 \text{ cup} = 8 \text{ fl oz}$$

NOTE

We do not see pints or quarts in this list. That is because these are considered to be part of the apothecaries' system.

EXAMPLE 3-28: A person at home drank $3\frac{1}{2}$ glasses of water. How many ounces did this individual consume?

$$3\frac{1}{2} \text{ glasses} \left(\frac{8 \text{ fl oz}}{1 \text{ glass}} \right) = \frac{7}{2} \times 8 = 28 \text{ fl oz}$$

 ## Using Your Calculator

$$3 \boxed{a^b/_c} \; 1 \boxed{a^b/_c} \; 2 \boxed{\times} \; 8 \boxed{=}$$

EXAMPLE 3-29: A patient drank 1 teacup of juice, a glass of water, and 16 fl oz of coffee. What was the total fluid intake, in fluid ounces, for this patient?

1 teacup = 6 fl oz and 1 glass = 8 fl oz. Therefore, this patient drank a total of

$$6 + 8 + 16 = 30 \text{ fl oz.}$$

EXAMPLE 3-30: How many tablespoons are in 12 oz?

$$12 \text{ oz} \left(\frac{2 \text{ tbs}}{1 \text{ oz}} \right) = 24 \text{ tbs}$$

The following are some of the fundamental conversions between various systems:

4 mL = 1 dram
1 g = 15 grains
60 mg = 1 grain
1 g = 1,000 mg
2.2 lb = 1 kg
1 tsp = 5 mL
1 tbs = 15 mL
1 tbs = 3 tsp
1 cup = 240 mL
1 mL = 16 minims
1 pt = 16 oz
1 fl oz = 30 mL
1 cup = 8 fl oz
1 qt = 32 fl oz
1 mL = 1 cc

PRACTICE PROBLEMS: Section 3.3

Perform the following conversions.

1. 5 fl oz = _____ fl dr

2. 5 fl dr = _____ minims

3. 2 fl dr = _____ fl oz

4. 200 minims = _____ dr

5. $5\frac{1}{4}$ glasses = _____ fl oz

6. 81 fl oz = _____ teacups

7. $\frac{1}{2}$ tbs = _____ tsp

8. $\frac{1}{2}$ tbs = _____ drops

9. 12 fl oz = _____ tsp

10. 25 fl oz = _____ mL

11. 16 fl oz = _____ mL

12. 100 mL = _____ fl oz

13. 250 mL = _____ tsp

14. 28 mL = _____ tsp

15. $\frac{1}{2}$ tsp = _____ mL

16. 75 tsp = _____ mL

17. $\frac{3}{4}$ mL = _____ minims

18. 15.4 g = _____ grains

19. A patient drank 2 glasses of soda water, 1 teacup of coffee, and 4 fluid ounces of juice. What is the total fluid intake (in ounces) of this patient?

20. A patient drank 1 glass of soda, 2 teacups of coffee, and 8 fluid ounces of juice in one day. What is the total fluid intake (in ounces) of this patient for that day?

3.4 – TEMPERATURE CONVERSIONS

The three scales used for temperature are **Fahrenheit**, **Celsius**, and **Kelvin**. Like the metric system, the Celsius system is based on powers of 10. Celsius uses the fundamental properties of water, at sea level, to create its relationship. It simply defines 0°C to equal the freezing point of water at sea level and 100°C to equal the boiling point of water at sea level. We will not take the time to derive the formulas; we will simply state them.

Celsius versus Fahrenheit

Following is the formula for converting a given temperature in Celsius to Fahrenheit:

$$°F = \left(°C \times \frac{9}{5} \right) + 32°$$

Note that $\frac{9}{5} = 1.8$. If we use 1.8 instead of $\frac{9}{5}$, we have

$$°F = (°C \times 1.8) + 32°.$$

Either of these formulas works; however, we will use the formula containing 1.8.

EXAMPLE 3-31: How many degrees Fahrenheit is 0°C?

Substitute 0° into the preceding formula.

$$°F = (0° \times 1.8) + 32° = 0° + 32° = 32°$$

Because 0°C is the temperature at which water freezes at sea level, 32°F is also the freezing point of water at sea level.

EXAMPLE 3-32: How many degrees Fahrenheit is 100°C?

$$°F = (100° \times 1.8) + 32° = 180° + 32° = 212°$$

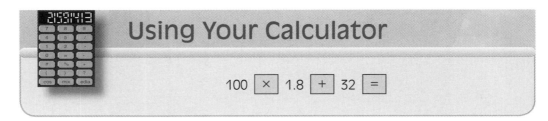

Using Your Calculator

100 × 1.8 + 32 =

It is common knowledge in the United States that 212°F is the boiling point of water.

EXAMPLE 3-33: How many degrees Fahrenheit is 37°C?

$$°F = (37° \times 1.8) + 32° = 66.6° + 32° = 98.6°$$

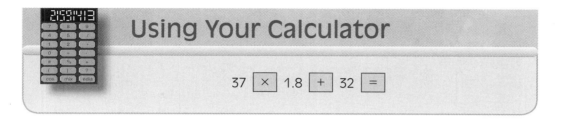

Using Your Calculator

37 [×] 1.8 [+] 32 [=]

Most people know that 98.6°F is normal body temperature. Therefore, in Celsius, 37° is normal body temperature.

EXAMPLE 3-34: How many degrees Fahrenheit is −40°C?

$$°F = (−40° \times 1.8) + 32° = −72° + 32° = −40°$$

These results tell us that −40° is the temperature at which Celsius and Fahrenheit are equal.

We can use the formula that we have just been using to derive the formula that converts a temperature in Fahrenheit to its equivalent temperature in Celsius. All we have to do is solve the equation we have just been using for °C.

We know that

$$°F = (°C \times 1.8) + 32°.$$

Subtracting 32° from both sides, we get

$$°F − 32 = °C \times 1.8.$$

Dividing both sides by 1.8, we get

$$\frac{°F − 32°}{1.8} = °C,$$

which is the same as

$$°C = \frac{°F − 32°}{1.8}.$$

EXAMPLE 3-35: How many degrees Celsius is 75°F?

Substituting 75° into the previous equation, we get

$$°C = \frac{°75 - 32°}{1.8} = \frac{43°}{1.8} = 23.9°.$$

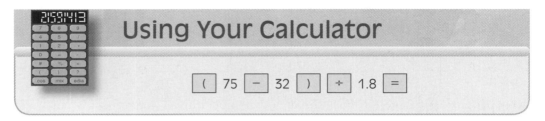

EXAMPLE 3-36: How many degrees Celsius is −25.8°F?

$$°C = \frac{-25.8° - 32°}{1.8} = \frac{-57.8°}{1.8} = -32.1°$$

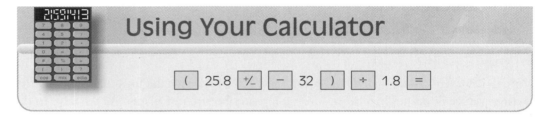

Kelvin

A man by the name of Lord Kelvin developed the kelvin (the k is supposed to be low-ercase) temperature scale, and it has a very simple relationship with the Celsius scale. The formula for converting a given temperature in Celsius to kelvin is

$$°K = °C + 273.15°.$$

From this equation, we can see that when °C = −273.15, °K = 0. This temperature is referred to as **absolute zero.** This is a theoretical temperature and is supposedly the coldest temperature in the universe.

From the kelvin equation, note that subtracting 273.15 from both sides yields

$$°C = °K - 273.15.$$

Clearly, we could use this formula to convert a given temperature in kelvin to Celsius.

EXAMPLE 3-37: Convert 100°C to °K.

Simply substitute this value into the formula $°K = °C + 273.15°$.

$$°K = 100° + 273.15° = 373.15°$$

We know from our earlier discussions in this section that $°C = \frac{°F - 32°}{1.8}$. Substituting this into the formula $°K = °C + 273.15°$, we obtain

$$°K = \frac{°F - 32°}{1.8} + 273.15°.$$

To solve this equation for °F, first subtract 273.15 from both sides, yielding

$$°K - 273.15° = \frac{°F - 32°}{1.8}.$$

Multiplying both sides by 1.8, we get

$$1.8(°K - 273.15°) = \frac{°F - 32°}{1.8}(1.8).$$

Reducing the 1.8s on the right-hand side and distributing the 1.8 on the left-hand side, we get

$$1.8°K - 491.67° = °F - 32°.$$

Adding 32 to both sides, we get

$$1.8°K - 491.67° + 32° = °F - 32° + 32°,$$

and simplifying we get

$$1.8°K - 459.67° = °F.$$

Rearranging we have

$$°F = 1.8°K - 459.67°.$$

This formula is used to convert a temperature in kelvin to degrees Fahrenheit. It can also be solved for °K and then used to convert a given temperature in Fahrenheit to kelvin.

EXAMPLE 3-38: Convert 300°K to °F.

Substitute 300 into the preceding formula and simplify.

$$°F = 1.8(300°) - 459.67° = 80.33°$$

EXAMPLE 3-39: Convert 98.6°F to °K.

Substitute this into the formula °F = 1.8°K − 459.67° and then solve for °K.

$$98.6° = 1.8°K - 459.67°$$

Adding 459.67 to both sides, we get

$$558.27° = 1.8°K.$$

Dividing both sides by 1.8, we obtain

$$°K = 310.15.$$

PRACTICE PROBLEMS: Section 3.4

Perform the temperature conversions.

1. 150°C = _____ °F	7. 50°F = _____ °C	13. 32°F = _____ °K
2. 25°C = _____ °F	8. 100°F = _____ °C	14. 200°K = _____ °F
3. 90°C = _____ °F	9. 150°F = _____ °C	15. 50°C = _____ °K
4. −15°C = _____ °F	10. 72°F = _____ °C	16. 150°K = _____ °C
5. −25°C = _____ °F	11. −30°F = _____ °C	17. 250°K = _____ °C
6. −5°C = _____ °F	12. −50°F = _____ °C	18. 212°F = _____ °K

CHAPTER SUMMARY

- To perform conversions correctly, you must be very familiar with Table 3–1. If you thoroughly understand this table, you will be able to perform conversions no matter which method you use. Understanding relationships such as how many centiliters are in a liter and how many liters are in a centiliter makes setting up a conversion straightforward.
- When setting up a conversion, keep in mind that you want all the units to cancel with the exception of the units to which you are converting.
- Conversions *within* the metric system can be done by using the horizontal format.
- The apothecaries' system is often used in calculating drug dosages, and the household system is used when administering medications in the home.
- Following are the three main temperature formulas:

$$°F = (°C \times 1.8) + 32°$$

$$°C = \frac{°F - 32°}{1.8}$$

$$°K = °C + 273.15°$$

CHAPTER TEST

1. Perform the metric conversions.

   a) $25 \text{ nL} = \rule{2cm}{0.4pt} \text{ mL}$

   b) $10 \ \mu\text{L} = \rule{2cm}{0.4pt} \text{ nL}$

   c) $4 \text{ cm} = \rule{2cm}{0.4pt} \text{ km}$

   d) $15 \text{ ng} = \rule{2cm}{0.4pt} \text{ kg}$

   e) $6 \ \mu\text{g} = \rule{2cm}{0.4pt} \text{ mg}$

   f) $12 \text{ mg} = \rule{2cm}{0.4pt} \text{ cg}$

   g) $20 \ ^{\text{mg}}\!/_{\text{dL}} = \rule{2cm}{0.4pt} \ ^{\text{g}}\!/_{\text{L}}$

   h) $25 \ ^{\mu\text{g}}\!/_{\text{mL}} = \rule{2cm}{0.4pt} \ ^{\text{g}}\!/_{\text{dL}}$

2. Perform the conversions.

   a) $28 \text{ lb} = \rule{2cm}{0.4pt} \text{ mg}$

   b) $1.5 \text{ gal} = \rule{2cm}{0.4pt} \text{ L}$

   c) $5.0 \text{ mg} = \rule{2cm}{0.4pt} \text{ lb}$

   d) $10 \text{ oz} = \rule{2cm}{0.4pt} \text{ mg}$

   e) $0.1 \text{ qt} = \rule{2cm}{0.4pt} \text{ mL}$

3. How many cubic centimeters are in 3 cups of water?

4. Six cups equals how many glasses?

5. Convert: 50 drops = _____ tbs

6. Convert: 30 mL = _____ fl oz

7. Convert: 8 cc = _____ mL

8. Perform the following temperature conversions.
    a) 40°C = _____ °F
    b) −10°C = _____ °F
    c) 105°F = _____ °C
    d) 75°F = _____ °C
    e) 50°K = _____ °F
    f) 150°K = _____ °F

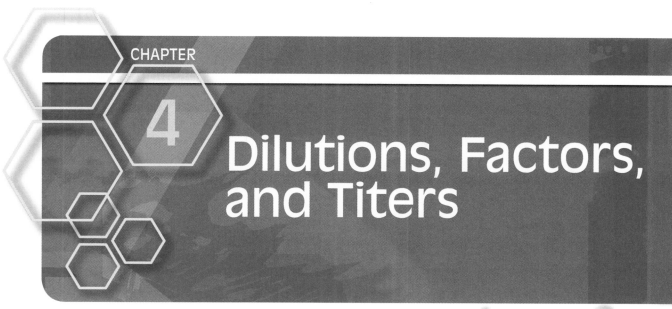

Dilutions, Factors, and Titers

INTRODUCTION

In the clinical laboratory, we are constantly mixing a concentrated solution, called a **concentrate**, with a solvent, referred to as the **diluent**, to decrease the concentration. For example, concentrated hydrochloric acid might need to be "watered down" because it is too strong in its concentrated form. If this concentrated hydrochloric acid is added to water, the hydrochloric acid would be the *concentrate* and the water would be the *diluent*. In the medical laboratory, serum is often the concentrate, and it is diluted with a saline solution or water. In this case the serum is the concentrate and the saline solution or water is the diluent. While these cases involve one dilution, sometimes it is necessary to perform several successive dilutions. These are referred to as *serial dilutions*. Serial dilutions are a necessary part when performing a *titer analysis,* which is the topic of Section 4.3.

EXAMPLE 4-1: Let's say we have a solution containing 1 μL of serum and 6 μL of saline. Clearly, this solution has a total volume of 7 μL. Recall from Chapter 2, the *ratio* of serum to saline would be $\frac{1}{6}$ (or 1:6), the ratio of serum to total volume would be $\frac{1}{7}$ (or 1:7), and the saline to total volume ratio would be $\frac{6}{7}$ (or 6:7).

Dilutions simply represent parts of concentrate in total volume. Therefore, in the previous example, the dilution would be $\frac{1}{7}$ because the concentrate is serum (and we had 1 μL of serum) and the total volume is 7 μL. We say there is a 1 in 7 dilution of serum in saline. Be careful because people often mistakenly think this means there is 1 part serum and 7 parts saline when it actually means 1 part serum and 7 total parts solution. We can also think of this as 1 part serum plus 6 parts saline gives us the total number of 7 parts solution. One of the main concepts to understand here is the mathematical equation that relates the concentrate with the diluent. Remember, dilution is defined as parts concentrate in total volume. But how do we get the total volume? We add a certain amount of diluent to the concentrate to get our total volume. Therefore,

> Parts concentrate + Parts diluent = Total volume.

This is the primary formula we use in the next section when doing calculations involving dilutions.

4.1 – SINGLE DILUTION CALCULATIONS AND FACTORS

Example 4-1 illustrated a procedure involving one dilution. We had a concentrate (serum), and we diluted it down by adding it to a diluent (saline). We will now continue with more examples that entail a single dilution.

EXAMPLE 4-2: We need to make a 1 in 10 dilution of serum in saline. The total volume must be 180 μL.

    a)   What volume of serum is needed?
    b)   What volume of diluent is needed?

Use the following diagram to visualize a 1 in 10 dilution of serum. The dark circle is the serum particle and the lighter circles are the saline particles. Notice there is 1 dark particle and 9 lighter particles to give a total of 10 particles.

    a)   To determine what volume of serum is needed, we simply set up a proportion.

$$\frac{1 \text{ part serum}}{10 \text{ parts total volume}} = \frac{x \text{ parts serum}}{180 \text{ parts total volume}}$$

Cross multiplying we get

$$10x = 180.$$

Dividing both sides by 10, we get

$$x = 18.$$

Therefore, we need 18 parts of serum. The units involved here are μL, so we need 18 μL of serum.

b) To figure out the volume of diluent, use the driving equation.

$$\text{Parts concentrate} + \text{Parts diluent} = \text{Total volume}$$

In part a we found the amount of concentrate (serum) needed, and the problem asks for a total solution amount of 180 μL. Substituting these into the driving equation, we get

$$18 + x = 180.$$

Solving this by subtracting 18 from both sides, we get

$$x = 162.$$

Therefore, we need 162 μL of saline to make this solution. Because the total volume is 180 μL, we would take 18 μL serum and add it to 162 μL of saline to get our total volume of 180 μL of solution. Notice the dilution for this is

$$\frac{\text{Parts serum}}{\text{Total volume}} = \frac{18\ \mu\text{L}}{180\ \mu\text{L}} = \frac{18}{180} = \frac{1}{10}.$$

And a 1 in 10 dilution is exactly what we wanted (and got).

EXAMPLE 4-3: We need to make a 1 in 9 dilution of sodium hydroxide in water. The total volume must be 225 μL.

a) What volume of sodium hydroxide is needed?
b) What volume of diluent is needed?

a) To solve this, set up a proportion.

$$\frac{1\,\text{part sodium hydroxide}}{9\,\text{parts total volume}} = \frac{x\,\text{parts sodium hydroxide}}{225\,\text{parts total volume}}$$

Cross multiplying we get

$$9x = 225.$$

Dividing both sides by 9, we find $x = 25$.

b) From part a we know we need 25 μL of sodium hydroxide.

$$\text{Sodium hydroxide} + \text{Diluent} = \text{Total volume}$$

$$25 + x = 225$$

Subtracting 25 from both sides, we get

$$x = 200.$$

Therefore, we need 200 μL of diluent.

NOTE

The dilution is $\dfrac{25}{225} = \dfrac{\cancel{25} \times 1}{\cancel{25} \times 9} = \dfrac{1}{9}$, which is exactly what we want.

EXAMPLE 4-4: Find the quantity of hydrogen peroxide in water in 160 μL of solution if the dilution is 1 in 8.

$$\frac{1\,\text{hydrogen peroxide}}{8\,\text{total volume}} = \frac{x\,\text{hydrogen peroxide}}{160\,\text{total volume}}$$

Cross multiplying we get

$$8x = 160.$$

Dividing by 8 we find

$$x = 20.$$

> **NOTE**
>
> $\dfrac{\overset{1}{\cancel{20}}}{\underset{8}{\cancel{160}}} = \dfrac{1}{8}$ and 20 μL hydrogen peroxide + 140 μL water = 160 μL total

EXAMPLE 4-5: A solution totaling 45 μL is made by diluting a glucose solution 1:9. How much of the original glucose solution was used in the dilution?

$$\frac{1\,\text{glucose}}{9\,\text{total volume}} = \frac{x\,\text{glucose}}{45\,\text{total volume}}$$

Cross multiplying we get

$$9x = 45.$$

Dividing by 9 we find

$$x = 5.$$

> **NOTE**
>
> $\dfrac{5}{45} = \dfrac{1}{9}$ and 5 μL glucose + 40 μL water = 45 μL total

EXAMPLE 4-6: For a 3 in 10 dilution, what is the ratio of serum to saline?

By the definition of dilution, Part serum/Total volume = $\dfrac{3}{10}$, and the governing equation is

$$\text{Serum} + \text{Diluent} = \text{Total volume}.$$

Therefore,

$$3 + x = 10$$

and

$$x = 7 \text{ (remember, this is the amount of saline).}$$

Thus, the serum to saline ratio is $\dfrac{3}{7}$.

EXAMPLE 4-7: For a 2 in 15 dilution, what is the ratio of ammonia to water?

By the definition of dilution, Part ammonia/Total volume, the governing equation is

$$\text{Ammonia} + \text{Water} = \text{Total volume.}$$

Therefore,

$$2 + x = 15.$$

Solving we find

$$x = 13 \text{ (remember, this is the amount of water).}$$

Thus, the ammonia to water ratio is $\dfrac{2}{13}$.

Final Concentrations

Concentration refers to the amount of a particular substance in a given volume. Therefore, the more substance in a given volume, the more concentrated the solution. Likewise, the less substance in a given volume, the less concentrated the solution. Now, suppose we have a 10% solution. That means 10% of the entire solution is made of some substance. Let's say we wish to dilute this in half. That is, we want the concentration to be half as strong or the dilution to be $\dfrac{1}{2}$. Clearly, half of 10% is 5%. But we can also see that

$$10\% \times \frac{1}{2} = \frac{10\%}{1} \times \frac{1}{2} = \frac{10\%}{2} = 5\%.$$

Therefore,

Original concentration × Dilution = Final concentration.

EXAMPLE 4-8: Find the final concentration if we dilute a saline solution consisting of 10% NaCl using a $\frac{1}{8}$ dilution.

$$\text{Original concentration} \times \text{Dilution} = \text{Final concentration}$$

$$10\% \times \frac{1}{8} = \frac{10\%}{8} = 1.25\%$$

EXAMPLE 4-9: Find the final concentration if we dilute a saline solution consisting of 18% KCl using a $\frac{1}{12}$ dilution.

$$\text{Original concentration} \times \text{Dilution} = \text{Final concentration}$$

$$18\% \times \frac{1}{12} = \frac{18\%}{12} = 1.50\%$$

EXAMPLE 4-10: An 8% solution is diluted $\frac{1}{100}$. What is the final concentration?

$$8\% \times \frac{1}{100} = \frac{8\%}{100} = 0.08\%$$

Factors

In the laboratory the scientist is often trying to find an "answer" about a patient's specimen. However, it is often necessary to dilute the specimen first to properly analyze it. When diluting a specimen and then analyzing it, always remember to make the appropriate correction for the results obtained from the diluted specimen. For example, if you are trying to find the glucose concentration of a blood sample and you dilute the sample, the glucose concentration of the diluted sample will have a lower value than that of the original specimen. If you dilute the specimen using a $\frac{1}{10}$ dilution, then the glucose value of the diluted specimen will be $\frac{1}{10}$ of the original specimen. Therefore, remember to make an appropriate adjustment. To make this correction, you use a dilution factor. The **dilution factor** is the reciprocal of the dilution. For example, if the dilution is $\frac{1}{10}$, the dilution factor would be 10 since $\frac{1}{10} \times 10 = 1$. This should make sense because if the dilution is $\frac{1}{10}$, the concentration of the diluted sample will be $\frac{1}{10}$ of the original concentration; therefore, we must compensate by multiplying our results (of the diluted sample) by 10.

EXAMPLE 4-11: Instruments used in the laboratory to measure glucose values can typically detect values less than 800 $^{mg}/_{dL}$. One patient's glucose value was more than 800 $^{mg}/_{dL}$, and the instrument could not read the value correctly. Therefore, the patient's glucose specimen was diluted as follows: 20 μL of serum was added to 80 μL of diluent for a total diluted volume of 100 μL. This diluted sample was then examined and its glucose value was found to be 190 $^{mg}/_{dL}$. What is the dilution factor and what glucose value should be submitted as the patient's actual glucose value?

The dilution that was carried out was

$$\frac{20\ \mu L}{20\ \mu L + 80\ \mu L} = \frac{20\ \mu L}{100\ \mu L} = \frac{1}{5}$$

The dilution factor is the reciprocal of the dilution, so the dilution factor is 5.

Multiply the glucose value of the diluted sample by this dilution factor to get

$$190\ ^{mg}\!/_{dL} \times 5 = 950\ ^{mg}\!/_{dL}.$$

The glucose value that should be submitted as the patient's actual glucose value is $950\ ^{mg}\!/_{dL}$.

EXAMPLE 4-12: A serum dilution is made using a 1 to 6 ratio of serum to diluent. The glucose concentration of the diluted specimen was found to be $140\ ^{mg}\!/_{dL}$. What is the dilution factor and what glucose value should be reported for the serum?

The dilution that was carried out was

$$\frac{1\ part\ serum}{1\ part\ serum + 6\ parts\ diluent} = \frac{1}{7}.$$

The dilution factor is the reciprocal of the dilution, so the dilution factor is 7.

We multiply the glucose value of the diluted sample by this dilution factor to get

$$140\ ^{mg}\!/_{dL} \times 7 = 980\ ^{mg}\!/_{dL}.$$

Thus, the glucose value that should be reported is $980\ ^{mg}\!/_{dL}$.

EXAMPLE 4-13: A sample had a highly elevated cholesterol level; therefore, a dilution with a 1 to 3 ratio of serum to diluent is made. The cholesterol value of the diluted specimen was found to be $95\ ^{mg}\!/_{dL}$. What is the dilution factor and what cholesterol value should be reported?

The dilution that was carried out was

$$\frac{1\ part\ serum}{1\ part\ serum + 3\ parts\ diluent} = \frac{1}{4}.$$

The dilution factor is the reciprocal of the dilution, so the dilution factor is 4.

Therefore, we multiply the cholesterol value of the diluted sample by this dilution factor to get

$$95\ ^{mg}\!/_{dL} \times 4 = 380\ ^{mg}\!/_{dL}.$$

Thus, the cholesterol value that should be submitted is $380\ ^{mg}\!/_{dL}$.

PRACTICE PROBLEMS: Section 4.1

1. To obtain the desired concentration, 2 mg of substance is required to make 6 mL of solution. How much substance is needed to make 10 mL of solution?

2. To obtain the desired concentration, 3 mg of substance is needed to make 10 mL of solution. How much substance is needed to make 50 mL of solution?

3. To obtain the desired concentration, 4 mg of substance is needed to make 60 mL of solution. How much substance is needed to make 100 mL of solution?

4. To obtain the desired concentration, 8 mg of substance is required to make 20 mL of solution. How much substance is needed to make 250 mL of solution?

5. For a 2 in 7 dilution, what is the ratio of serum to saline? What is the ratio of serum to total volume?

6. For a 3 in 10 dilution, what is the ratio of urine to water? What is the ratio of water to total volume?

7. For a 4 in 15 dilution, what is the ratio of urine to water? What is the ratio of water to total volume?

8. For a 5 in 12 dilution, what is the ratio of serum to saline? What is the ratio of saline to total volume?

9. One microliter of serum is added to 6 μL of diluent. Give the dilution of the solution. What is the serum to total volume ratio?

10. Three milliliters of urine is added to 11 mL of diluent. Give the dilution of the solution. What is the urine to total volume ratio?

11. Two milliliters of urine is added to 15 mL of diluent. Give the dilution of the solution. What is the urine to total volume ratio?

12. Five milliliters of serum is added to 18 mL of diluent. Give the dilution of the solution. What is the serum to total volume ratio?

13. The serum to water ratio is 2 to 3. Find the solution dilution.

14. The alcohol to water ratio is 5 to 8. Find the solution dilution.

15. The alcohol to water ratio is 1 to 10. Find the solution dilution.

16. The serum to water ratio is 3 to 10. Find the solution dilution.

17. Explain how a laboratorian would make 270 mL of a urine in water solution if the dilution is to be 9/15.

18. Explain how a lab technician would make 100 mL of a urine in water solution if the dilution is to be 2/5.

19. Explain how a laboratorian would make 50 mL of a urine in water solution if the dilution is to be 5/8.

20. If 3 parts serum is added to 9 parts water, find the solution dilution.

21. If 2 parts urine is added to 12 parts water, find the solution dilution.

22. If 2 parts serum is added to 5 parts water, find the solution dilution.

23. A lab technician needs to make a 1 in 8 dilution of serum. The total volume must be 120 μL. What volume of serum is needed? What volume of diluent is needed?

24. Four milliliters of urine is to be used to make a 2 in 9 dilution. What will be the total volume of the solution? What volume of diluent is needed?

25. A laboratorian needs to make a 1 in 15 dilution of serum. The total volume is to be 150 μL. What volume of serum is needed? What volume of diluent is needed?

26. Three milliliters of urine is to be used to make a 2 in 8 dilution. What will be the total volume of the solution? What volume of diluent is needed?

27. How would a scientist make 500 mL of a 3/5 dilution of concentrate?

28. How would a scientist make 400 μL of a 2/5 dilution of concentrate?

29. We have 50 μL of a 1/4 dilution of serum. How much serum would be present?

30. How would a scientist make 250 μL of a 1/2 dilution of concentrate?

31. We have 20 μL of a 1/10 dilution of serum. How much serum would be present?

32. Five milliliters of concentrate will make how much of a 2/5 dilution?

33. A 15% solution is diluted $\frac{1}{10}$. Find the final concentration.

34. A 20% solution is diluted $\frac{1}{10}$ and then again by $\frac{1}{100}$. Find the final concentration.

35. A solution whose concentration is 8% is diluted $\frac{1}{2}$ and then again by $\frac{1}{4}$. Find the final concentration.

36. A solution whose concentration is 12% is diluted $\frac{1}{8}$. Find the final concentration.

37. An instrument used in the laboratory to measure cholesterol values has a certain range of values it can measure. A 1/2 dilution of serum in saline is carried out and then reanalyzed. What dilution factor should be used to determine the correct amount of cholesterol in the original specimen?

38. A 1 to 3 ratio of serum to diluent is carried out on a specimen and then reanalyzed. What is the dilution factor needed in this case to obtain the correct amount of cholesterol in the original specimen?

39. An instrument used in the laboratory to measure glucose values has a certain range of values it can measure. One patient's glucose value was too high and the instrument could not read the value correctly. Therefore, the patient's glucose specimen was diluted as follows: 15 μL of serum was added to 90 μL of diluent. This diluted sample was then reanalyzed and its glucose value was found to be 150 $^{mg}\!/_{dL}$. What is the dilution factor and what glucose value should be submitted as the patient's actual glucose value?

Continues

PRACTICE PROBLEMS: Section 4.1 *(continued)*

40. An instrument used in the laboratory to measure cholesterol values has a certain range of values it can measure. A 1/10 dilution of serum in saline is carried out and then reanalyzed. What is the dilution factor needed in this case to obtain the correct amount of cholesterol in the original specimen?

41. To dilute a patient's specimen, 30 μL of serum is added to 150 μL of diluent. What is the dilution factor needed to obtain the correct amount of glucose in the original specimen?

42. A 1 to 4 ratio of serum to diluent is carried out to dilute a specimen. The diluted sample is then reanalyzed. The result is 185 $\frac{mg}{dL}$ of glucose. What is the dilution factor and what glucose value should be submitted?

43. A 1/20 dilution of serum in saline is carried out on a specimen and then the specimen is reanalyzed. What is the dilution factor needed in this case to obtain the correct amount of glucose in the original specimen?

44. The glucose value of a sample of serum is outside the range of the instrument being used to analyze the sample. A 1 to 3 ratio of serum to diluent is used to dilute the specimen. The diluted sample is then reanalyzed. The result is 230 $\frac{mg}{dL}$ of glucose. What is the dilution factor and what glucose value should be submitted?

4.2 – SERIAL DILUTIONS

A series of dilutions is obtained by taking a solution and successively diluting that solution in a given number of steps. A series of dilutions is referred to as **serial dilutions.** In the laboratory this is usually done with test tubes. One reason we might perform such an involved procedure is to estimate the amount of antibodies present in a patient's specimen, a topic discussed in the next section.

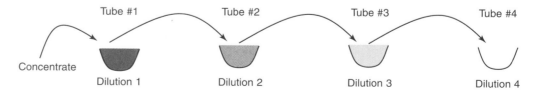

| Tube #1 | Tube #2 | Tube #3 | Tube #4 |

Concentrate

| Dilution 1 | Dilution 2 | Dilution 3 | Dilution 4 |

To find the concentration, dilution, and so on in each test tube, simply apply the same procedures learned in Section 4.1 and repeat until you are at the last test tube. This is demonstrated in the following examples.

EXAMPLE 4-14: An original serum sample contains a substance that has a concentration of $32 \,^{mg}\!/_{dL}$. It is then serially diluted $\dfrac{1}{2}, \dfrac{1}{4}, \dfrac{1}{8},$ and $\dfrac{1}{16}$, each representing the dilution being made.

    a) Find the concentration in each test tube.

    b) In test tube #2, 1 part serum was added to how many parts diluent?

    c) Give the final dilution for the system also known as the **solution dilution**.

    d) Give the final concentration for the system.

We first write this problem in picture format. The number under each tube is the dilution factor.

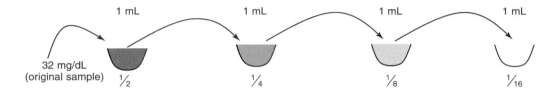

    a) We know from section 4.1 that Original concentration × Dilution = Final concentration.

        Applying this formula, the concentration in the first tube would then be

$$32 \times \frac{1}{2} = 16 \,^{mg}\!/_{dL}.$$

        The concentration in the second tube would be

$$16 \times \frac{1}{4} = 4 \,^{mg}\!/_{dL}.$$

        The concentration in the third tube would be

$$4 \times \frac{1}{8} = \frac{4}{8} = 0.5 \,^{mg}\!/_{dL}.$$

        The concentration in the fourth (and last) tube would be

$$0.5 \times \frac{1}{16} = \frac{0.5}{16} = 0.03125 \,^{mg}\!/_{dL}.$$

    b) The dilution of tube #2 is $\dfrac{1}{4}$. Remember, because serum is the concentrate, the dilution is

$$\frac{\text{Serum}}{\text{Total volume}} = \frac{1}{4}.$$

        Also remember that Serum + Diluent = Total volume, so

$$1 + x = 4, \text{ which means } x = 3.$$

Therefore, in tube #2, for every 1 part diluted serum from tube #1, we need 3 parts diluent. Specifically, we would use 1/4 mL from tube #1 and 3/4 mL diluent to get 1 mL.

c) The solution dilution is nothing more than the product of all the dilutions.

$$\frac{1}{2} \times \frac{1}{4} \times \frac{1}{8} \times \frac{1}{16} = \frac{1}{1,024} \, ^{mg}\!/_{dL}$$

d) The final concentration is simply the last result in part a or $0.03125 \, ^{mg}\!/_{dL}$.

NOTE

Check the answer in Part d by using the equation

$$\text{Original concentration} \times \text{Dilution} = \text{Final concentration}.$$

In this example the original concentration is $32 \, ^{mg}\!/_{dL}$ and the dilution of the entire system is 1 in 1,024. Plugging these into the preceding equation, we get

$$32 \, ^{mg}\!/_{dL} \times \frac{1}{1,024} = \frac{32}{1,024} \, ^{mg}\!/_{dL} = \frac{32^1}{1,024^{32}} \, ^{mg}\!/_{dL} = \frac{1}{32} \, ^{mg}\!/_{dL} = 0.03125 \, ^{mg}\!/_{dL}.$$

At this point let's examine how to multiply the dilutions in part c. The first tube is diluted by $\frac{1}{2}$. Then that is diluted again by $\frac{1}{4}$, which gives us an overall dilution in tube #2 of $\frac{1}{2} \times \frac{1}{4} = \frac{1}{8}$. Now in tube #3 we dilute again by $\frac{1}{8}$; therefore, the overall dilution in tube #3 is

$$\frac{1}{8} \times \frac{1}{8} = \frac{1}{64}.$$

In tube #4 we dilute again by $\frac{1}{16}$; thus, the overall dilution is

$$\frac{1}{64} \times \frac{1}{16} = \frac{1}{1,024}.$$

But this is nothing more than

$$\frac{1}{2} \times \frac{1}{4} \times \frac{1}{8} \times \frac{1}{16} = \frac{1}{1,024}.$$

10-Fold Series

EXAMPLE 4-15: A urine sample has a protein concentration of $300 \, ^{mg}\!/_{dL}$. A dilution series is to be carried out by diluting this sample $\frac{1}{10}$, $\frac{1}{10}$, and again $\frac{1}{10}$, each representing the dilution being made.

 a) Find the concentration in each tube.

 b) Find the solution dilution (final dilution of the system).

 c) Find the final concentration.

As a picture we are looking at

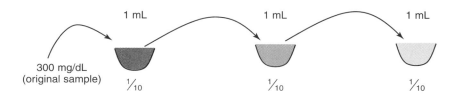

 a) Concentration in tube #1: $300 \times \dfrac{1}{10} = 30 \, ^{mg}\!/_{dL}$

 Concentration in tube #2: $30 \times \dfrac{1}{10} = 3 \, ^{mg}\!/_{dL}$

 Concentration in tube #3: $3 \times \dfrac{1}{10} = 0.3 \, ^{mg}\!/_{dL}$

 b) Solution dilution: $\dfrac{1}{10} \times \dfrac{1}{10} \times \dfrac{1}{10} = \dfrac{1}{1,000} \, ^{mg}\!/_{dL}$

 c) Final concentration: from part a we see it is $0.3 \, ^{mg}\!/_{dL}$

 As a check: $300 \times \dfrac{1}{1,000} = \dfrac{300}{1,000} = \dfrac{3}{10} = 0.3 \, ^{mg}\!/_{dL}$

Doubling

EXAMPLE 4-16: A urine sample has a protein concentration of $400 \, ^{mg}\!/_{dL}$. A dilution series is then carried out with the following dilutions for each tube: $\frac{1}{2}$, $\frac{1}{2}$, $\frac{1}{2}$, $\frac{1}{2}$, and $\frac{1}{2}$, each representing the dilution being made.

 a) Find the concentration in each test tube.

 b) In test tube #2, 1 part urine was added to how many parts diluent?

 c) Give the solution dilution for the system.

 d) Give the final concentration for the system.

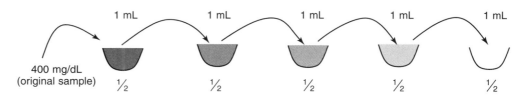

a) Concentration in tube #1: $400 \times \dfrac{1}{2} = 200 \ ^{mg}\!/\!_{dL}$

Concentration in tube #2: $200 \times \dfrac{1}{2} = 100 \ ^{mg}\!/\!_{dL}$

Concentration in tube #3: $100 \times \dfrac{1}{2} = 50 \ ^{mg}\!/\!_{dL}$

Concentration in tube #4: $50 \times \dfrac{1}{2} = 25 \ ^{mg}\!/\!_{dL}$

Concentration in tube #5: $25 \times \dfrac{1}{2} = 12.5 \ ^{mg}\!/\!_{dL}$

b) The dilution of tube #2 is $\dfrac{1}{2}$. Since urine is the concentrate, the dilution is

$$\frac{\text{Urine}}{\text{Total volume}} = \frac{1}{2}$$

We must also remember that Urine + Diluent = Total volume. So

$$1 + x = 2, \text{ which means } x = 1.$$

Therefore in tube #2, for every 1 part diluted urine from tube # 1, we need 1 part diluent. Specifically, we would use 1/2 mL from tube #1 plus 1/2 mL diluent to get a total of 1 mL.

c) The solution dilution for the system is

$$\frac{1}{2} \times \frac{1}{2} \times \frac{1}{2} \times \frac{1}{2} \times \frac{1}{2} = \frac{1}{32}$$

d) The final concentration is the result from part a, which is $12.5 \ ^{mg}\!/\!_{dL}$.

As a check, the final concentration can also be calculated by

$$400 \times \frac{1}{32} = 12.5 \ ^{mg}\!/\!_{dL}.$$

PRACTICE PROBLEMS: Section 4.2

1. Work the series dilution problem.

   An original serum sample contains a substance that has a concentration of 10 $^{mg}\!/_{dL}$. Following are the dilutions for each tube:

   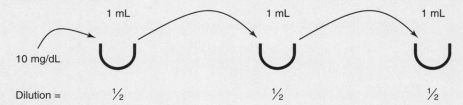

   a) Find the concentration in each tube.

   b) Find the final dilution for the system (solution dilution).

   c) Find the final concentration.

2. An original serum sample contains a substance that has a concentration of 20 $^{mg}\!/_{dL}$. Following are the dilutions for each tube:

   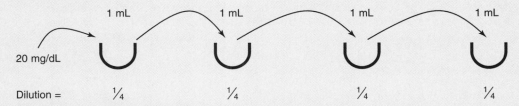

   a) Find the concentration in each tube.

   b) Find the final dilution for the system (solution dilution).

   c) Find the final concentration.

3. A serum sample contains a substance that has a concentration of 50 $^{mg}\!/_{dL}$. Following are the dilutions for each tube:

   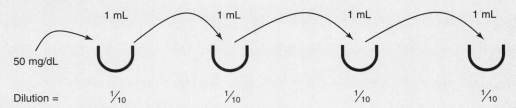

   a) Find the concentration in each tube.

   b) Find the final solution for the system (solution dilution).

   c) Find the final concentration.

Continues

PRACTICE PROBLEMS: Section 4.2 *(continued)*

4. A urine sample has a concentration of $600\,^{mg}\!/_{dL}$. A dilution series is then carried out with the following dilutions for each tube: $\frac{1}{4}, \frac{1}{4}, \frac{1}{4}, \frac{1}{4}$, and $\frac{1}{4}$.

   a) Find the concentration in each test tube.

   b) In test tube #2, 1 part urine was added to how many parts diluent?

   c) Give the solution dilution for the system.

   d) Give the final concentration for the system.

5. A urine sample has a concentration of $400\,^{mg}\!/_{dL}$. A dilution series is then carried out with the following dilutions for each tube: $\frac{1}{2}, \frac{1}{4}, \frac{1}{8}$, and $\frac{1}{16}$.

   a) Find the concentration in each test tube.

   b) In test tube #2, 1 part urine was added to how many parts diluent?

   c) Give the solution dilution for the system.

   d) Give the final concentration for the system.

6. A serum sample contains a substance that has a concentration of $30\,^{mg}\!/_{dL}$. Following are the dilutions for each tube:

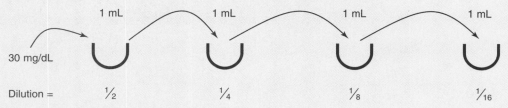

   a) Find the concentration in each tube.

   b) Find the final dilution for the system (solution dilution).

   c) Find the final concentration.

7. A serum sample contains a substance that has a concentration of $150\,^{mg}\!/_{dL}$. Following are the dilutions for each tube:

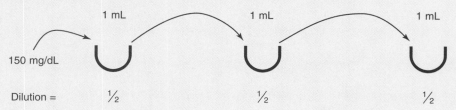

   a) Find the concentration in each tube.

   b) Find the final dilution for the system (solution dilution).

   c) Find the final concentration.

8. A serum sample contains a substance that has a concentration of 90 $^{mg}/_{dL}$. Following are the dilutions for each tube:

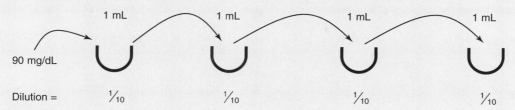

a) Find the concentration in each tube.

b) Find the final dilution for the system (solution dilution).

c) Find the final concentration.

9. A urine sample has a concentration of 500 $^{mg}/_{dL}$. A dilution series is then carried out with the following dilutions for each tube: $\frac{1}{2}, \frac{1}{2}, \frac{1}{2}, \frac{1}{2}$, and $\frac{1}{2}$.

a) Find the concentration in each test tube.

b) In test tube #2, 1 part urine was added to how many parts diluent?

c) Give the solution dilution for the system.

d) Give the final concentration for the system.

10. A urine sample has a concentration of 460 $^{mg}/_{dL}$. A dilution series is then carried out with the following dilutions for each tube: $\frac{1}{10}, \frac{1}{10}, \frac{1}{10}$, and $\frac{1}{10}$.

a) Find the concentration in each test tube.

b) In test tube #2, 1 part urine was added to how many parts diluent?

c) Give the solution dilution for the system.

d) Give the final concentration for the system.

11. A solution that contains 0.8 $^{mg}/_{dL}$ serum is diluted $\frac{1}{2}$, then $\frac{1}{4}$, then $\frac{1}{8}$, and then again $\frac{1}{16}$ in a series. Determine the following.

a) Final concentration

b) Solution dilution

12. A solution that contains 60 $^{mg}/_{dL}$ serum is diluted $\frac{1}{2}$, then $\frac{1}{4}$, then $\frac{1}{8}$, and then again $\frac{1}{16}$ in a series. Determine the following.

a) Final concentration

b) Solution dilution

13. A solution that contains 1.6 $^{mg}/_{dL}$ serum is diluted $\frac{1}{2}$, then $\frac{1}{2}$, then $\frac{1}{2}$, and then again $\frac{1}{2}$ in a series. Determine the following.

a) Final concentration

b) Solution dilution

Continues

PRACTICE PROBLEMS: Section 4.2 *(continued)*

14. A solution contains 45 $\%$. It is diluted $\frac{1}{10}$ and then $\frac{1}{5}$ (serial dilution). What is the concentration of the final solution?

15. A solution contains 60 $\frac{mg}{dL}$ of concentrate. It is diluted $\frac{1}{2}$ and then again by $\frac{1}{2}$ (serial dilution). What is the concentration of the final solution?

16. A solution contains 50 $\%$. It is diluted $\frac{1}{2}$ and then $\frac{1}{4}$ (serial dilution). What is the concentration of the final solution?

4.3 – TITERS

In the medical laboratory, one reason (and certainly not the only reason) we create a series of dilutions is to detect antibody reactivity in a patient's specimen. Antibodies are proteins produced by the immune system. If a patient has a bacterial infection, antibodies are produced to attack the bacteria. To find the antibody reactivity of antibodies present in a patient's specimen, we perform a titer analysis, usually by adding an antigen to each test tube. Adding an antigen to each tube will lead to either a positive or a negative reaction in each tube. The word **titer** refers to the estimation of the amount of a substance in a solution. In our case titer refers to the *last* dilution that produces a positive reaction. The titer is often given as the reciprocal of the last dilution that produces a positive reaction. This idea can be more easily understood by doing some concrete examples.

EXAMPLE 4-17: A Lyme disease antibody titer analysis was prepared by creating a series of dilutions on a patient's serum, with each test tube containing the following dilutions, respectively:

$$\frac{1}{2}, \frac{1}{4}, \frac{1}{8}, \frac{1}{16}, \frac{1}{32}.$$

An examination for the presence of an antibody was then made on each test tube by adding a Lyme disease antigen. It was found to be positive for the $\frac{1}{2}$ and $\frac{1}{4}$ dilutions and negative for the $\frac{1}{8}$, $\frac{1}{16}$, and $\frac{1}{32}$ dilutions. Expressing this a little bit differently, we have

$\frac{1}{2}$	$\frac{1}{4}$	$\frac{1}{8}$	$\frac{1}{16}$	$\frac{1}{32}$
Positive	Positive	Negative	Negative	Negative

The highest concentration that produced a change from positive to negative is $\frac{1}{4}$, so the patient's titer is 4 because the reciprocal of $\frac{1}{4}$ is 4.

EXAMPLE 4-18: A hepatitis A antibody titer analysis was prepared on a blood sample. The serum dilutions were $\frac{1}{2}, \frac{1}{8}$, and $\frac{1}{32}$, respectively. A test for the presence of an antibody was then made by adding a hepatitis A antigen to each of the tubes, and it was found to be positive for the $\frac{1}{2}$ and $\frac{1}{8}$ dilutions and negative for the $\frac{1}{32}$ dilution. Therefore, the patient's hepatitis A titer is 8 since $\frac{1}{8}$ was the highest positive dilution.

PRACTICE PROBLEMS: Section 4.3

1. A dilution series was carried out with a dilution of $\frac{1}{4}, \frac{1}{8}, \frac{1}{16}, \frac{1}{32}$, respectively. Each test tube was then tested for a hepatitis A antibody by adding a hepatitis A antigen to each tube, and the results are as follows:

Tube:	#1	#2	#3	#4
Dilution:	1/4	1/8	1/16	1/32
Test results:	Positive	Positive	Negative	Negative

   What is the titer for this test?

2. A dilution series was executed. Each test tube was then tested for a mononucleosis antibody by adding a mononucleosis antigen to each tube. The results are as follows:

Tube:	#1	#2	#3	#4	#5
Dilution:	1/2	1/4	1/8	1/10	1/20
Test results:	Positive	Positive	Positive	Negative	Negative

   What is the titer for this test?

3. A hepatitis A antibody titer analysis was executed on a blood sample. The dilutions tested were $\frac{1}{4}, \frac{1}{8}, \frac{1}{32}$, and $\frac{1}{64}$. A test for the presence of an antibody was then made by adding a hepatitis A antigen to each of the tubes. Positive reactions were seen in the $\frac{1}{4}, \frac{1}{8}$, and $\frac{1}{32}$ dilutions and negative in the $\frac{1}{64}$ dilution. Find the antibody titer.

4. A dilution series was executed. Each test tube was then tested for a mononucleosis antibody. The results are as follows:

Tube:	#1	#2	#3	#4	#5
Dilution:	1/2	1/4	1/8	1/16	1/32
Test results:	Positive	Positive	Positive	Positive	Negative

   What is the titer for this test?

CHAPTER SUMMARY

- The fundamental formula used when calculating parts concentrate and parts diluent in total volume is

    Parts concentrate + Parts diluent = Total volume.

- Dilutions represent parts of concentrate in total volume.
- A formula used to calculate final concentration is

    Original concentration × Dilution = Final concentration.

- The dilution factor is the reciprocal of the dilution.
- A series of dilutions is referred to as serial dilutions.
- The solution dilution is the product of all the dilutions in a series.
- Titer is the reciprocal of the highest dilution that produces a positive reaction.

CHAPTER TEST

1. We need to make a 1 in 12 dilution of vinegar in water. The total volume must be 300 μL. What volume of vinegar is needed? What volume of diluent is needed?

2. If 4 mg of concentrate will make 30 mL of solution, how much concentrate is needed to make 100 mL of solution?

3. For a 1 in 10 dilution, what is the ratio of serum to saline?

4. If 5 mL of urine is added to 16 mL of diluent, what is the dilution of the solution? What is the ratio of urine to total volume?

5. The alcohol to water ratio is 4 to 15. Find the solution dilution.

6. If 2 parts serum is added to 7 parts water, find the solution dilution.

7. How would a scientist make 600 mL of a 3/4 dilution of concentrate?

8. We have 15 μL of a 1/2 dilution of serum. How much serum would be present?

9. A solution whose concentration is 80% is diluted $\frac{1}{10}$ and then again by $\frac{1}{10}$. Find the final concentration.

10. The glucose value of a sample of serum is outside the range of the instrument being used to analyze the sample. A 1 to 8 ratio of serum to diluent is used to dilute the specimen so the glucose value falls within the range of the instrument being used. The glucose value of the diluted specimen was found to be 120 $^{mg}\!/_{dL}$. What is the dilution factor and what glucose value should be reported?

11. A urine sample has a protein concentration of 280 $^{mg}\!/_{dL}$. A dilution series is to be carried out by diluting this sample $\frac{1}{10}$, $\frac{1}{10}$, and again $\frac{1}{10}$. Find the protein concentration in each tube. Find the solution dilution (final dilution of the system). Find the final concentration.

12. The original serum has a concentration of 40 $^{mg}\!/_{dL}$. Following are the dilutions for each tube:

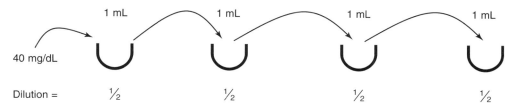

a) Find the concentration in each tube.
b) Find the final dilution for the system (solution dilution).
c) Find the final concentration.

13. A urine sample has a concentration of 420 $^{mg}\!/_{dL}$. A dilution series is then carried out with the following dilutions for each tube: $\frac{1}{10}$, $\frac{1}{10}$, $\frac{1}{10}$, and $\frac{1}{10}$.

a) Find the concentration in each test tube.
b) In test tube #3, 1 part urine was added to how many parts diluent?
c) Give the solution dilution for the system.
d) Give the final concentration for the system.

14. An antibody titer analysis was performed on a dilution series of the patient's serum with the following dilutions carried out on each of the test tubes, respectively: $\frac{1}{2}$, $\frac{1}{4}$, $\frac{1}{8}$, $\frac{1}{16}$, $\frac{1}{32}$.

A test for the presence of an antibody was then made by adding an antigen to each test tube. It was found to be positive for the $\frac{1}{2}$, $\frac{1}{4}$, and $\frac{1}{8}$ dilutions and negative for the $\frac{1}{16}$ and $\frac{1}{32}$ dilutions. Find the titer.

5

Standard Curves, Rate of Change, and Variation

INTRODUCTION

In many courses within the medical and clinical science curriculums, graphs are used to show how two quantities are related. The graphs will be straight lines in some cases and curved lines in others. In either case, to create a graph, the *coordinate plane* is used. Once a graph has been created, we need to be able to read and interpret it. We must also be able to calculate the slope and determine relationships between the plotted quantities. As we will see, the relationship between the two quantities is sometimes *direct* and sometimes *inverse*.

5.1 – THE COORDINATE PLANE

Most often a graph is plotted on the **Cartesian plane**, also known as the **coordinate plane**, illustrated in Figure 5–1. Graph paper used in the laboratory may look a little different, but the idea is the same.

The solid horizontal line is called the **x-axis**, and the solid vertical line is called the **y-axis**. The point where these two lines cross is called the **origin**. At the origin, both x and y equal zero. This coordinate system is a two-dimensional system because any point on this plane can be represented with two pieces of information, namely the x-value, also called the **abscissa**, and the y-value, also called the **ordinate**. These two values are most often written together as an **ordered pair** (x, y). Note the x always comes first and the y always comes second. As an example, $(3, 4)$ is the point at which x is equal to 3 and y is equal to 4. The location of this point is illustrated in Figure 5–2 with a dark point.

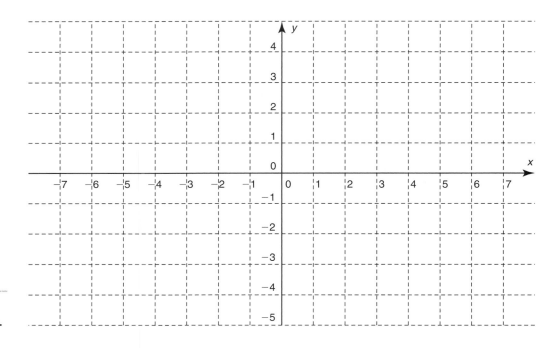

FIGURE 5-1
The coordinate plane.

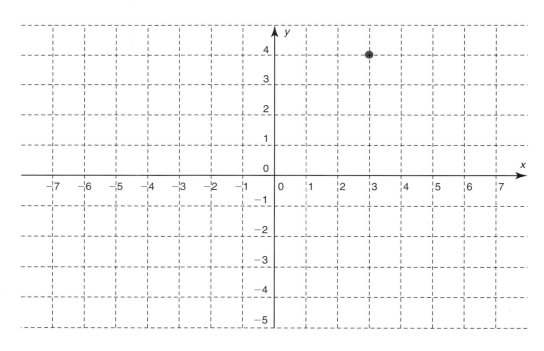

FIGURE 5-2
Location of $(3, 4)$.

Note that the coordinate plane is divided into four regions. These regions are called quadrants, as illustrated in the Figure 5–3.

Another important concept to understand when working with the coordinate plane is that the x-axis and y-axis are usually labeled with some other letter or word. As discussed in the introduction to this chapter, we might want to show how the concentra-

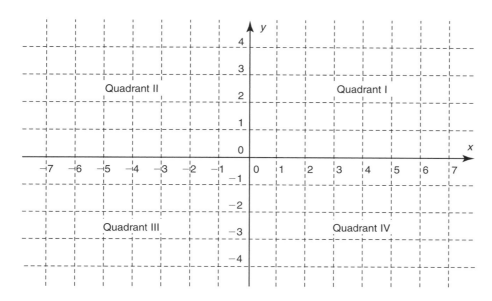

FIGURE 5–3
Quadrants of the coordinate plane.

tion of a solution changes over time. In this case we would label the *x*-axis as time and the *y*-axis as concentration.

Because of the nature of the quantities we use in the laboratory such as concentration, time, volume, and so on, graphs involving these quantities lie entirely in the first quadrant. The reason is because time is never negative nor are volumes or concentrations. Therefore, we often show only the first quadrant, and in such cases the coordinate plane would look like Figure 5–4. Keep in mind, in the laboratory the *x*-axis might be time and the *y*-axis concentration. How the axes are labeled depends upon the experiment being performed.

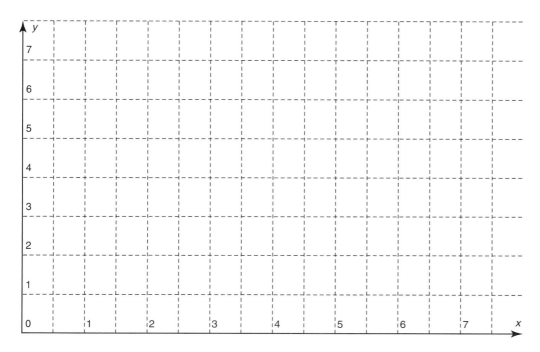

FIGURE 5–4 The first quadrant.

PRACTICE PROBLEMS: Section 5.1

1. Determine which quadrant the following points lie in.

   a) (−8, 12)

   b) (−1, −20)

   c) (50, −10)

   d) (20, 150)

   e) (5, −4)

   f) (−10, −10)

2. Plot the following points on the coordinate plane.

   a) (4, −6)

   b) (5, 1)

   c) (−2, 4)

   d) (−5, −5)

   e) (2, 0)

   f) (0, −4)

   g) (0, 0)

   h) (−3, 0)

3. Express the origin as an ordered pair.

5.2 – SLOPE AND RATE OF CHANGE

Another important property of a graph is the **slope**. Before discussing why this property is so important, we need to understand what it is and how it is defined. The slope is defined as

$$\text{Slope} = m = \frac{\text{change in } y}{\text{change in } x} = \frac{\Delta y}{\Delta x}$$

The letter m is universally used in mathematics to notate slope, and the delta symbol, Δ, is used to notate "change." Therefore, $\Delta y/\Delta x$ can be read as either "the change in y over the change in x" or "delta y over delta x." Many people think of the slope as "the rise over the run" because y is the vertical axis (rise) and x is the horizontal axis (run). Let's take a closer look at what the slope is.

As discussed in Section 5.1, in many situations instead of using x and y, we use some other letters or words such as time and concentration. However, before doing some examples involving time and concentration, let's first look at an example involving time and distance in order to get a better understanding of slope. Let's say the x-axis is labeled as time and the y-axis is labeled as distance. In this case the slope would be

m = Change in distance/Change in time. For example, if a car is traveling down a high-way at 60 mph, the change in distance would be 60 miles and the change in time would be 1 hour. In this case we would then have m = 60 miles/1 hour. This is nothing more than the rate at which the car is traveling—60 miles per hour. Thus, the slope tells us the rate at which things are changing.

If we look at concentration versus time, with concentration as the y-axis and time as the x-axis, the slope would be Change in concentration/Change in time. In this case the slope would be giving us information about the rate at which the concentration is changing over time.

Next we determine the slope of a straight line given its graph. A straight line is often re-ferred to as a **linear function**.

EXAMPLE 5-1: Determine the slope of the following graph in which the concentration is given in multiples of 10 with units of mmol/L and the time is in seconds.

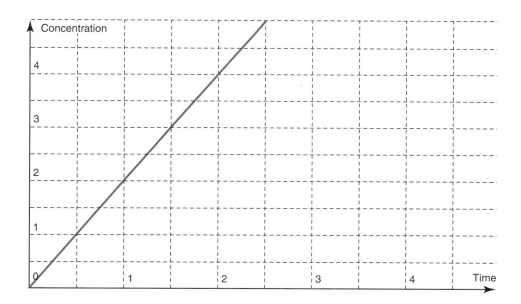

To determine the slope, keep in mind what the definition is—the change in y over the change in x. However, in this case it is the change in concentration over the change in time. To go from one point on the line to another point on the same line, we need to determine how much we go up (change in concentration) and how much we go over (change in time). Begin by picking two points that lie on this line. We will pick the points $(1, 2)$ and $(2, 4)$. Starting at the point $(1, 2)$ in order to get to the point $(2, 4)$, we can go up 2 and then over 1 as illustrated in the following graph.

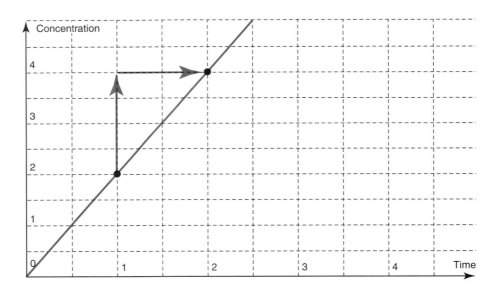

Be careful when counting how much to go up and over. Each dotted line does not represent one unit. For this graph it represents half a unit. Because the change in concentration is 2 and the change in time is 1, we can write the slope as $\frac{2}{1} = 2.$

Therefore, the slope of this line is 2. However, remember the numbers associated with the concentration axis are multiples of 10. Thus, the slope is actually 20 mmol/1 sec. It is easy to see that this is the rate at which the concentration is changing—it is increasing by 20 mmol every 1 second.

How would our answer be affected if we picked the points $(0, 0)$ and $(2, 4)$ to determine the slope instead? As illustrated in the following graph, the number of points we go up is 4, and the number of points we go over is 2. Therefore, the slope in this case is $\frac{4}{2} = 2$. We get the same answer. Therefore, to determine the slope, it does not matter which points are selected on the line.

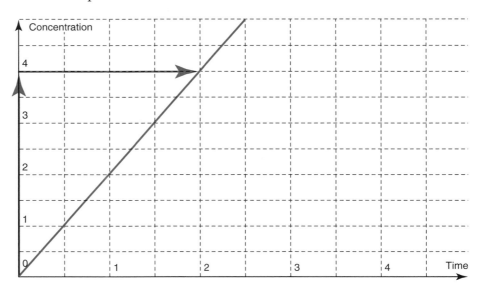

NOTE

When a line rises to the right, it has a positive slope. In this case the slope indicates that the concentration is increasing with time. In general, any curve rising to the right indicates that the quantity on the y-axis is increasing as the quantity on the x-axis increases.

EXAMPLE 5-2: Determine the slope of the following graph.

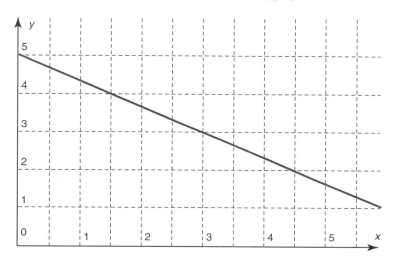

Beginning at the point $(0, 5)$, notice we must move down 2. Moving down corresponds to a decrease in the value of the y. Therefore, the change in y will be -2. We move to the right 3, which corresponds to an increase in x. Therefore, the change in x will be 3. Thus, the slope is

$$m = \frac{\Delta y}{\Delta x} = \frac{-2}{3} = -\frac{2}{3}.$$

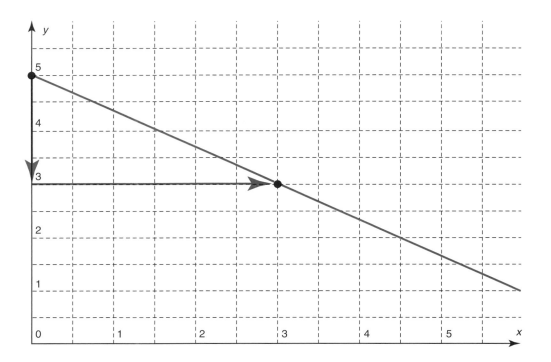

NOTE

When a line falls to the right, it has a negative slope. In general, any graph falling to the right indicates that the quantity on the *y*-axis is decreasing as the quantity on the *x*-axis increases.

In the last two examples, we learned how to determine the slope of a straight line given a graph. However, in many applications instead of a graph we are given two data points. What then do we do to find the change in *y* and the change in *x*? Let's first take a closer look at the real number line. Keep in mind that the *x*-axis and *y*-axis are nothing more than two *real* number lines crossed at a 90-degree angle. So before we discuss how to find the distance between *any* two *x* values or *any* two *y* values, we first look at how to determine the distance between any two points on the real number line.

EXAMPLE 5-3: What is the distance between 3 and 7 on the following number line?

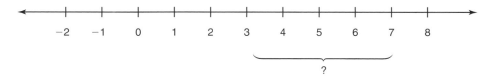

To find the distance between 3 and 7, subtract: $7 - 3 = 4$. Thus, the distance between 3 and 7 is 4. If we think of this number line as the x-axis where 3 and 7 are two different x values, then to find the distance between any two x values, we simply subtract. In mathematics, to indicate two different x values, we use the notation x_1 and x_2. So 3 would be x_1 and 7 would be x_2. In general, to find the distance between any two x values x_1 and x_2, we subtract: $x_2 - x_1$. Therefore, the change in x is simply $x_2 - x_1$. Likewise, the change in y is $y_2 - y_1$. Therefore, the slope would be

$$m = \frac{\text{Change in } y}{\text{Change in } x} = \frac{\Delta y}{\Delta x} = \frac{y_2 - y_1}{x_2 - x_1}.$$

EXAMPLE 5-4: Find the slope of the straight line that contains the two points $(2, 4)$ and $(3, 7)$.

First, label the points. Keep in mind that the first number in each ordered pair is an x value and the second number in each ordered pair is a y value. Therefore,

$$(2, 4) \qquad (3, 7)$$
$$\uparrow \uparrow \qquad \uparrow \uparrow$$
$$x_1 y_1 \qquad x_2 y_2$$

To find the slope, just plug these values into the slope formula where $x_1 = 2$, $x_2 = 3$, $y_1 = 4$, and $y_2 = 7$.

Therefore, the slope is

$$m = \frac{y_2 - y_1}{x_2 - x_1} = \frac{7 - 4}{3 - 2} = \frac{3}{1} = 3.$$

EXAMPLE 5-5: Find the slope of the straight line containing the points $(3, 30)$ and $(7, 60)$.

First, label each point.

$$(3, 30) \qquad (7, 60)$$
$$x_1 \ y_1 \qquad x_2 \ y_2$$

Second, plug these values into the slope formula.

$$m = \frac{y_2 - y_1}{x_2 - x_1} = \frac{60 - 30}{7 - 3} = \frac{30}{4} = \frac{15}{2}$$

EXAMPLE 5-6: Find the slope of the straight line containing the points $(0, 15)$ and $(10, 5)$.

First, label each point.

$$\underset{x_1 \; y_1}{(0, 15)} \qquad \underset{x_2 \; y_2}{(10, 5)}$$

Second, plug these values into the slope formula.

$$m = \frac{y_2 - y_1}{x_2 - x_1} = \frac{5 - 15}{10 - 0} = \frac{-10}{10} = -1$$

EXAMPLE 5-7: At the beginning of an experiment, the concentration of a solution was $25 \, {}^{\text{mmol}}\!/_{\text{dL}}$. Three seconds later the concentration was $54 \, {}^{\text{mmol}}\!/_{\text{dL}}$. Find the rate at which the concentration is changing, given that the rate of change is linear. Use these results to predict what the concentration would be after 12 seconds.

At the beginning of any experiment, the time is zero. Therefore, the first data point is $(0, 25)$. We are given that 3 seconds later the concentration is 54. Thus, the second data point is $(3, 54)$. To find the slope, first label each point.

$$\underset{x_1 \; y_1}{(0, 25)} \qquad \underset{x_2 \; y_2}{(3, 54)}$$

Substituting these values into the slope formula, we find the rate at which the concentration is changing to be

$$m = \frac{y_2 - y_1}{x_2 - x_1} = \frac{54 - 25}{3 - 0} = \frac{29 \; {}^{\text{mmol}}\!/_{\text{dL}}}{3 \; \text{sec}} = 9.7 \, {}^{\text{mmol}}\!/_{\text{dL·sec}}.$$

This result is telling us that the concentration is increasing by $9.7 \, {}^{\text{mmol}}\!/_{\text{dL}}$ every second. If the original concentration is 25, then if we let t represent the number of seconds that have passed, the concentration, C, after t seconds would be

$$C = 25 + 9.7t.$$

Thus, after 12 seconds the concentration should be

$$C = 25 + 9.7(12) = 25 + 116.4 = 141.4 \, {}^{\text{mmol}}\!/_{\text{dL}}.$$

Enzyme Kinetics

Enzyme kinetics involves the examination of the rate at which enzymes react. Enzymes are often used as catalysts to make a reaction occur at a particular rate. Often enzyme kinetics is studied by observing the concentration of a substrate that is available to the enzyme. A **substrate** is the substance the enzyme is acting upon. Typically an enzyme is added to a test tube containing a substrate and the rate at which the substrate is consumed by the enzyme is observed. As a result, a product is formed. It turns out that the amount of product formed is directly proportional to the activity of the enzyme and the amount of time the reaction is given to take effect. As a mathematical equation (this will be explained more thoroughly in section 5.5), we can write this relationship as

$$P = A \cdot t$$

where P is the amount of product formed, A is the activity of the enzyme, and t is the length of time we let the reaction occur.

In the equation $P = A \cdot t$, if we divide both sides by t, we get

$$\frac{P}{t} = \frac{A\,t}{t}.$$

Thus, the enzyme activity A is

$$A = \frac{P}{t}.$$

This is telling us that the activity of the enzyme is equal to the amount of product formed over the amount of time. But the amount of product formed from the beginning of the experiment to the end of the experiment can also be thought of as the change in product. Likewise, the beginning to the end is the change in time. In other words, $A = \Delta P / \Delta t =$ Change in product/Change in time, and this is simply the rate at which the product is changing with respect to time, which is nothing more than the slope. It should be mentioned that enzyme activity is characteristically reported as U or units.

PRACTICE PROBLEMS: Section 5.2

1. Find the slope of the line through (0, 20) and (4, 36).
2. Find the slope of the line through (5, 20) and (3, 50).
3. Find the slope of the line through (20, 60) and (30, 40).
4. Find the slope of the line through (0, 10) and (50, 120).
5. Find the slope of the line through (10, 20) and (20, 10).
6. Find the slope of the line through (10, 100) and (50, 200).
7. Find the slope of the line through (0, 60) and (20, 20).

Continues

PRACTICE PROBLEMS: Section 5.2 *(continued)*

8. Find the slope of the line where the *y*-axis is concentration given in multiples of 10 with units of mmol/L and the *x*-axis is time given in seconds.

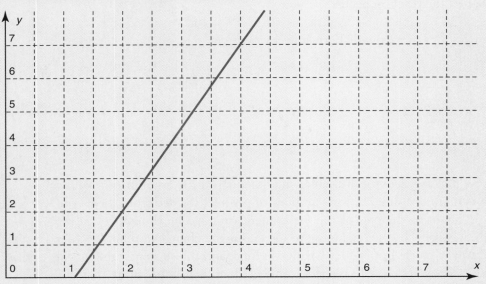

9. Find the slope of the line where the *y*-axis is concentration given in multiples of 10 with units of mmol/L and the *x*-axis is time given in seconds.

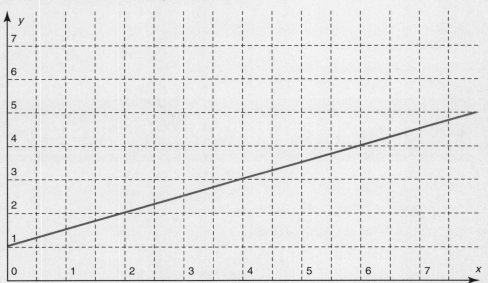

10. Find the slope of the line where the *y*-axis is concentration given in multiples of 10 with units of mmol/L and the *x*-axis is time given in seconds.

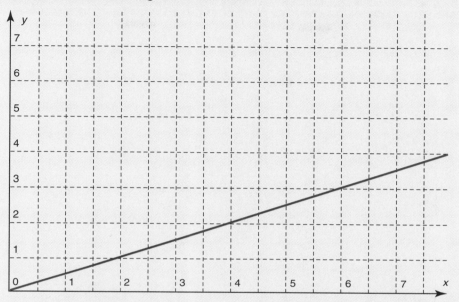

11. Find the slope of the line where the *y*-axis is concentration given in multiples of 10 with units of mmol/L and the *x*-axis is time given in seconds.

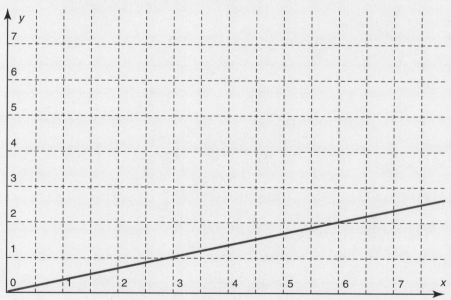

Continues

PRACTICE PROBLEMS: Section 5.2 *(continued)*

12. Find the slope of the line.

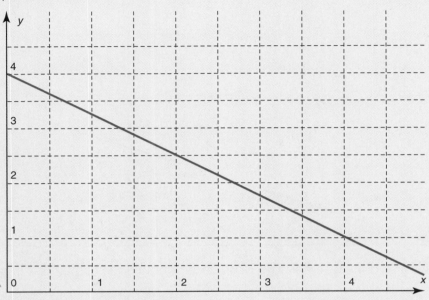

13. Find the slope of the line.

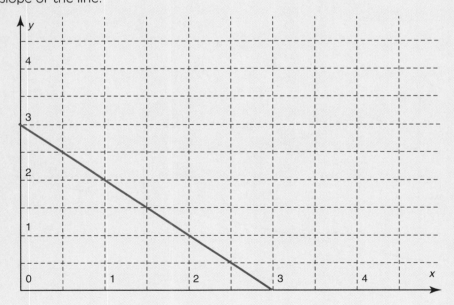

14. Find the slope of the line where the *y*-axis is concentration given in multiples of 10 with units of mmol/L and the *x*-axis is time given in seconds.

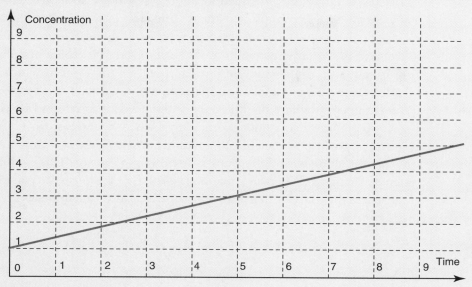

15. Find the slope of the line.

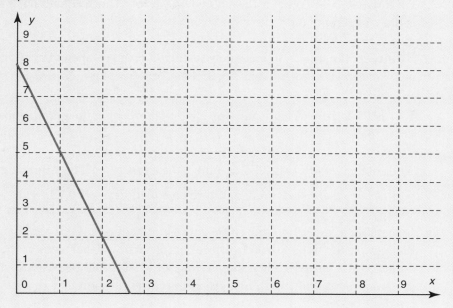

5.3 – LINEAR EQUATIONS AND GRAPHING

As discussed in the previous section, a linear graph is a straight line. A **linear equation** is any equation whose graph is a straight line. The basic form, or **standard form**, of any linear equation is $Ax + By = C$. However, in applications of linear equations, it is often convenient to write the equation in the form given in the blue box that follows. This form is called the **slope-intercept form** and will be the form in which we write linear equations from this point forward. In the equation $y = mx + b$, m is the slope of the line and b is the point where the line crosses the y-axis; b is referred to as the **y-intercept**. This form of a linear equation is commonly used for a few reasons. The primary reason, however, is because when a linear equation is written in this form we can immediately see what the slope is, and the slope is important because it tells us the rate at which a system is changing. When an equation is written in this form, we can identify the slope because it is the number in front of the x. This is also called the **coefficient of x**.

$$y = mx + b$$

EXAMPLE 5-8: What is the slope of the graph whose equation is $y = 3x - 7$? What is the y-intercept?

By inspection, we can immediately see that 3 is the coefficient of x; therefore, the slope is 3. We can also immediately see that the y-intercept is -7.

EXAMPLE 5-9: What is the slope and y-intercept of the graph whose equation is $y = 0.75x$?

The coefficient of x is 0.75 or $\frac{3}{4}$; thus, the slope is $\frac{3}{4}$. The y-intercept is 0 (or the origin) because we can think of the given equation as $y = 0.75x + 0$.

Being able to determine the slope and y-intercept of a given equation makes it easy to then graph the line of that equation. Simply start on the y-axis at the point where the y-intercept is located. Then, depending on what the slope is, go up and over to find a second point on the line. Then just connect the two points with a straight line and you are done.

EXAMPLE 5-10: Graph the portion of $y = 2x + 1$ that lies in the first quadrant.

To begin, first identify the slope and y-intercept. By inspection we see the slope is $m = 2$ or $\frac{2}{1}$ (it is easier if we think of 2 as a fraction because now we see that the rise is 2 and the run is 1). We can also see that the y-intercept is $b = 1$, or $(0, 1)$ as an ordered pair. Therefore, to graph this begin at 1 on the y-axis, then from that point go up

2 points and over 1 point taking you to the point $(1, 3)$. Connecting the two points $(0, 1)$ and $(1, 3)$ gives the following graph.

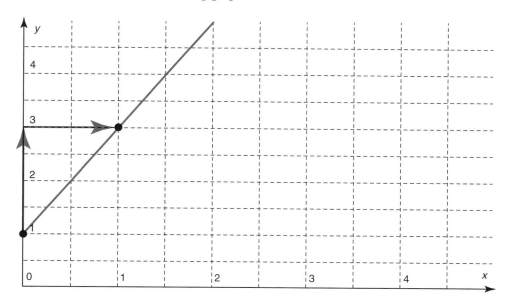

EXAMPLE 5-11: Graph the portion of $y = \frac{2}{3}x$ that lies in the first quadrant.

We can see the slope is $\frac{2}{3}$ and the y-intercept is 0. Therefore, go to 0 on the y-axis (or the origin). Starting at that point, we go up 2 and over 3 leaving us at the point $(3, 2)$. Connecting these two points with a straight line gives the following graph.

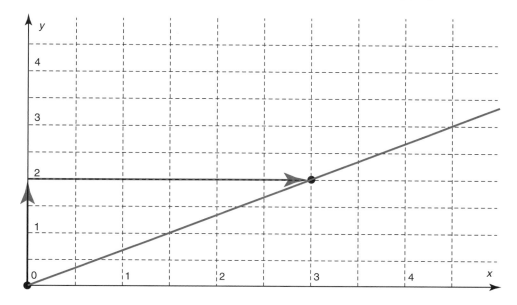

EXAMPLE 5-12: Graph the portion of the line in the first quadrant passing through the point $(2, 1)$ whose slope is 3.

We begin at the point (2, 1) because we are told the line goes through this point. Starting at this point, move up 3 and over 1 because it is given that the slope is 3. Connect these two points with a line.

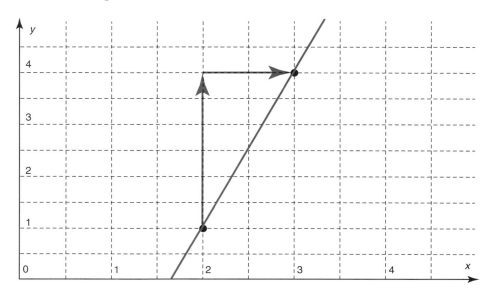

EXAMPLE 5-13: Graph the portion of $y = -2x + 4$ that lies in the first quadrant.

To begin, we must first identify the slope and y-intercept. By inspection we see that the slope is $m = -2$ or $\frac{-2}{1}$ (thinking of -2 as a fraction leads us to see that the rise is actually a fall because of the negative 2). We can also see that the y-intercept is $b = 4$, or $(0, 4)$ as an ordered pair. Therefore, to graph this we begin at 4 on the y-axis, then from that point we go down 2 (because of the negative) and 1 to the right, taking us to the point $(1, 2)$. Connecting the two points $(0, 4)$ and $(1, 2)$, we obtain the following graph.

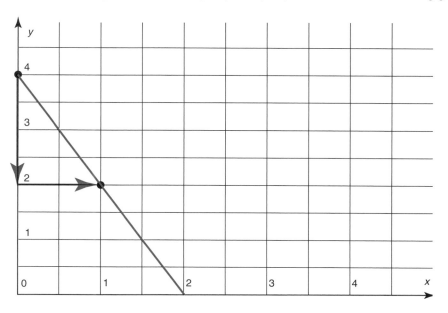

PRACTICE PROBLEMS: Section 5.3

1. Graph the portion of $y = \frac{3}{4}x + 3$ that lies in the first quadrant.

2. Graph the portion of $y = \frac{1}{3}x + 4$ that lies in the first quadrant.

3. Graph the portion of $y = 0.5x$ that lies in the first quadrant. (Hint: Convert the slope, which is in decimal form, to fraction form.)

4. Graph the portion of $y = 0.75x + 1$ that lies in the first quadrant.

5. Graph the portion of $y = 0.2x + 2$ that lies in the first quadrant.

6. Graph the portion of $y = -3x + 5$ that lies in the first quadrant.

7. Graph the portion of $y = -\frac{1}{3}x + 6$ that lies in the first quadrant.

8. Graph the portion of $y = -\frac{3}{5}x + 7$ that lies in the first quadrant.

9. Graph the portion of $y = -0.4x + 8$ that lies in the first quadrant.

10. Graph the line through (2, 1) with a slope of $\frac{3}{4}$.

11. Graph the line through (1, 4) with a slope of -3.

12. Graph the line through (2, 3) with a slope of 0.4.

13. Graph the line through the origin with a slope of 0.5.

14. Graph the line through (0, 10) with a slope of -5.

15. Graph the line through (0, 0) with a slope of $\frac{1}{5}$.

16. Graph the line through (0, 10) with a slope of $-\frac{4}{5}$.

5.4 – READING AND INTERPRETING STANDARD CURVES

A **standard curve** is a graph that is typically used to help determine the concentration of some substance. As we mentioned earlier, the graph paper used in the lab may look a little different from the graph paper used here, but the concept is the same. When we create a standard curve, we use the graph to analyze how values, given by an instrument or some test procedure, behave relative to variations in the concentration. In the laboratory many standard curves take the form of a straight line (linear equation). There are certainly many that do not, but reading and interpreting a graph in either case involves the same concept.

EXAMPLE 5-14: Based on the standard curve that follows, what is the concentration (given in hundreds of milligrams per deciliter) when the time is 4 seconds?

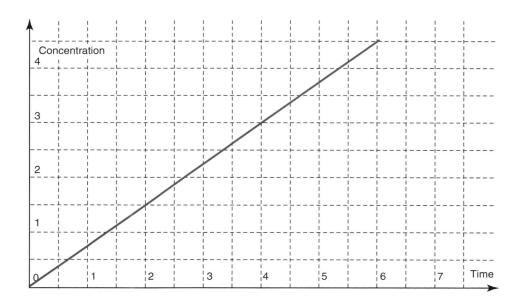

First, go to 4 on the horizontal time axis. Starting at that point, go straight up until you hit the graph as illustrated in Figure 5–5.

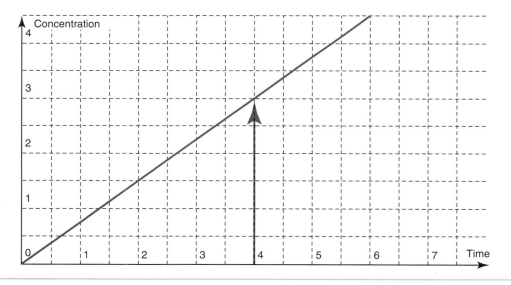

FIGURE 5-5 Determining the concentration beginning with the horizontal axis.

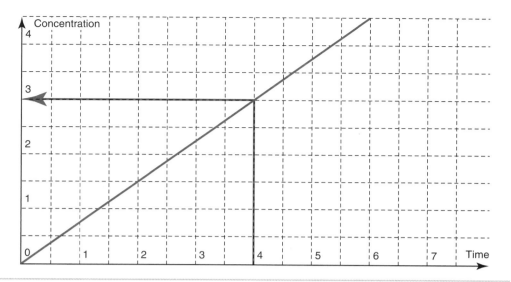

FIGURE 5-6 Solving the concentration.

Next, move directly to the left until you hit the concentration axis as illustrated in Figure 5–6.

We end up at 3 on the concentration axis, and this tells us that the concentration is $300 \, ^{mg}\!/_{dL}$ when the time is 4 seconds.

EXAMPLE 5-15: In the standard curve that follows, the horizontal axis is concentration (given in hundreds of milligrams per deciliter), and the vertical axis is percent transmittance (in tens). **Percent transmittance** tells us about how much light can shine through a solution. Based on the graph that follows, what is the percent transmittance when the concentration is $100 \, ^{mg}\!/_{dL}$? Interpret the behavior of this graph.

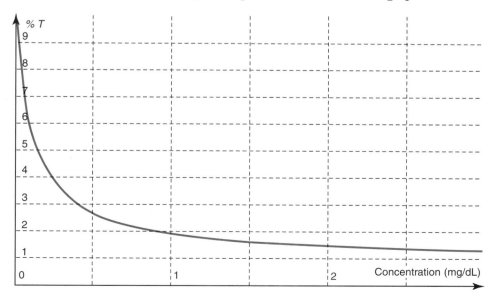

Starting on the concentration axis at 1 (which represents $100 \, ^{mg}/_{dL}$), we move straight up until we hit the graph and then move to the left until we hit the percent transmittance axis, and we find the percent transmittance is 2, which is actually 20% because the % T axis is in tens. This is illustrated on the following graph.

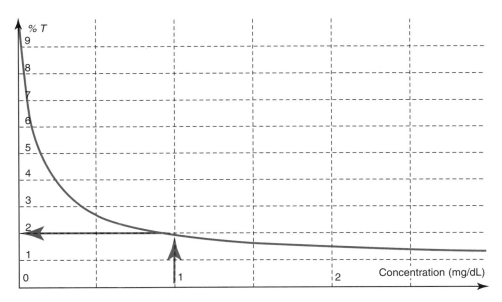

Interpreting this graph we see that as the concentration increases, the percent transmittance decreases. This makes sense because as the concentration of a solution increases, the amount of light able to pass through the solution decreases.

PRACTICE PROBLEMS: Section 5.4

1. The following graph is a plot of time versus concentration where the time is in seconds and the concentration is in tens with units of mmol/L. What is the value of the concentration when the time is 2? What is the value of the concentration when the time is 5? What is the time when the concentration is 30 mmol/L? What is the time when the concentration is 70 mmol/L?

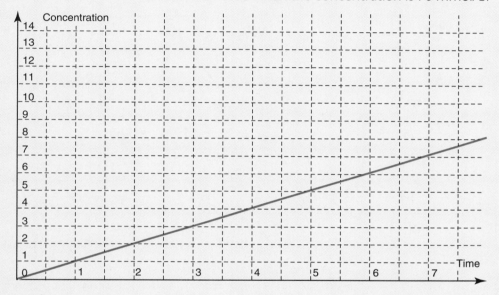

2. In the following graph, the horizontal axis is concentration (given in hundreds) and the vertical axis is percent transmittance (in tens). Based on the following graph, what is the percent transmittance when the concentration is $100\,^{mg}\!/_{dL}$? What is the concentration when T is 10%?

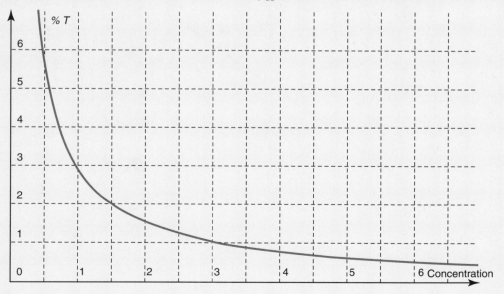

Continues

PRACTICE PROBLEMS: Section 5.4 *(continued)*

3. The following graph is a plot of time versus population where the time is in hours and the population is in hundreds. What is the approximate value of the population when the time is 4? What is the approximate value of the population when the time is 3? What is the approximate time when the population is 200? What is the approximate time when the population is 1,200?

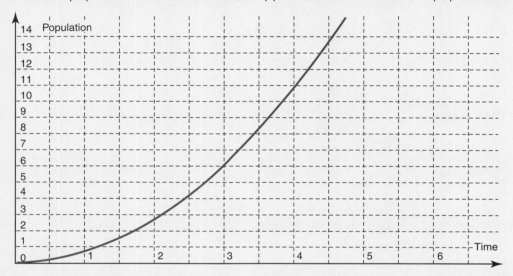

4. The following graph is a plot of time versus concentration where the time is in seconds and the concentration is in tens with units of mmol/L. What is the value of the concentration when the time is 4? What is the value of the concentration when the time is 1? What is the time when the concentration is 70? What is the time when the concentration is 100?

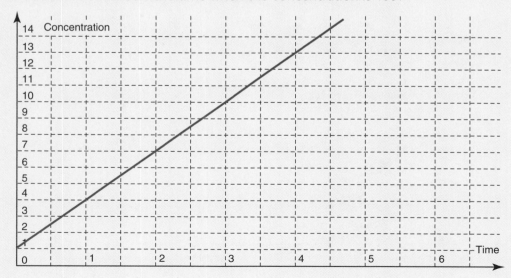

5. The following graph is a plot of the amount of reactant versus absorbance where the absorbance is in tenths. What is the approximate value of the absorbance when the amount of reactant is 1? What is the approximate value of the absorbance when the amount of reactant is 3? What is the approximate amount of reactant when the absorbance is 0.6? What is the approximate amount of reactant when the absorbance is 0.5?

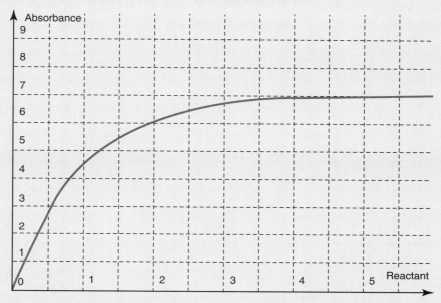

6. The following graph is a plot of the amount of reactant versus absorbance where the absorbance is in tenths. What is the value of the absorbance when the amount of reactant is 1.5? What is the value of the absorbance when the amount of reactant is 3? What is the amount of reactant when the absorbance is 0.6? What is the amount of reactant when the absorbance is 0.3?

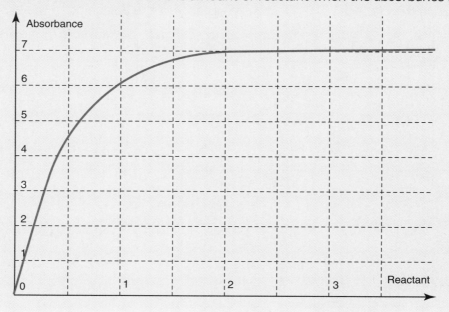

Continues

PRACTICE PROBLEMS: Section 5.4 (continued)

7. The following graph is a plot of concentration (given in hundreds) versus percent transmittance (given in tens). Based on the graph, what is the approximate percent transmittance when the concentration is 300 $\frac{mg}{dL}$? What is the approximate concentration when T is 20%?

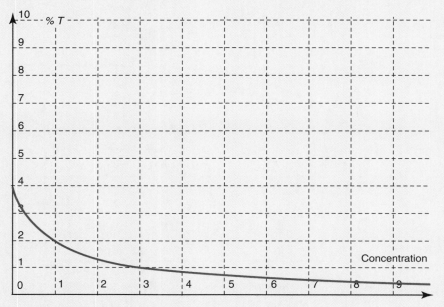

8. The following nonstandard graph is a plot of time versus distance (in tens). What is the value of the distance when the time is 7? What is the value of the distance when the time is 1? What is the time when the distance is 41? What is the distance at the beginning of the experiment?

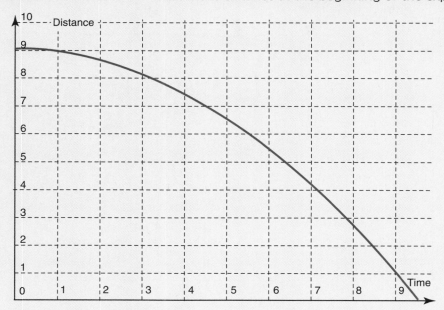

5.5 – VARIATION

In the laboratory scientists often need to know about the behavior of two related quantities. The relationship between two related quantities is often a direct or indirect relationship. If y varies directly with x, then y increases as x increases or if y decreases then x also decreases. This is called a direct relationship. If y varies inversely with x, then y increases as x decreases or visa versa.

If y **varies directly with** x, then it is expressed mathematically as

$$y = kx$$

where k is some nonzero variation constant, called the proportionality constant, to be determined. A simple example of two quantities that vary directly is the concentration of a solution and the amount of concentrate within the solution. The more concentrate in a solution, the more concentrated the solution. Likewise, the less concentrate in a solution, the less concentrated the solution.

EXAMPLE 5-16: If y varies directly with x and if $y = 12$ when $x = 6$, determine the proportionality constant k.

The basic equation is $y = kx$.

However, in this example we are given that $y = 12$ when $x = 6$. Substituting these values into the basic equation, we get

$$12 = k(6).$$

Dividing both sides by 6, we find

$$k = 2.$$

EXAMPLE 5-17: If y varies directly with x and if $y = 15$ when $x = 3$, determine the proportionality constant k. Then find the value of y when $x = 8$.

First, find k by substituting 15 for y and 3 for x.

$$15 = k \cdot 3$$

Dividing by 3, we find

$$k = 5.$$

Substituting this into the direct variation equation, $y = kx$, we get

$$y = 5x.$$

To find the value of y when x is 8, simply plug in 8 for x and solve.

$$y = 5(8) = 40$$

Therefore, $y = 40$ when $x = 8$.

EXAMPLE 5-18: When light is shone through a solution, the absorbance tells us about how much light is absorbed by the solution. The absorbance varies directly with the total protein concentration of a solution. It was found that the absorbance is 0.20 when the protein concentration is 40 $^{mg}\!/_{mL}$. Find the absorbance when the concentration is 60 $^{mg}\!/_{mL}$. Find the protein concentration when the absorbance is 0.10.

Because the absorbance, A, varies directly with the concentration, C, the equation relating these quantities will be

$$A = kC.$$

We are also given that $A = 0.20$ when $C = 40$ $^{mg}\!/_{mL}$. Substituting these values into the equation, we get

$$0.20 = k(40).$$

Dividing both sides by 40, we get

$$k = \frac{0.20}{40} = 0.005.$$

Substituting this value of k into $A = kC$, we have

$$A = 0.005C.$$

To find the absorbance when the concentration is 60, simply substitute 60 for C.

$$A = 0.005(60) = 0.3$$

To find the protein concentration when the absorbance is 0.10, substitute 0.10 for A and solve for C.

$$0.10 = 0.005C$$

Dividing both sides by 0.005, we find

$$C = 20 \; ^{mg}\!/_{mL}.$$

EXAMPLE 5-19: The absorbance varies directly with the glucose concentration of a solution. It was found that the absorbance is 0.25 when the glucose concentration is 100 $^{mg}\!/_{dL}$. Find the absorbance when the concentration is 300 $^{mg}\!/_{dL}$. Find the glucose concentration when the absorbance is 0.50.

Because the absorbance, A, varies directly with the concentration, C, the equation relating these quantities will be

$$A = kC.$$

We are also given that $A = 0.25$ when $C = 100 \, ^{mg}/_{dL}$. Substituting these values into the equation, we get

$$0.25 = k(100).$$

Dividing both sides by 100, we get

$$k = \frac{0.25}{100} = 2.5 \times 10^{-3}.$$

Substituting this value of k into $A = kC$, we have

$$A = 2.50 \times 10^{-3} \, C.$$

To find the absorbance when the concentration is 300, simply substitute 300 for C.

$$A = 2.50 \times 10^{-3}(300) = 0.75$$

To find the glucose concentration when the absorbance is 0.50, substitute 0.50 for A and solve for C.

$$0.50 = 2.50 \times 10^{-3} \, C$$

Dividing both sides by 2.50×10^{-3}, we find

$$C = 200 \, ^{mg}/_{dL}.$$

Now that we have discussed direct variation, we continue with inverse variation. If **y varies inversely with x**, it is expressed mathematically as

$$y = \frac{k}{x}.$$

Again, k is a nonzero variation constant. If a gas (at a constant temperature) is compressed, the volume decreases as the pressure increases—this is an example of two quantities that vary inversely, and the relationship can be expressed mathematically as

$$V = \frac{k}{P}$$

where V is the volume, P is the pressure, and k is some nonzero constant.

EXAMPLE 5-20: The pressure exerted on a gas is 45 pounds per square inch (psi) when the volume is 0.4 ft³. What pressure is required to have a volume of 0.2 ft³?

Substituting the given values into $V = \frac{k}{P}$, we have

$$0.4 = \frac{k}{45}.$$

Multiplying both sides by 45, we find

$$k = 18.$$

Therefore,

$$V = \frac{18}{P}.$$

To find the pressure for a volume of 0.2, substitute 0.2 for the volume and solve for the pressure.

$$0.2 = \frac{18}{P}$$

Multiply both sides by P.

$$0.2P = 18$$

Divide by 0.2.

$$P = \frac{18}{0.2} = 90$$

Thus, the pressure would be 90 psi.

EXAMPLE 5-21: If y varies inversely with x and if $y = 8$ when $x = 2$, find y when $x = 4$.

Because y varies inversely with x,

$$y = \frac{k}{x}.$$

Substituting the values of 8 and 2 for y and x, respectively, we get

$$8 = \frac{k}{2}.$$

Multiply both sides by 2.

$$k = 16$$

Substitute this into the inverse variation equation, $y = \frac{k}{x}$.

$$y = \frac{16}{x}$$

Lastly, we are asked to find y when $x = 4$. Plugging 4 in for x, we get

$$y = \frac{16}{4} = 4.$$

PRACTICE PROBLEMS: Section 5.5

1. If the number of molecules varies directly with the volume and there are 3×10^8 molecules in 1.5 ft^3, how many molecules will be in 5 ft^3?

2. The absorbance varies directly with the concentration of an unknown substance, and the absorbance is 0.3 when the concentration is 100 $\frac{mg}{dL}$. Find the absorbance when the concentration is 200 $\frac{mg}{dL}$. Find the concentration when the absorbance is 0.15.

3. The absorbance varies directly with the glucose concentration, and the absorbance is 0.9 when the glucose concentration is 300 $\frac{mg}{dL}$. Find the absorbance when the glucose concentration is 400 $\frac{mg}{dL}$. Find the glucose concentration when the absorbance is 1.5.

4. The absorbance varies directly with the concentration of an unknown substance, and the absorbance is 0.2 when the concentration is 20 $\frac{mg}{dL}$. Find the absorbance when the concentration is 50 $\frac{mg}{dL}$. Find the concentration when the absorbance is 0.6.

5. The absorbance varies directly with the protein concentration, and the absorbance is 0.4 when the protein concentration is 2.5 $\frac{mg}{mL}$. Find the absorbance when the protein concentration is 1.0 $\frac{mg}{mL}$. Find the protein concentration when the absorbance is 0.1.

6. The absorbance varies directly with the concentration of an unknown substance, and the absorbance is 0.7 when the concentration is 90 $\frac{mg}{dL}$. Find the absorbance when the concentration is 70 $\frac{mg}{dL}$. Find the concentration when the absorbance is 0.4.

7. If the temperature is constant, the volume of gas varies inversely with the pressure. If the pressure on 3 ft^3 of gas is 15 lb per square foot, what is the pressure when the volume is 4.5 ft^3?

8. If the temperature is constant, the volume of gas varies inversely with the pressure. If the pressure on 5 ft^3 of gas is 30 lb per square foot, what is the pressure when the volume is 10 ft^3?

9. If the temperature is constant, the volume of gas varies inversely with the pressure. If the pressure on 2 ft^3 of gas is 20 lb per square foot, what is the volume when the pressure is 8 ft^3?

10. If y varies inversely as x and if $y = 9$ when $x = 5$, what is y when $x = 3$?

11. If a varies inversely as c and if $a = 12$ when $c = 2$, what is a when $c = 10$?

12. If y varies inversely as x and if $y = 9$ when $x = 50$, what is x when $y = 75$?

13. If y varies directly as x and if $y = 12$ when $x = 2$, what is y when $x = 10$?

14. If y varies directly with x and if $y = 15$ when $x = 3$, what is y when $x = 15$?

15. If y varies directly with x and if $y = 30$ when $x = 4$, what is y when $x = 20$?

16. If r varies inversely as A and if $r = 6$ when $A = 30$, what is A when $r = 12$?

17. If y varies directly with x and if $y = 4.8$ when $x = 0.6$, what is y when $x = 9.8$?

CHAPTER SUMMARY

- Slope $= m = \dfrac{\text{Change in } y}{\text{Change in } x} = \dfrac{\Delta y}{\Delta x}$. Many remember this formula as $m = \dfrac{\text{Rise}}{\text{Run}}$.

- $m = \dfrac{y_2 - y_1}{x_2 - x_1}$

- Slope gives us information about the rate of change.

- The slope-intercept form of a linear equation is $y = mx + b$ where m is the slope and b is the y-intercept.

- When one of the axes of a graph is concentration, the graph is called a standard curve.

- Interpreting graphs is a common practice in the laboratory sciences.

- If y varies directly with x, then $y = kx$.

- If y varies inversely with x, then $y = \dfrac{k}{x}$.

CHAPTER TEST

1. Determine the slope of the line passing through the points $(10, 35)$ and $(20, 50)$.

2. Determine the slope of the line passing through the points $(0, 15)$ and $(5, 5)$.

3. Determine the slope of the following line.

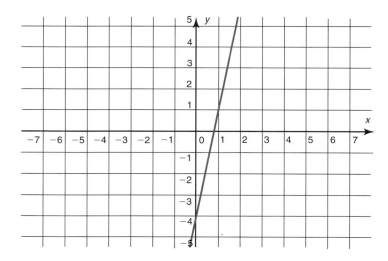

4. Determine the slope of the following line.

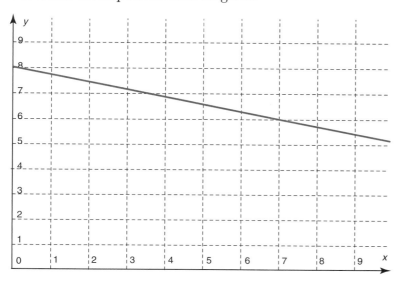

5. What is the slope of the graph of $y = \dfrac{1}{3}x - 2$?

6. What is the slope of the graph of $y = -0.7x + 20$?

7. Graph the portion of $y = 0.2x + 1$ that lies in the first quadrant.

8. Graph the portion of $y = -0.8x + 10$ that lies in the first quadrant.

9. Graph the line through $(1, 2)$ with a slope of 0.6.

10. Graph the line through $(0, 9)$ with a slope of $-\dfrac{2}{3}$.

11. Referring to the following graph, find the value of y when $x = 1$. Find the value of y when $x = -1$. What is the value of x when $y = 3$?

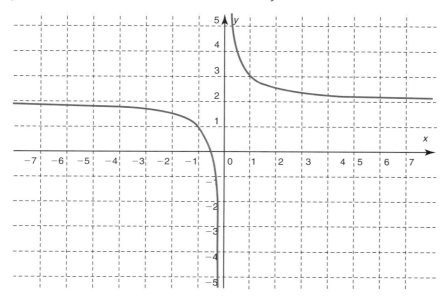

12. The following graph is a plot of the amount of reactant versus absorbance where the absorbance is in tenths. What is the value of the absorbance when the amount of reactant is 1? What is the value of the absorbance when the amount of reactant is 7? What is the amount of reactant when the absorbance is 0.3? What is the amount of reactant when the absorbance is 0.2?

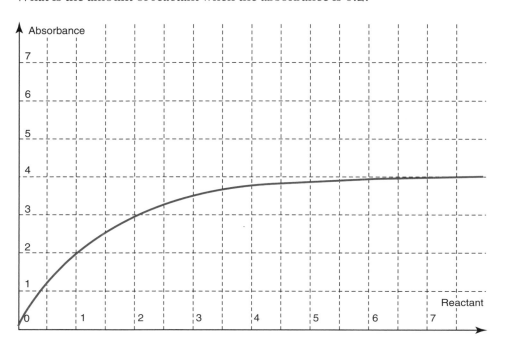

13. The pressure exerted on a gas is 36 pounds per square inch (psi) when the volume is 0.5 ft³. What pressure is required to have a volume of 0.3 ft³?

14. If y varies directly with x and if $y = 10$ when $x = 15$, determine the proportionality constant k. Then find the value of y when $x = 30$.

15. If y varies inversely with x and if $y = 40$ when $x = 20$, determine the proportionality constant k. Then find the value of y when $x = 40$.

Solutions

INTRODUCTION

It is common practice in the laboratory to take a solution and dilute it down by adding it to water or some other diluent. The resulting solution will have a decreased concentration and a different volume. The formula that relates the two volumes and two concentrations is

$$V_1 \times C_1 = V_2 \times C_2$$

where V_1 and C_1 are the original volume and concentration and V_2 and C_2 are the volume and concentration of the diluted solution (or vice versa). In addition, we will also study solutions that involve percents along with the very basics of molarity, normality, and specific gravity.

6.1 – VARYING CONCENTRATIONS AND VOLUMES

When we dilute a solution, the concentration of the resulting solution decreases to create an inverse relationship between the volume and the concentration. Remember, if it were a direct variation, the equation would be

$$\frac{V_1}{V_2} = \frac{C_1}{C_2}.$$

However, because dilutions have an inverse relationship, the governing equation is

$$\frac{V_1}{V_2} = \frac{C_2}{C_1}.$$

NOTE

If y varies inversely with x, then $y = \dfrac{1}{x}$. Thus,

$$\frac{1}{C_1/C_2} = 1 \div \frac{C_1}{C_2} = 1 \times \frac{C_2}{C_1} = \frac{C_2}{C_1}$$

Because the equation $\dfrac{V_1}{V_2} = \dfrac{C_2}{C_1}$ is a proportion, we can cross multiply to get

$$V_1 \times C_1 = V_2 \times C_2$$

Therefore, when a solution's concentration and volume change as a result of adding a diluent, the formula $V_1 \times C_1 = V_2 \times C_2$ can be used to find the volume and concentration of the original and resulting solutions.

EXAMPLE 6-1: If $V_1 = 8\ \mu\text{L}$, $V_2 = 12\ \mu\text{L}$, and $C_1 = 40\%$, find C_2 in the following equation.

$$V_1 \times C_1 = V_2 \times C_2$$

Substituting the given values into the equation, we get

$$8 \times 40\% = 12 \times C_2.$$

Writing 40% as a decimal, we get

$$8 \times 0.40 = 12 \times C_2.$$

Simplify the left-hand side.

$$3.20 = 12 \times C_2$$

Divide both sides by 12.

$$\frac{3.20}{12} = C_2$$

Simplifying, we find that

$$C_2 = 0.2\overline{66} \approx 26.7\%.$$

EXAMPLE 6-2: Calculate the concentration if 12 μL of a 2.5% solution is diluted up to 75 μL.

Let $V_1 = 12$, $C_1 = 2.5\% = 0.025$, and $V_2 = 75$. Substituting into the equation

$$V_1 \times C_1 = V_2 \times C_2,$$

we get

$$12 \times 0.025 = 75C_2.$$

Simplifying the left-hand side, we get

$$0.300 = 75C_2.$$

Dividing both sides by 75, we get

$$C_2 = \frac{0.300}{75} = 0.004.$$

Therefore, the concentration of the diluted solution is $0.004 = 0.004 \times 100\% = 0.40\%$.

EXAMPLE 6-3: Calculate the volume needed to get $30.0~\mu$L with a concentration of 2.0% if a 6.0% solution is used in the dilution process.

As we just discussed, we must use the equation

$$V_1 \times C_1 = V_2 \times C_2.$$

In this example we will let

$$V_1 = 30.0~\mu\text{L}, C_1 = 2.0\%, \text{ and } C_2 = 6.0\%.$$

Thus, we need to find V_2. Plugging these values into the equation, we get

$$30.0 \times 0.02 = V_2 \times 0.06.$$

Simplifying the left-hand side, we get

$$0.6 = V_2 \cdot 0.06.$$

Dividing both sides by 0.06, we find

$$V_2 = 10.0.$$

So we would take $10.0~\mu$L of the 6.0% solution and dilute it up to $30.0~\mu$L.

EXAMPLE 6-4: How many milliliters of a 6% KCl solution are needed to make 400 mL of a 3% KCl solution? How would the solution be prepared?

Again, we must use the formula $V_1 \times C_1 = V_2 \times C_2$.

So $V_1 = 400$, $C_1 = 3\%$, $C_2 = 6\%$, and V_2 is what we are trying to find. Substituting these into our governing equation, we get

$$400 \times 0.03 = V_2 \times 0.06.$$

Simplifying the left-hand side, we get

$$12 = V_2 \times 0.06.$$

Dividing both sides by 0.06, we get

$$V_2 = 200 \text{ mL.}$$

Therefore, we must take 200 mL of the 6% KCl solution and dilute it up to a total of 400 mL by adding 200 mL of diluent.

EXAMPLE 6-5: A scientist poured a 4% NaCl solution into a flask already containing a NaCl solution of unknown concentration. If the total volume of the mixed solution in the flask is 200 mL and its concentration is 2.5%, how many milliliters of the 4% NaCl solution were poured into the flask?

Let $C_1 = 4\%$, $C_2 = 2.5\%$, $V_2 = 200$ mL, and V_1 is what we are trying to find.

Substituting these values into $V_1 \times C_1 = V_2 \times C_2$, we get

$$V_1 \times 0.04 = 200 \times 0.025.$$

Simplifying the right-hand side,

$$0.04 V_1 = 5.$$

Dividing by 0.04 we find $V_1 = 125$ mL.

PRACTICE PROBLEMS: Section 6.1

1. How many milliliters of a 5% KCl solution are needed to make 500 mL of a 4% KCl solution?

2. We need a total of 200 mL of a 6% NaCl solution. However, all we have is a 7% solution of sodium chloride. To make 200 mL of the 6% solution, how many milliliters of the 7% NaCl solution are needed?

3. How many milliliters of a 9% NaCl solution are needed to make 300 mL of a 7% NaCl solution?

4. We need 1,200 mL of a 7% NaCl solution by diluting a 12% solution of sodium chloride. How many milliliters of the 12% NaCl solution are needed?

5. A total of 1,000 mL of a 7% NaCl solution is needed. However, all we have is a 10% solution of sodium chloride. To make 1,000 mL of the 7% solution, how many milliliters of the 10% NaCl solution are needed?

6. We need to dilute 60.0 mL of a 2.50% solution up to 120 mL. What is the concentration of the diluted 120 mL solution?

7. We need to dilute 50.0 mL of a 3.00% solution up to 300 mL. What is the concentration of the diluted 300 mL solution?

8. We need to dilute 80.0 mL of a 3.50% solution up to 160 mL. What is the concentration of the diluted 160 mL solution?

9. If 40.0 mL of a 4.50% solution must be diluted up to 240 mL, what is the concentration of the diluted 240 mL solution?

10. We need to dilute 100.0 mL of a 2.00% solution up to 500 mL. What is the concentration of the diluted 500 mL solution?

11. A scientist poured a 5% NaCl solution into a flask already containing a NaCl solution. The total volume of the mixed solution in the flask is 300 mL and its concentration is 4.5%. How many milliliters of the 5% NaCl solution were poured into the flask?

12. A scientist poured a 10% NaCl solution into a flask already containing a NaCl solution. If the total volume of the mixed solution in the flask is 400 mL and its concentration is 6%, how many milliliters of the 10% NaCl solution were poured into the flask?

13. A scientist poured a 9% KCl solution into a test tube already containing a KCl solution. If the total volume of the mixed solution in the test tube is 300 mL and its concentration is 5%, how many milliliters of the 9% KCl solution were poured into the flask?

14. A scientist poured a 7% NaCl solution into a flask already containing a NaCl solution. The total volume of the mixed solution in the flask is 200 mL and its concentration is 5.5%. How many milliliters of the 7% NaCl solution were poured into the flask?

6.2 – SOLUTIONS INVOLVING PERCENTS

Recall from our discussion about percents in Chapter 1 that percent means "per 100." Keeping this in mind, let's define some percent solutions.

A **percent weight per unit weight**, % w/w, is defined as

$$\% \text{ w / w} = \frac{\text{Unit weights of solute}}{100 \text{ unit weights of solution}} = \frac{\text{Grams of solute}}{100 \text{ grams of solution}}.$$

In the preceding formula, the solute is the substance being dissolved in the solution. To understand this a little better, 5% w/w means that 5% of the total mass of the entire solution is the mass of the solute.

EXAMPLE 6-6: How would a laboratorian make 150 grams of a 20% w/w NaCl solution?

Using the % w/w formula, we have

$$0.20 = \frac{x \text{ grams of NaCl}}{100 \text{ grams of solution}}.$$

Multiplying both sides by 100, we find

$$x = 20 \text{ grams.}$$

Therefore, to make 100 grams of solution, the laboratorian would need 20 g of NaCl. To find how to make 150 g, we use proportions because we want the concentration to remain the same.

$$\frac{20 \text{ g NaCl}}{100 \text{ g solution}} = \frac{x \text{ g NaCl}}{150 \text{ g solution}}$$

Cross multiplying we get

$$100x = 3{,}000.$$

Dividing by 100 we find

$$x = 30.$$

Therefore, to make 150 grams of solution, the laboratorian would take 30 g NaCl and mix it with 120 grams of diluent to get a total of 150 grams.

A **percent weight per unit volume**, % w/v, is defined as

$$\% \text{ w / v} = \frac{\text{Grams of solute}}{100 \text{ mL of solution}} = \frac{\text{Grams of solute}}{1 \text{ dL of solution}}.$$

To understand this better, 5% w/v means that a 100 mL solution would contain 5 grams of solute.

EXAMPLE 6-7: How would a laboratorian make 350 mL of a 12% w/v HCl solution?

Using the % w/v formula, we have

$$0.12 = \frac{x \text{ grams}}{100 \text{ mL}}.$$

Solving, we find

$$x = 12 \text{ g.}$$

Therefore, the laboratorian would take 12 grams of HCl and dissolve it in 100 mL (or 1 deciliter) of diluent (water) to get 100 mL. However, we want 350 mL. Again, we use proportions to solve.

$$\frac{12 \text{ g}}{100 \text{ mL}} = \frac{x \text{ g}}{350 \text{ mL}}$$

Cross multiplying we get

$$100x = 4{,}200.$$

Dividing by 100 we find

$$x = 42.$$

Therefore, dissolve 42 grams of HCl in 350 mL of diluent.

A **percent volume per unit volume**, % v/v, is defined as

$$\% \text{ v/v} = \frac{\text{mL of concentrate}}{100 \text{ mL of solution}} = \frac{\text{mL of concentrate}}{1 \text{ dL of solution}}.$$

To understand this better, 5% v/v means that 5% of the entire solution is the solute.

EXAMPLE 6-8: How would a laboratorian make 50 mL of a 60% v/v solution of HNO_3 (nitric acid) in water?

Using the % v/v formula,

$$0.60 = \frac{x \text{ mL of } HNO_3}{100 \text{ mL of solution}}.$$

Therefore $x = 60$ and the laboratorian would take 60 mL of HNO_3 and add it to 40 mL of water to get a 100 mL solution having a 60% v/v. To find out how to make 50 mL, use proportions.

$$\frac{60 \text{ mL}}{100 \text{ mL}} = \frac{x \text{ mL}}{50 \text{ mL}}$$

Cross multiplying and solving, we find

$$x = 30.$$

Thus, the laboratorian would take 30 mL of HNO_3 and add it to 20 mL of water to get a 50 mL solution having a 60% v/v.

EXAMPLE 6-9: How many milliliters of alcohol are in 40 mL of a 60% v/v solution?

The concentration remains the same, so this is solved by using proportions.

$$\frac{60 \text{ mL alcohol}}{100 \text{ mL solution}} = \frac{x \text{ mL alcohol}}{40 \text{ mL solution}}$$

Cross multiplying we get

$$100x = 2,400.$$

Dividing by 100 we find

$$x = 24.$$

Therefore, there are 24 mL of alcohol in 40 mL of a 60% v/v solution.

NOTE

24 is 60% of 40 since $\frac{24}{40} = 0.6 = 60\%$. The amount of solution does not really matter. What matters is the percentage. That is, 24 L of alcohol in 40 L of solution is still a 60% v/v solution.

EXAMPLE 6-10: How many grams of NaCl are in 25 mL of a 12% w/v NaCl solution?

From our knowledge of percents, we know that a 12% w/v NaCl solution contains v12 grams of NaCl in every 100 mL of solution. The concentration is the same, so we again solve by using proportions.

$$\frac{12 \text{ g NaCl}}{100 \text{ mL solution}} = \frac{x \text{ grams NaCl}}{25 \text{ mL solution}}$$

Cross multiplying we have

$$100x = 300.$$

Dividing by 100 we find

$$x = 3.$$

Therefore, there are 3 grams of NaCl in 25 mL of a 12% w/v NaCl solution.

NOTE

$$\frac{3}{25} = 0.12 = 12\%$$

EXAMPLE 6-11: How many grams of NaOH are in 6 dL of a 20% w/v NaOH solution?

First, convert 6 dL to mL.

$$6 \text{ dL}\left(\frac{100 \text{ mL}}{1 \text{ dL}}\right) = 600 \text{ mL}$$

Setting up the proportion, we have

$$\frac{20 \text{ g NaCl}}{100 \text{ mL solution}} = \frac{x \text{ grams NaCl}}{600 \text{ mL solution}}.$$

Cross multiplying we have

$$100x = 12{,}000.$$

Dividing by 100 we see

$$x = 120.$$

NOTE

$$\frac{120}{6\ dL} = \frac{120}{600\ mL} = 0.2 = 20\%$$

We could have also solved this using the fact that % w/v is also defined as

$$\% \ w/v = \frac{\text{Grams of solute}}{1\ \text{deciliter}}$$

Attacking the problem this way, we would have

$$\frac{20\ g\ NaCl}{1\ dL\ \text{solution}} = \frac{x\ \text{grams}\ NaCl}{6\ dL\ \text{solution}}.$$

Cross multiplying we have $x = 120$.

PRACTICE PROBLEMS: Section 6.2

1. How would a laboratorian make 125 g of an 18% w/w NaOH solution?
2. How would a laboratorian make 250 g of a 15% w/w NaOH solution?
3. How would a laboratorian make 75 g of a 9% w/w NaCl solution?
4. How would a laboratorian make 300 g of a 30% w/w NaCl solution?
5. How would a technician make 150 mL of a 25% w/v NaCl solution?
6. How would a technician make 200 mL of a 6% w/v NaCl solution?
7. How would a technician make 50 mL of a 2% w/v NaCl solution?
8. How would a technician make 125 mL of a 12% w/v HCl solution?
9. How would a technician make 150 mL of a 14% w/v HCl solution?
10. How would a laboratorian make 250 mL of an 18% v/v solution of alcohol in water?
11. How would a laboratorian make 200 mL of a 20% v/v solution of alcohol in water?

Continues

PRACTICE PROBLEMS: Section 6.2 *(continued)*

12. How would a laboratorian make 225 mL of a 10% v/v solution of alcohol in water?

13. How many milliliters of ethanol are in 70 mL of a 70% v/v solution?

14. How many milliliters of HNO_3 are in 2 dL of a 50% v/v solution?

15. How many milliliters of ethanol are in 40 dL of a 30% v/v solution?

16. How would a laboratorian make a 30% v/v solution of alcohol in water?

17. How would a laboratorian make a 12% v/v solution of alcohol in water?

18. How many grams of NaCl are in 10 dL of a 15% w/v NaCl solution?

19. How many grams of NaCl are in 45 mL of a 30% w/v NaCl solution?

20. How many grams of NaCl are in 20 mL of a 10% w/v NaCl solution?

6.3 – MOLARITY, NORMALITY, AND SPECIFIC GRAVITY

Molarity

A **mole** is the amount of an element or compound equal to its molecular or atomic weight in grams. This is expressed as an equation as

$$\text{Mole} = \frac{\text{Gram weight}}{\text{Molecular weight}} = \frac{\text{Gram weight}}{\text{Atomic weight}}.$$

Mole is abbreviated as mol. The atomic weight of any element can easily be determined by referring to the periodic table. To find the gram molecular weight of any compound, simply add the atomic weights of the elements making up the compound.

No matter what compound or element we have, 1 mole of that compound or element will contain approximately 6.02×10^{23} atoms. This number is known as **Avogadro's number**. If we took a mole of a substance, or a mole of solute, and dissolved it in some solution, the resulting solution would have a certain concentration. The more moles we put in, the more concentrated the solution. The **molarity**, M, of a solution tells us about the level of concentration. Molarity can be expressed as

$$\text{Molarity (M)} = \frac{\text{Number of moles of solute}}{\text{Unit volume of solution}}.$$

EXAMPLE 6-12: One liter of a solution is made by using 3.0 moles of potassium chloride. Find the molarity.

$$\text{Molarity} = \frac{\text{Number of moles of solute}}{\text{Unit volume of solution}} = \frac{3.0 \text{ moles KCl}}{1.0 \text{ L of solution}} = 3.0$$

If the unit volume of solution is 1.0 L, then as we increase the number of moles of solute, the numerical value of the molarity also increases. This should make sense because molarity is one way of measuring concentration.

Normality

Normality is another way to measure concentration. However, normality is measured by the number of equivalent weights per unit volume where the **equivalent weight** is the molecular weight divided by the valence. Valence is a number associated with each element and will be discussed thoroughly in your chemistry class. The mathematical equation for normality is

$$\text{Normality} = \frac{\text{Number of equivalent weights}}{\text{Unit volume}} = \frac{\left(\dfrac{\text{Number of grams of solute}}{\text{Gram equivalent weight of solute}}\right)}{\text{Unit volume}}.$$

EXAMPLE 6-13: Find the normality of 1.50 liters of solution whose number of equivalent weights is

$$\frac{85.0 \text{ g of solute}}{38.2 \text{ geqw of solute}}$$

$$\text{Normality} = \frac{\left(\dfrac{\text{Number of grams of solute}}{\text{Gram equivalent weight of solute}}\right)}{\text{Unit volume}} = \frac{\left(\dfrac{85.0 \text{ g}}{38.2 \text{ geqw}}\right)}{1.50 \text{ L}} = 1.48 \text{ eqw}$$

As the number of grams of solute increases, so will the normality.

Specific Gravity

Density tells us how much matter is in a given volume or the amount of mass per volume.

$$\text{Density} = \frac{\text{Mass of material}}{\text{Volume occupied by material}}$$

Specific gravity is typically used to measure the amount of change in the density. **Specific gravity** is the ratio of the density of a liquid to the density of pure water at some specific temperature. At an air temperature of 4°C, pure water has a density of 1.000 g/mL.

$$\text{Specific gravity} = \frac{\text{Density of some liquid}}{\text{Density of pure water at some specific temperature}}$$

A substance whose specific gravity is 1.080 is 8% heavier than an equal volume of pure water. Likewise, a substance whose specific gravity is 1.120 is 12% heavier than an equal volume of pure water. In addition, because both the numerator and denominator are given as density, the units will cancel. Therefore, specific gravity is a number with no units associated with it. Finally, as we see from the definition, the specific gravity of any substance will change with the temperature.

EXAMPLE 6-14: A chemical has a specific gravity of 1.05. Find the density of this chemical.

Substituting the given information into the specific gravity formula, we obtain

$$1.05 = \frac{x}{1.000 \text{ g/mL}}.$$

Multiplying both sides by 1.000 g/mL we find

$$x = 1.05 \text{ g/mL}.$$

EXAMPLE 6-15: A 100 mL container of phosphoric acid has a specific gravity of 1.7 and a 50% purity. Interpret this information. (Note: The term *50% purity* is often stated as 50% assay or assay 50%.)

A specific gravity of 1.7 means 1 mL of this phosphoric acid has a mass of 1.7 g. An assay of 50% means of the 1.7 g, 50% is phosphoric acid. As we can see, this is a % w/w solution. Because 50% of 1.7 is $(0.500)(1.7) = 0.85$, there are 0.85 grams of phosphoric acid per milliliter of solution. Because this container has 100 mL, this specific container has $(0.85)(100) = 85$ g of phosphoric acid.

EXAMPLE 6-16: How would a scientist make 500 mL of a 20% w/v nitric acid solution using an 80% assay nitric acid with a specific gravity of 1.42?

We can find the number of grams per milliliter in the 80% assay as follows:

$$(1.42)(0.80) = 1.136.$$

Therefore, in 1.0 mL of an 80% solution of nitric acid, there are 1.136 grams of nitric acid. However, we want 500 mL of a 20% assay, which means in 100 mL there will be 20 g of nitric acid. To find the number of grams in 500 mL, use proportions.

$$\frac{20 \text{ g}}{100 \text{ mL}} = \frac{x \text{ g}}{500 \text{ mL}}$$

Cross multiplying we get

$$100x = 10,000.$$

Dividing by 100 we find

$$x = 100.$$

This tells us there are 100 g of nitric acid in 500 mL of a 20% assay. Next we need to determine how many milliliters of the 80% assay contain 100 g of nitric acid. Again, you can find this by using proportions.

$$\frac{1.136 \text{g}}{1.0 \text{ mL}} = \frac{100 \text{ g}}{x \text{ mL}}$$

Cross multiplying and solving, we find

$$x = 88.0.$$

Thus, if we take 88.0 mL of the 80% solution and dilute it up to 500 mL, the result would be a 500 mL solution with a 20% assay.

PRACTICE PROBLEMS: Section 6.3

1. Find the molarity of a 2.0 L solution containing 2.0 moles of potassium chloride.

2. Find the molarity of a 1.0 L solution containing 5.0 moles of potassium chloride.

3. A 3.0 L solution was made by using 9.0 moles of potassium chloride. Find the molarity.

4. A 2.0 L solution was made by using 6.0 moles of potassium chloride. Find the molarity.

5. Find the normality of a 2.50 L solution whose number of equivalent weights is $\frac{68.0 \text{ g of solute}}{27.5 \text{ geqw of solute}}$.

6. Find the normality of a 3.00 L solution whose number of equivalent weights is $\frac{52.3 \text{ g of solute}}{33.2 \text{ geqw of solute}}$.

7. Find the normality of a 5.00 L solution whose number of equivalent weights is $\frac{48.2 \text{ g of solute}}{24.1 \text{ geqw of solute}}$.

8. Find the normality of a 4.00 L solution whose number of equivalent weights is $\frac{70.5 \text{ g of solute}}{38.6 \text{ geqw of solute}}$.

9. How many grams of nitric acid are in 1.00 mL of a 60% assay with specific gravity of 1.30?

10. How many grams of nitric acid are in 2.00 mL of a 90% assay with specific gravity of 1.45?

11. How many grams of nitric acid are in 2.50 mL of a 70% assay with specific gravity of 1.40?

12. How would a scientist make 500 mL of a 10% w/v nitric acid solution using a 60% assay given that nitric acid has a specific gravity of 1.42?

13. How would a scientist make 1,000 mL of a 20% w/v phosphoric acid solution using a 70% assay given that this phosphoric acid has a specific gravity of 1.70?

Continues

PRACTICE PROBLEMS: Section 6.3 (continued)

14. How would a scientist make 1 L of a 15% w/v phosphoric acid solution using a 90% assay given that this phosphoric acid has a specific gravity of 1.75?

15. How would a scientist make 1 L of a 10% w/v nitric acid solution using a 70% assay given that this nitric acid has a specific gravity of 1.45?

16. A chemical has a specific gravity of 1.15. Find the density of this chemical.

17. A chemical has a specific gravity of 1.20. Find the density of this chemical.

18. A chemical has a specific gravity of 1.10. Find the density of this chemical.

CHAPTER SUMMARY

- When a solution's concentration and volume change as a result of adding a diluent, the formula $V_1 \times C_1 = V_2 \times C_2$ can be used to find the volume and concentration of the original and resulting solutions.

- A percent weight per unit weight, % w/w, is

$$\% \text{ w/w} = \frac{\text{Unit weights of solute}}{100 \text{ unit weights of solution}} = \frac{\text{Grams of solute}}{100 \text{ grams of solution}}.$$

- A percent weight per unit volume, % w/v, is

$$\% \text{ w/v} = \frac{\text{Grams of solute}}{100 \text{ mL of solution}} = \frac{\text{Grams of solute}}{1 \text{ dL of solution}}.$$

- A percent volume per unit volume, % v/v, is

$$\% \text{ v/v} = \frac{\text{mL of concentrate}}{100 \text{ mL of solution}} = \frac{\text{mL of concentrate}}{1 \text{ dL of solution}}.$$

- $\text{Mole} = \dfrac{\text{Gram weight}}{\text{Molecular weight}} = \dfrac{\text{Gram weight}}{\text{Atomic weight}}$

- $\text{Molarity} = \dfrac{\text{Number of moles of solute}}{\text{Unit volume of solution}}$

- $\text{Normality} = \dfrac{\text{Number of equivalent weights}}{\text{Unit volume}} = \dfrac{\left(\dfrac{\text{Number of grams of solute}}{\text{Gram equivalent weight of solute}} \right)}{\text{Unit volume}}$

- $\text{Specific gravity} = \dfrac{\text{Density of some liquid}}{\text{Density of pure water at some specific temperature}}$

CHAPTER TEST

1. If 15 μL of a 4.0 % solution is diluted up to 50 μL, what is the concentration of the resulting solution?

2. We need to make 1,000 mL of a 7% NaCl solution using an 11% solution of sodium chloride. To make 1,000 mL of the 7% solution, how many milliliters of the 11% NaCl solution are needed?

3. We need to dilute 80.0 mL of a 2.50% solution up to 340 mL. What is the concentration of the diluted 340 mL solution?

4. How many grams of NaOH are in 8 dL of a 30% w/v NaOH solution?

5. How would a laboratorian make 50 g of a 10% w/w NaOH solution?

6. How many milliliters of ethanol are in 50 mL of a 40% v/v solution?

7. Find the molarity of 2.0 liters of solution containing 4.0 moles of potassium chloride.

8. A chemical has a specific gravity of 1.05. Find the density of this chemical.

9. Find the normality of a 6.00 L solution whose number of equivalent weights is $\frac{42.5 \text{ g of solute}}{23.8 \text{ geqw of solute}}$.

7

Chemistry, Logarithms, and Spectrophotometry

INTRODUCTION

This chapter briefly discusses ions, logarithms, pH, and spectrophotometry. Logarithms will be encountered in courses within the clinical science curriculum, especially when working with pH. By definition, pH involves the concentration of hydrogen ions in a solution. Because spectrophotometry and colorimetry are extensively used in the laboratory to measure characteristics of a specimen, we also discuss these topics.

7.1 – IONS, LOGARITHMS, AND pH

Logarithms

Recall from Chapter 2 that $10^2 = 100$, $10^3 = 1,000$, $10^4 = 10,000$, and so on. When quantities can be expressed as exponentials of 10, the quantities tend to be either very large or very small. In such cases *logarithms* can be incorporated to make the calculations involving these quantities easier to work with. The mathematical notation for a logarithm is $\log x$ and is read as "the logarithm base 10 of x." When you are working with logarithms in base 10 and an exponential of 10 is being evaluated, the answer is the value of the exponent associated with the 10. For example, $\log 10,000 = 4$ because $\log 10,000 = \log 10^4$. To understand why logarithms behave in this manner, let's continue with the definition of a **logarithm base 10**.

$$y = \log x \text{ if and only if } 10^y = x$$

If and only if means if $y = \log x$ is true, then $10^y = x$ is true and, likewise, if $10^y = x$ is true, then $y = \log x$ is true. This is essentially saying these two equations are the same thing. In mathematics *if and only if* is usually notated with the symbol $\leftrightarrow$.

EXAMPLE 7-1: Determine the value of y without using a calculator.

$$y = \log 100$$

From the first part of the definition, $y = \log x$, we can see that $x = 100$. Plugging this into the second part of the definition, $10^y = x$, we get $10^y = 100$. We know that $10^2 = 100$, thus $y = 2$. Also notice that $\log(100)$ could be written as $\log(10^2)$. In general,

$$\log(10^y) = y.$$

Follow up by entering $\log 100$ into your calculator to see that the answer is indeed 2.

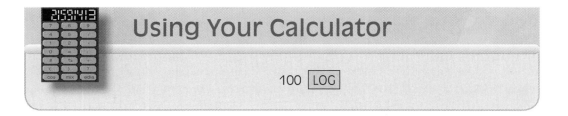

Using Your Calculator

100 $\boxed{\text{LOG}}$

EXAMPLE 7-2: Determine the value of y without using a calculator.

$$y = \log 1{,}000$$

Because 1,000 is the same as 10^3, this problem can be rewritten as $y = \log 10^3$. From the fact that $\log(10^y) = y$, we see y is equal to 3. Follow up by entering $\log 1{,}000$ into your calculator to see that the answer is indeed 3.

Following are some properties of logarithms:

1) $\log x > 0$ if $x > 1$
2) $\log x < 0$ if $0 < x < 1$
3) $\log(1) = 0$
4) $\log(A \times B) = \log(A) + \log(B)$
5) $\log\left(\dfrac{A}{B}\right) = \log(A) - \log(B)$
6) $-\log(A) = \log(A)^{-1} = \log\left(\dfrac{1}{A}\right)$
7) Logarithms of negative numbers do not exist.

Following are the values, rounded to four decimals, of log(1) through log(9).

$$\log(1) = 0$$
$$\log(2) = 0.3010$$
$$\log(3) = 0.4771$$
$$\log(4) = 0.6021$$
$$\log(5) = 0.6990$$
$$\log(6) = 0.7782$$
$$\log(7) = 0.8451$$
$$\log(8) = 0.9031$$
$$\log(9) = 0.9542$$

In the examples that follow, we use these values together with the properties of logarithms to determine the value of a given logarithm.

EXAMPLE 7-3: Determine the value of log(500) without using a calculator.

$$\log(500) = \log(5 \times 10^2)$$

By property 4, $\log(A \times B) = \log(A) + \log(B)$, so we can rewrite $\log(5 \times 10^2)$ as

$$\log(5 \times 10^2) = \log(5) + \log(10^2).$$

From the list of values, we know $\log(5) = 0.6990$, and from our previous discussions, we know $\log(10^2) = 2$. Therefore,

$$\log(500) = \log(5) + \log(10^2) = 0.6990 + 2 = 2.6990.$$

Use your calculator to verify that this answer is correct.

Using Your Calculator

500 $\boxed{\text{LOG}}$

If we round the answer appearing on the calculator to four decimal places, we get 2.6990.

EXAMPLE 7-4: Find the value of log(0.0007) without using a calculator.

$$\log(0.0007) = \log(7 \times 10^{-4}) = \log(7) + \log(10^{-4}) = 0.8451 + (-4) = -3.1549$$

Notice we could have calculated this by using the properties of exponents along with property 5 of logarithms as illustrated in the following.

$$\log(0.0007) = \log(7 \times 10^{-4}) = \log\left(\frac{7}{10^4}\right) = \log(7) - \log(10^4) = 0.8451 - 4 = -3.1549$$

EXAMPLE 7-5: Find the value of $-\log\left(\dfrac{7}{10^{-3}}\right)$ without using a calculator.

By property 5 we have

$$-\log\left(\frac{7}{10^{-3}}\right) = -[\log 7 - \log 10^{-3}].$$

By the definition of logarithm, we know $\log 10^{-3} = -3$. Substituting this we have

$$-[\log 7 - (-3)].$$

Simplifying we get

$$-[\log(7) + 3].$$

Substituting the value of $\log 7$ from the list of values, we get

$$-[0.8451 + 3] = -3.8451.$$

pH

Atoms and molecules contain protons and electrons. When an atom or molecule is positively charged or negatively charged, it is referred to as an **ion**. An **electrolyte** is a substance that forms ions. When an electrically neutral atom or molecule is transformed into either a positively or negatively charged atom or molecule, this process is called **ionization**. One typical solvent in which ionization occurs is water, H_2O or HOH. When a water molecule dissociates, it leads to the formation of two ions, the hydrogen ion H^+ and the hydroxide ion OH^- (notice they both have a charge). The concentration of hydrogen ions, in any solution, is directly related to the pH of the solution as the following example shows.

EXAMPLE 7-6: The **pH** of a solution is defined by the molar concentration of hydrogen ions, H^+, as $pH = \log\left(\dfrac{1}{H^+}\right)$. Show that pH could also be expressed as

$$pH = -\log(H^+).$$

By the properties of exponents, we know

$$\log\left(\frac{1}{H^+}\right) = \log(H^+)^{-1}.$$

By property 6 we know

$$\log(H^+)^{-1} = -\log(H^+).$$

EXAMPLE 7-7: In some applications of pH, the following formula is used (the relevance of a and b will be discussed in courses that follow). Simplify this formula so it contains only a and b and no factor of 10.

$$pH = -\log(a \times 10^{-b})$$

Using property 4 we have

$$pH = -[\log(a) + \log(10^{-b})].$$

By the definition of logarithm, we know $\log 10^{-b} = -b$. Substituting we have

$$pH = -[\log a + (-b)].$$

Distributing the negative sign, we get

$$pH = -\log(a) + b.$$

Rearranging we have

$$pH = b - \log(a).$$

Acids and Bases

Notice as the pH increases, the H^+ concentration decreases. A **base** is a substance that can receive a hydrogen ion. Therefore, bases have a "high" pH because they accept the hydrogen ions, thus making the H^+ concentration decrease. On the other hand, **acids** are substances that donate hydrogen ions, thus increasing the H^+ concentration. As a result acids have lower pH values. A pH of 7.0 is considered neutral. Substances with a pH higher than 7.0 are considered basic, and those below 7.0 are considered acidic. Overall, substances have a pH between 0 and 14.

EXAMPLE 7-8: For a pH of 4, what would be the H^+ molar concentration? What is the H^+ concentration for a pH of 9?

Using the formula given in Example 7-6, $pH = -\log(H^+)$, we have

$$4 = -\log(H^+).$$

Multiplying both sides by -1, we get

$$-4 = \log(H^+).$$

If we let $H^+ = 10^y$, our equation becomes

$$-4 = \log(10^y).$$

From our previous discussions, we know $y = -4$. Therefore, the molar concentration of hydrogen ions is

$$H^+ = 10^{-4} = 0.0001.$$

For a pH of 9, we have

$$9 = -\log(H^+).$$

Multiplying both sides by -1, we get

$$-9 = \log(H^+).$$

Again, if we let $H^+ = 10^y$, our equation becomes

$$-9 = \log(10^y).$$

And we know in this case that $y = -9$. Therefore, the hydrogen ion concentration for a pH of 9 is

$$H^+ = 10^{-9} = 0.000000001.$$

One common measurement of pH in the medical laboratory is the urine dipstick. Urinary pH can take on a wide range of values depending on the health of the patient. It can be as low as 4.5 and as high as 9.0.

The Henderson-Hasselbach Equation

The Henderson-Hasselbach equation relates the pH of a buffer to the concentration of a weak acid and its conjugate base. We will not take the time to derive the Henderson-Hasselbach equation. We simply state it and draw some conclusions using this equation.

To begin our discussion, one format of the Henderson-Hasselbach equation is

$$pH = pK_a - \log\left(\frac{HA}{A^-}\right)$$

where HA is the concentration of a weak acid, A^- is the concentration of its conjugate base, and pK_a is an ionization constant of the weak acid.

Using the rules of logarithms and exponents, we could express this equation as

$$pH = pK_a + \log\left(\frac{HA}{A^-}\right)^{-1} = pK_a + \log\frac{A^-}{HA}$$

Therefore, a second format of the Henderson-Hasselbach equation is

$$pH = pK_a + \log\frac{A^-}{HA}.$$

It is also a fact that a buffer solution is at its greatest buffering capacity when the pH of the solution is equal to the pK_a of the weak acid. Keeping this in mind, if we subtract pK_a from both sides of the preceding equation, we obtain

$$pH - pK_a = \log\frac{A^-}{HA}.$$

However, if the solution is at its greatest buffering capacity, the pH is equal to pK_a, and this equation becomes

$$0 = \log \frac{A^-}{HA}.$$

But we know that $\log 1 = 0$. Therefore, $\frac{A^-}{HA}$ must equal 1, which means the concentration of the weak acid must equal the concentration of its conjugate base. Thus, for a buffer to be at its greatest buffering capacity, HA must equal A^-.

Using the Calculator to Evaluate Logarithms

EXAMPLE 7-9: Evaluate $\log\left(\dfrac{32}{30 \times 0.06}\right)$ by using a calculator.

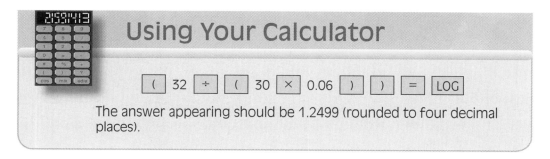

Using Your Calculator

(32 ÷ (30 × 0.06)) = LOG

The answer appearing should be 1.2499 (rounded to four decimal places).

Occasionally, a special type of logarithm arises called the natural logarithm. The **natural logarithm** is a logarithm whose base, instead of 10, is about 2.718. The derivation of this is beyond the scope of this course. However, we need to know what it looks like. First, the natural log of x is notated as

$$\ln x.$$

For the clinical science program, the student must be proficient in using the calculator to evaluate expressions involving $\ln x$. The natural log key, or ln key, is located next to the log key on the calculator. Following is an example.

EXAMPLE 7-10: Evaluate using a calculator: $\dfrac{\log(278)}{\ln(10) - \ln(8)}$

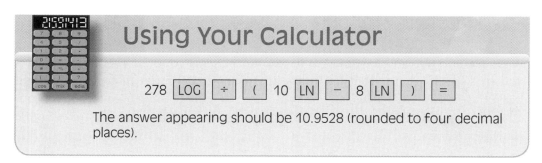

Using Your Calculator

278 LOG ÷ (10 LN − 8 LN) =

The answer appearing should be 10.9528 (rounded to four decimal places).

PRACTICE PROBLEMS: Section 7.1

1. Without the help of a calculator, determine the value of $\log(10)$.

2. Without the help of a calculator, determine the value of $\log(10{,}000)$.

3. Without the help of a calculator, determine the value of $\log(10{,}000{,}000)$.

4. Without the help of a calculator, determine the value of $\log(100{,}000{,}000)$.

5. Using a calculator, find the value of the following expressions.

   a) $(\log 240)^2$

   b) $\dfrac{\ln(98) - \ln(25)}{\log(5)}$

   c) $\log(5{,}680) - 2.4$

   d) $\log\left(\dfrac{45.9}{3.2 - 1.8}\right)$

   e) $\dfrac{\ln(2{,}500) + 4.7}{\ln(145)}$

6. Find the value of the logarithms without using a calculator.

   a) $\log(8{,}000)$

   b) $\log(90{,}000)$

   c) $\log(0.03)$

   d) $\log(0.000007)$

   e) $\log(0.6)$

f) $\log(10{,}000{,}000)$

g) $\log\left(\dfrac{3}{1{,}000}\right)$

h) $\log\left(\dfrac{5}{100{,}000}\right)$

i) $-\log(10^{-3})$

j) $-\log(10^{-5})$

k) $\log(9 \times 10^{-7})$

l) $-\log\left(\dfrac{2}{10^{-4}}\right)$

7. Find the pH of a solution where $H^+ = 10^{-2}$.

8. Find the pH of a solution where $H^+ = 10^{-8}$.

9. Find the pH of a solution where $H^+ = 10^{-5}$.

10. Find the pH of a solution where $H^+ = 10^{-10}$.

11. Find the pH of a solution where $H^+ = 10^{-9}$.

12. Evaluate using a calculator.

    a) $\log(3 \times 10^{12})$

    b) $\log\left(\dfrac{4.8}{2 \times 10^{-1}}\right)$

    c) $\log\left(\dfrac{6}{5 - 0.51}\right)$

    d) $\ln(4 \times 10^{-8})$

    e) $\dfrac{\ln(450)}{\log(600)}$

    f) $\log[(2 \times 10^3) \times (3 \times 10^4)]$

7.2 – SPECTROPHOTOMETRY AND COLORIMETRY

Spectrophotometry can be defined as the science of measuring the absorption of light by using a spectrophotometer. A spectrophotometer measures the intensity of the light after it travels through a solution. For example, if we were shining light through a copper sulfate solution, $CuSO_4$, we would encounter an observable fact illustrated in the following diagram.

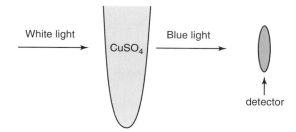

When the intensity of the light changes in this manner (from white to blue), we can presume the solution absorbed some of the energy from the light for this change to take place. Thus, *absorption* gives us information about how much energy a solution absorbs from the light while *transmittance* gives us information about the intensity of the light after it travels through the solution. There is a clear correspondence between absorption and transmittance, and we will discuss the formulas relating these two quantities shortly.

Colorimetry might best be defined as the science of colors. A colorimeter is an instrument that measures the depth of the color of a given solution as compared with the depth of the color of some standard solution. We can see that spectrophotometry and colorimetry are closely related. In the clinical laboratory, spectrophotometry is used to measure the amount of light a solution absorbs or transmits. Lambert Beer's Law provides us with a mathematical formula that tells us how much light is absorbed by a solution. This law asserts there are three factors that affect how much light a solution will absorb. Those three factors are the concentration of the solution, the path length the light travels through the solution, and an absorptivity constant. Mathematically the formula for Beer's Law is

$$A = \epsilon \cdot c \cdot l$$

where A is the absorbance, ϵ is a molar absorptivity constant, c is the concentration, and l is the path length in which the light travels through the solution. Depending on the characteristics of the light and what method is used, ϵ can take on a wide range of values. However, it is always going to be a constant. In the case of the clinical lab, the molar absorptivity constant will typically be about 3×10^3. Analyzing this equation we see there is a direct variation relationship between the absorbance A and both the concentration and the distance the light travels through the solution. This makes sense because as the concentration increases, the amount of light absorbed will also increase. Likewise, as the distance in which the light travels through the solution increases, the more particles the light will hit and thus the more light will be absorbed. Sometimes, instead of using Beer's Law, we use another equation that involves transmittance instead of absorbance.

Transmittance tells us about how much light can shine through a solution, as opposed to absorbance, which tells us how much light is absorbed. The more concentrated the solution, the less light can shine through. We can also see that the more light a solution absorbs, the less will be transmitted. Therefore, there is an inverse relationship between the absorbance and the transmittance. We will see this behavior manifest in the formulas to come. However, before introducing the formula that relates absorbance with transmittance, let's first cover some preliminaries.

The strength or intensity of the light before it shines through the solution we will notate as I_0, and the intensity of the light after it shines through the solution we will notate as I. The following diagram illustrates this phenomenon.

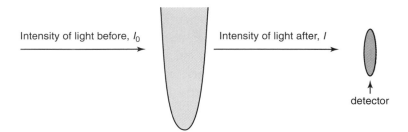

Transmittance, T, is defined as

$$T = \frac{I}{I_0}.$$

Notice the transmittance will always be less than 1—the intensity of the light I_0 before it shines through a solution will always be greater than the intensity after it shines through because some of the intensity of the light will inevitably be absorbed by the solution. Therefore, I_0 is greater than I and thus $\frac{I}{I_0} < 1$.

A mathematical formula that relates the absorbance, A, with transmittance is

$$A = \log\frac{I_0}{I}.$$

But $T = \frac{I}{I_0}$. If we multiply both sides of $T = \frac{I}{I_0}$ by $\frac{I_0}{I}$, we get

$$\frac{I_0}{I} \cdot T = \frac{I}{I_0} \cdot \frac{I_0}{I},$$

which simplifies to

$$\frac{I_0}{I} \cdot T = 1.$$

Lastly, if we divide both sides by T, we get $\frac{I_0}{I} = \frac{1}{T}$.

Now if we substitute $\frac{1}{T}$ for $\frac{I_0}{I}$ in the equation $A = \log\frac{I_0}{I}$, we get

$$A = \log\frac{1}{T}$$

where A is the absorbance and T is the transmittance. Again, notice this is an inverse relationship. If we apply the properties of logarithms to this formula, we get

$$A = \log 1 - \log T.$$

But we know from Section 7.1 that $\log 1 = 0$. Therefore, this formula becomes

$$A = -\log T.$$

This equation is convenient when we are given the transmittance and are trying to find the absorbance. All we do is plug in the transmittance and we can find the absorbance. To find the transmittance given the absorbance, we can use a modified version of this formula. To get this modified version, multiply both sides of this equation by -1 and it becomes

$$-A = \log T.$$

Keeping in mind the definition of a logarithm, which is

$$y = \log x \leftrightarrow x = 10^y,$$

we can express the equation $-A = \log T$ as

$$T = 10^{-A}.$$

This equation is convenient to use when we are given the absorbance and want to find the transmittance. Remember, Beer's Law states

$$A = \epsilon \cdot c \cdot l,$$

and if we substitute this into the equation $T = 10^{-A}$, we get $T = 10^{-\epsilon c l}$.

NOTE

Absorbance and transmittance are often calculated to three decimal places.

EXAMPLE 7-11: Find the absorbance if the transmittance is 68%.

As a decimal $68\% = 0.680$. Substituting this for T in the formula $A = -\log T$, we get

$$A = -\log(0.680).$$

Using a calculator and rounding to three decimal places, we get

$$A = -(-0.167) = 0.167.$$

EXAMPLE 7-12: Find the transmittance if the absorbance is 0.175.

Because we are given the absorbance, use the formula $T = 10^{-A}$. Substituting the given value for the absorbance into this formula, we get

$$T = 10^{-0.175}.$$

Using our calculator we find that

$$T = 0.668.$$

EXAMPLE 7-13: Find the transmittance if the absorbance is 0.459.

Because we are given the absorbance, we want to use the formula $T = 10^{-A}$. Substituting the given value for the absorbance into this formula, we get

$$T = 10^{-0.459}.$$

Using our calculator we find that

$$T = 0.348.$$

Beer's Formula

If we know the value of ϵ in Beer's formula, we can then find the concentration of a solution by first finding the absorbance. If we solve Beer's formula for the concentration, c, we obtain

$$c = \frac{A}{\epsilon \times l},$$

as illustrated in the following.

$$A = \epsilon \times c \times l$$

Dividing both sides by $\epsilon \times l$, we get

$$\frac{A}{\epsilon \times l} = c.$$

Now the path length, l, in which the light travels, is a controlled distance, and thus we know this value. We can also use a spectrophotometer to find the absorption, A. As we are assuming, we also know the value of ϵ. Thus, we know, or can find, the value of all the variables in the right-hand side of the equation

$$c = \frac{A}{\epsilon \times l},$$

and therefore we can find the concentration of a solution if we know the value of ϵ.

The units associated with ϵ and l are usually $^{L}/_{mol \cdot cm}$ and cm, respectively. Therefore, the denominator of the equation

$$c = \frac{A}{\epsilon \times l}$$

will have units of

$$\frac{L}{mol \cdot cm} \cdot cm = \frac{L}{mol}.$$

Thus, the concentration, in terms of units, will equal

$$c = \frac{A}{L/mol} = A \div \frac{L}{mol} = A \cdot \frac{mol}{L}.$$

A is a constant, so c will have units of mol/L.

EXAMPLE 7-14: The molar absorptivity constant of a particular solution is 2.5×10^3. A spectrophotometer was used to determine the absorbance, and it was found to be 0.345. If the path length is 1.50 cm, find the concentration.

Substituting these values into the formula

$$c = \frac{A}{\epsilon \times l},$$

we obtain

$$c = \frac{0.345}{2.5 \times 10^3 \times 1.50} = 9.2 \times 10^{-5} \, mol/L.$$

EXAMPLE 7-15: The molar absorptivity constant of a particular solution is 1.8×10^3. A spectrophotometer was used to determine the absorbance, and it was found to be 0.694. If the path length is 2.00 cm, find the concentration.

Substituting these values into the formula

$$c = \frac{A}{\epsilon \times l},$$

we obtain

$$c = \frac{0.694}{1.8 \times 10^3 \times 2.00} = 1.9 \times 10^{-4} \, mol/L$$

Using Proportions in Spectrometry

In some applications of spectrophotometry, proportions can be implemented to solve a problem. This is because the absorbance of a solution is directly proportional to its concentration. When using this approach we must be careful to have solutions of different concentrations that contain the same chemical and are measured under the same conditions, specifically, the same wavelength and path length. When all of these conditions are satisfied, we can use the proportion equation

$$\frac{A_1}{A_2} = \frac{c_1}{c_2}.$$

EXAMPLE 7-16: A solution with a concentration of 3×10^{-5} $^{mol}/_{L}$ is found to have an absorbance of 0.281 by using a spectrophotometer with a light whose wavelength is 350 nm and path length was 1 cm. A second solution with the same chemical properties was measured under the same conditions and was found to have an absorbance of 0.340. Find the concentration of the second solution.

We are given the concentration and absorbance of the first solution and only the absorbance of the second solution. Therefore, we know that

$$c_1 = 3 \times 10^{-5} \ ^{mol}/_{L} \qquad A_1 = 0.281 \qquad A_2 = 0.340$$

Plugging these values into the proportion equation

$$\frac{A_1}{A_2} = \frac{c_1}{c_2},$$

we get

$$\frac{0.281}{0.340} = \frac{3 \times 10^3}{c_2}.$$

Cross multiplying we obtain

$$0.281 c_2 = (0.340)(3 \times 10^3).$$

Simplifying the right-hand side, we get

$$0.281 c_2 = 1.020 \times 10^3.$$

Dividing both sides by 0.281, we find

$$c_2 = \frac{1.020 \times 10^3}{0.281} = 3.6 \times 10^{3} \ ^{mol}/_{L}.$$

EXAMPLE 7-17: A solution with a concentration of 1.3×10^{-4} $^{mol}/_{L}$ is found to have an absorbance of 0.112. A second solution with the same chemical properties was measured under the same conditions and was found to have an absorbance of 0.185. Find the concentration of the second solution.

We are given that

$$c_1 = 1.3 \times 10^{-4} \ ^{mol}/_{L} \qquad A_1 = 0.112 \qquad A_2 = 0.185$$

Substituting these into the proportion equation, we get

$$\frac{0.112}{0.185} = \frac{1.3 \times 10^{-4}}{c_2}.$$

Cross multiplying we get

$$0.112 c_2 = (0.185)(1.3 \times 10^{-4}).$$

Simplifying the right-hand side, we get

$$0.112c_2 = 2.405 \times 10^{-5}.$$

Dividing both sides by 0.112, we find

$$c_2 = 2.1 \times 10^{-4} \,\mathrm{mol/L}.$$

PRACTICE PROBLEMS: Section 7.2

1. Find the absorbance if the transmittance is 0.723.

2. Find the absorbance if the transmittance is 66.2%.

3. Find the absorbance if the transmittance is 58.8%.

4. Find the absorbance if the transmittance is 0.686.

5. Find the transmittance if the absorbance is 0.377.

6. Find the transmittance if the absorbance is 0.237.

7. Find the transmittance if the absorbance is 0.288.

8. Find the transmittance if the absorbance is 0.082.

9. Find the transmittance if the absorbance is 0.302.

10. The molar absorptivity constant of a particular solution is 1.4×10^3. A spectrophotometer was used to determine the absorbance, and it was found to be 0.179. If the path length is 1.0 cm, find the concentration.

11. The molar absorptivity constant of a particular solution is 6.7×10^3. A spectrophotometer was used to determine the absorbance, and it was found to be 0.425. If the path length is 1.5 cm, find the concentration.

12. The molar absorptivity constant of a particular solution is 4.1×10^3. A spectrophotometer was used to determine the absorbance, and it was found to be 0.215. If the path length is 1.0 cm, find the concentration.

13. The molar absorptivity constant of a particular solution is 5.9×10^3. A spectrophotometer was used to determine the absorbance, and it was found to be 0.382. If the path length is 1.5 cm, find the concentration.

14. Given that $\epsilon = 1.7 \times 10^3$, the absorbance is 0.257, and the path length is 1.5 cm, find the concentration.

15. Given that $\epsilon = 2.2 \times 10^3$, the absorbance is 0.292, and the path length is 16 mm, find the concentration.

16. Given that $\epsilon = 2.8 \times 10^3$, the absorbance is 0.392, and the path length is 14 mm, find the concentration.

Continues

PRACTICE PROBLEMS: Section 7.2 (continued)

17. Given that $\epsilon = 2.5 \times 10^3$, the absorbance is 0.315, and the path length is 15 mm, find the concentration.

18. Given that $\epsilon = 1.9 \times 10^3$, the absorbance is 0.263, and the path length is 1.4 cm, find the concentration.

19. Given the concentration is 6×10^{-5} $\frac{mol}{L}$, the absorbance is 0.238, and the path length is 15 mm, find the value of ϵ.

20. Given the concentration is 5×10^{-5} $\frac{mol}{L}$, the absorbance is 0.220, and the path length is 14 mm, find the value of ϵ.

21. Given the concentration is 6×10^{-5} $\frac{mol}{L}$, the absorbance is 0.255, and the path length is 16 mm, find the value of ϵ.

22. A solution with a concentration of 5.9×10^{-5} $\frac{mol}{L}$ is found to have an absorbance of 0.524 by using a spectrophotometer with a light whose wavelength is 320 nm and path length was 2 cm. A second solution with the same chemical properties was measured under the same conditions and was found to have an absorbance of 0.826. Find the concentration of the second solution.

23. A solution with a concentration of 4×10^{-5} $\frac{mol}{L}$ is found to have an absorbance of 0.398 by using a spectrophotometer. A second solution with the same chemical properties was measured under the same conditions and was found to have an absorbance of 0.162. Find the concentration of the second solution.

24. A solution with a concentration of 4.8×10^{-5} $\frac{mol}{L}$ is found to have an absorbance of 0.720. A second solution with the same chemical properties was measured under the same conditions and was found to have an absorbance of 0.600. Find the concentration of the second solution.

25. A solution with a concentration of 5.2×10^{-5} $\frac{mol}{L}$ is found to have an absorbance of 0.496 by using a spectrophotometer with a light whose wavelength is 300 nm and path length was 2 cm. A second solution with the same chemical properties was measured under the same conditions and was found to have an absorbance of 0.797. Find the concentration of the second solution.

CHAPTER SUMMARY

- The definition of logarithm is $y = \log x$ if and only if $10^y = x$.
- Following are the properties of logarithms:
  - $\log x > 0$ if $x > 1$
  - $\log x < 0$ if $0 < x < 1$
  - $\log(1) = 0$
  - $\log(A \times B) = \log(A) + \log(B)$
  - $\log\left(\dfrac{A}{B}\right) = \log(A) - \log(B)$
  - $-\log(A) = \log(A)^{-1} = \log\left(\dfrac{1}{A}\right)$
  - Logarithms of negative numbers do not exist.
- $\mathrm{pH} = \log\left(\dfrac{1}{\mathrm{H}^+}\right)$
- The Henderson-Hasselbach equation relates the pH of a buffer to the concentration of a weak acid and its conjugate base.
- $A = -\log T$, where A is absorbance and T is transmittance.
- $T = 10^{-A}$, where A is absorbance and T is transmittance.
- Beer's Law is $A = \epsilon \cdot c \cdot l$, where A is the absorbance, ϵ is a molar absorptivity constant, c is the concentration, and l is the path length.
- The absorbance of a solution is directly proportional to its concentration.

CHAPTER TEST

1. Determine the value of $\log(900)$ without using a calculator.

2. Determine the value of $\log\left(\dfrac{7}{10,000}\right)$ without using a calculator.

3. Determine the value of $\log\left(\dfrac{1}{100,000}\right)$ without using a calculator.

4. Find the pH of a solution where $\mathrm{H}^+ = 10^{-7}$.

5. Find the pH of a solution where $\mathrm{H}^+ = 10^{-8}$.

6. Find the absorbance if the transmittance is 59.1%.

7. Find the absorbance if the transmittance is 0.613.

8. Find the transmittance if the absorbance is 0.311.

9. Find the transmittance if the absorbance is 0.425.

10. Given that $\epsilon = 2.1 \times 10^3$, the absorbance is 0.285, and the path length is 15 mm, find the concentration.

11. The molar absorptivity constant of a particular solution is 5.7×10^3. A spectrophotometer was used to determine the absorbance, and it was found to be 0.405. If the path length is 165 mm, find the concentration.

12. A solution with a concentration of 6×10^{-5} $^{mol}\!/\!_L$ is found to have an absorbance of 0.422 by using a spectrophotometer. A second solution with the same chemical properties was measured under the same conditions and was found to have an absorbance of 0.191. Find the concentration of the second solution.

Hematology Mathematics

INTRODUCTION

Hematology is the science of the study of blood. This chapter covers the mathematical concepts behind calculating the number of blood cells in a sample of blood in addition to some other topics encountered in hematology, including a brief discussion of transfusion medicine.

Remember from Chapter 2 that the formula for volume can be written as

$$V = (L \times W) \times H$$

where volume equals area times depth.

EXAMPLE 8-1: An instrument measured a blood sample and found it had 6,500 white blood cells per cubic millimeter. About how many white blood cells (WBCs) should a $1 \times 1 \times 0.1$ mm sample of this blood contain?

$1\,\text{mm} \times 1\,\text{mm} \times \dfrac{1}{10}\,\text{mm} = \dfrac{1}{10}\,\text{mm}^3$. Therefore this sample should have about

$$\frac{1}{10}\,\text{mm}^3 \times \frac{6{,}500\,\text{WBCs}}{\text{mm}^3} = \frac{6{,}500\,\text{WBCs}}{10} = 650\,\text{WBCs/mm}^3$$

8.1 – COUNTING CELLS

In the laboratory we often count blood cells by using a Neubauer counting chamber. This is a heavy glass slide with two chambers containing ruled areas each measuring 3×3 mm, or 9 mm². Each ruled area is 9 square millimeters, so there are 9 squares with each square measuring 1×1 mm. Figure 8–1 is a diagram of one of the ruled areas.

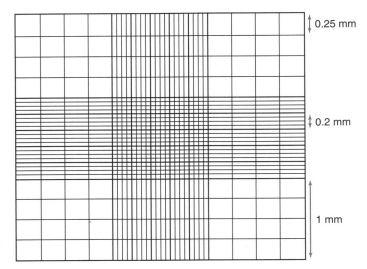

FIGURE 8-1
Diagram of a Neubauer
counting chamber.

As we see from the diagram, the 4 corner squares are typically divided further into 16 smaller squares, with each smaller square measuring 0.25×0.25 mm; the middle square is subdivided into 25 smaller squares, with each smaller square measuring 0.2×0.2 mm. The middle square is divided even further with each of the 25 smaller squares subdivided again into 16 even smaller squares as illustrated in Figure 8–1. This would leave the middle square consisting of $25 \times 16 = 400$ very small squares. The middle square is subdivided like this so when there is a very high cell count we can simply count the number of cells in some of these very small squares and then compensate by using an area factor when we do our calculations. The **area factor** is

$$\frac{1}{\text{Total area counted in mm}^2}$$

When we are given a specimen of blood, the white blood cell (WBC) count or the red blood cell (RBC) count is typically very high. Therefore, we often need to dilute the specimen before we try to count the number of cells. As a result, a **dilution factor** must be used to get the actual cell count of the original specimen. The dilution factor is the reciprocal of the dilution.

We often report the number of cells as the number per cubic millimeter. This can be represented mathematically as

$$\frac{\text{Number of cells}}{\text{mm}^3}$$

However, when we count the number of cells on a slide, we do not usually have a full cubic millimeter. So we also have a **depth factor**. Like the dilution factor, the depth factor is the reciprocal of the depth. In a Neubauer hemacytometer, the depth is $\frac{1}{10}$ of a millimeter (0.1 mm); therefore, the depth factor will always be 10.

Putting all of this together, the formula for calculating the number of cells per cubic millimeter is

$$\frac{\text{Number of cells}}{\text{mm}^3} = \text{No. of cells counted} \times \text{Area factor} \times \text{Depth factor} \times \text{Dilution factor}$$

$$= \text{No. of cells counted} \times \frac{1}{\text{Total area counted (in mm}^2)} \times \text{Depth factor} \times \text{Dilution factor}$$

Simplifying, this formula becomes

$$\frac{\text{Number of cells}}{\text{mm}^3} = \text{Total \# of cells counted} \times \frac{\text{Depth factor} \times \text{Dilution factor}}{\text{Total area counted (in mm}^2)}$$

EXAMPLE 8-2: A red blood cell count must be performed on a specimen of blood. Because the RBC count is typically between 4 million and 6 million per cubic millimeter, the cells were suspended in a $\frac{1}{500}$ dilution. Four hundred RBCs were then counted in the four small corners and the small middle square of the large middle square of both sides of the Neubauer counting chamber (see following diagram). Assume the depth is $\frac{1}{10}$ mm and calculate the number of RBCs per cubic millimeter of this blood sample.

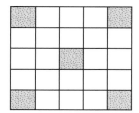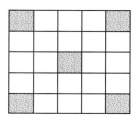

The number of RBCs counted was 400. The depth factor is 10 because the depth is $\frac{1}{10}$. The dilution factor is 500 because the dilution performed was $\frac{1}{500}$. The "hard" part is finding the total number of square millimeters we counted. In all we counted within 2 "big" squares; however, we did not count the entire square. We counted only the RBCs in the 5 smaller squares in each large middle square. Remember that each of the small squares is 0.2×0.2 mm. Each small square, therefore, has an area of $0.2 \times 0.2 = 0.04$ mm^2. We counted 5 small squares in each of the 2 middle squares, so we counted a total of 10 small squares. Thus, the total area counted is $10 \times 0.04 = 0.40$ mm^2. Plugging everything into the number-of-cells formula, we get

$$\frac{\text{Number of RBCs}}{\text{mm}^3} = 400 \times \frac{10 \times 500}{0.40} = 5,000,000.$$

Therefore, we would report that this blood specimen has a total RBC count of 4.00×10^6 RBCs per cubic millimeter.

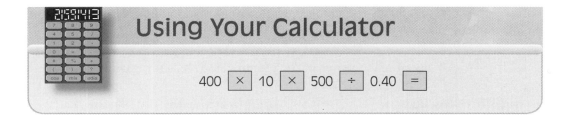

Using Your Calculator

400 $\boxed{\times}$ 10 $\boxed{\times}$ 500 $\boxed{\div}$ 0.40 $\boxed{=}$

EXAMPLE 8-3: A $\frac{1}{100}$ dilution was carried out on a blood specimen and then 180 WBCs were counted using the entire ruled area of both counting chambers. Determine the total count and assume the depth is 0.1 mm.

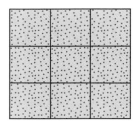
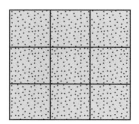

We are told that the total number of WBCs is 180. Because the depth is 0.1 or $\frac{1}{10}$, the depth factor is 10. A $\frac{1}{100}$ dilution was performed, so the dilution factor is 100. The total area counted is $9 + 9 = 18$ mm^2 since all the squares were counted in both chambers. Substituting these values into the number-of-cells formula, we get

$$\frac{\text{Number of WBCs}}{\text{mm}^3} = 180 \times \frac{10 \times 100}{18} = 10,000.$$

Therefore, this blood specimen has 10,000 WBCs per cubic millimeter.

EXAMPLE 8-4: A $\frac{1}{400}$ dilution was made from a blood specimen and then 150 RBCs were counted in the four small corners and the small middle square of the large middle square of one of the counting chambers. If the depth is $\frac{1}{10}$ mm, calculate the number of RBCs in this blood sample.

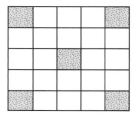

Because we counted the number of RBCs in five small squares of the large middle square, the area is 1 mm^2. Each small square has an area of 0.04 mm^2 and because we counted five small squares, the total area is 5×0.04 mm$^2 = 0.2$ mm^2. The dilution factor is 400, the depth factor is 10, and the number of RBCs was 150. Substituting all of this into the number-of-cells formula, we get

$$\frac{\text{Number of RBCs}}{\text{mm}^3} = 150 \times \frac{10 \times 400}{0.2} = 3,000,000.$$

Therefore, this specimen of blood has 3,000,000 RBCs per cubic millimeter.

PRACTICE PROBLEMS: Section 8.1

1. An instrument measured a blood sample and found it had 7,250 white blood cells per cubic millimeter. About how many white blood cells should a 1 × 2 × 0.1 mm sample of this blood contain?

2. An instrument measured a blood sample and found it had 8,500 white blood cells per cubic millimeter. About how many white blood cells should a 1 × 1 mm sample of this blood contain if the depth of the blood sample is 0.2 mm?

3. The RBCs were counted in the four corner squares and the middle square of the large middle square of one chamber. Find the area factor to be used when calculating the total number of RBCs in this manner.

4. The RBCs were counted in the four corner squares of the large upper right side square of both Neubauer counting chambers. Find the area factor to be used when calculating the total number of RBCs.

5. A lab technician is asked to find the WBC count for a blood specimen. A $\frac{1}{10}$ dilution was carried out and 80 WBCs were counted in each of the four corners in each of the two Neubauer counting chambers. Determine the total count and assume the depth is 0.1 mm.

6. A laboratorian is asked to find the WBC count for a blood specimen. A $\frac{1}{100}$ dilution is carried out and 35 WBCs were counted in two of the four corners in each of the two chambers. Determine the total count and assume the depth is 0.1 mm.

7. A laboratorian is asked to find the WBC count for a blood specimen with a low level of WBCs. A $\frac{1}{10}$ dilution is carried out. Sixty-five WBCs were then counted in each of the four corners in each of the two chambers. Determine the total count and assume the depth is 0.1 mm.

8. A laboratorian is asked to find the WBC count for a blood specimen. A $\frac{1}{100}$ dilution is carried out. Twenty WBCs were then counted in two of the four corners in one of the two chambers. Determine the total WBC count and assume the depth is 0.1 mm.

9. A laboratorian is asked to find the WBC count for a blood specimen. A $\frac{1}{10}$ dilution is carried out and a total of 45 WBCs were counted in each of the four corners in one of the two chambers. Determine the total WBC count and assume the depth is 0.1 mm.

Continues

PRACTICE PROBLEMS: Section 8.1 *(continued)*

10. A red blood cell count was to be performed on a specimen of blood and a $\frac{1}{200}$ dilution was used. A total of 1,200 RBCs were then counted in the four smaller corners of the large lower right corner square and the large lower left corner square of each chamber. Assume the depth is 0.1 mm and calculate the number of RBCs per cubic millimeter of this blood sample.

11. A red blood cell count was to be performed on a specimen of blood. Because the RBC count is typically between 4 million and 6 million per cubic millimeter, we used a $\frac{1}{200}$ dilution. A total of 975 RBCs were then counted in the four smaller corners of the large top right corner square of each chamber. Assume the depth is $\frac{1}{10}$ mm and calculate the number of RBCs per cubic millimeter of this blood sample.

12. A red blood cell count was to be performed on a specimen of blood and a $\frac{1}{200}$ dilution was used. A total of 1,025 RBCs were then counted in the four smaller corners of the large lower left corner square of each chamber. Assume the depth is $\frac{1}{10}$ mm and calculate the number of RBCs per cubic millimeter of this blood sample.

13. A red blood cell count was to be performed on a specimen of blood and a $\frac{1}{200}$ dilution was used. A total of 1,100 RBCs were counted in the four smaller corners of the large upper right corner square and the large upper left corner square of each chamber. Assume the depth is $\frac{1}{10}$ mm and calculate the number of RBCs per cubic millimeter of this blood sample.

14. A red blood cell count was to be performed on a specimen of blood and a $\frac{1}{200}$ dilution was used. A total of 550 RBCs were then counted in the four smaller corners of the large lower right corner square of each chamber. Assume the depth is $\frac{1}{10}$ mm and calculate the number of RBCs per cubic millimeter of this blood sample.

15. One hundred forty platelets were counted in the entire middle square of one of the chambers. A $\frac{1}{200}$ dilution was carried out on the original blood sample. Assume the depth is $\frac{1}{10}$ mm. Calculate the number of platelets in the original blood sample per cubic millimeter.

16. Two hundred fifty platelets were counted in the entire middle square of one of the chambers. A $\frac{1}{100}$ dilution was carried out on the original blood sample. Assume the depth is $\frac{1}{10}$ mm. Calculate the number of platelets in the original blood sample per cubic millimeter.

17. The platelets were counted in the entire middle square of both of the chambers. The total count was found to be 475 platelets. A $\frac{1}{100}$ dilution was carried out on the original blood sample. Assume the depth is $\frac{1}{10}$ mm. Calculate the number of platelets in the original blood sample per cubic millimeter.

8.2 – RED BLOOD CELL INDICES

Mean Corpuscular Volume

The calculation of the mean corpuscular volume (MCV) is often done in the clinical laboratory because the mean corpuscular volume tells us how much space a red blood cell occupies. The percentage of (packed) red blood cells that makes up the blood is called the **hematocrit**. The hematocrit (Hct) is commonly given as a percent. For example, if the hematocrit is 50%, this means half of the blood is occupied by red blood cells. On the other hand, to calculate the MCV, we divide the hematocrit (given as a percentage) by the number of RBCs. We then multiply this result by 10. Mathematically, the formula for the MCV is

$$MCV = \frac{Hct\,(\%)}{\#\,RBCs\,(in\,millions/\mu L)} \times 10$$

EXAMPLE 8-5: A laboratorian analyzed a blood sample to determine the counts given here. Find the MCV.

- Hct = 40%

- # RBCs = 4.5×10^6

$$MCV = \frac{40}{4.5} \times 10 \approx 89$$

EXAMPLE 8-6: Given that MCV = 100 and Hct = 55%, find the number of RBCs.

Substituting the given values into the formula, we have

$$100 = \frac{55}{x} \times 10.$$

Multiplying both sides by x, we get

$$100x = 550.$$

Dividing by 100 we find the number of RBCs to be 5.5 (million).

Mean Corpuscular Hemoglobin and Mean Corpuscular Hemoglobin Concentration

Other formulas are used to calculate the mean corpuscular hemoglobin (MCH) and the mean corpuscular hemoglobin concentration (MCHC). **Hemoglobin** is the oxygen-carrying protein that gives RBCs their color. MCH is in picograms (pg) and therefore tells us about the amount (weight) of hemoglobin per RBC, and the MCHC tells us about the hemoglobin concentration per RBC. MCHC is usually given as a percent.

The hemoglobin concentration (Hb) tells us about the amount of hemoglobin present relative to the size of the RBC. Following are the formulas for these two RBC indices.

$$MCH = \frac{Hb \, (g/dL)}{\# \, RBCs \, (in \, millions/\mu L)} \times 10$$

$$MCHC = \frac{Hb \, (g/dL)}{Hct \, (\%)} \times 100$$

EXAMPLE 8-7: A laboratorian analyzed a blood sample and obtained the following values. Find the MCH.

- Hb = 14

- # RBCs = 5.3×10^6

$$MCH = \frac{Hb \, (g/dL)}{\# \, RBCs \, (millions/\mu L)} \times 10 = \frac{14}{5.3} \times 10 = 26 \, pg$$

EXAMPLE 8-8: A laboratorian analyzed a blood sample and obtained the following values. Find the MCHC.

- Hb = 12

- Hct = 40%

$$MCHC = \frac{Hb \, (g/dL)}{Hct \, (\%)} \times 100 = \frac{12}{40\%} \times 100 = 30\%$$

PRACTICE PROBLEMS: Section 8.2

1. Find the MCV of a blood sample if its Hct = 45% and the RBC count is 5.5 million per microliter.
2. Find the MCV of a blood sample if its Hct is 40% and the RBC count is 4.0 million per microliter.
3. Find the MCV of a blood sample if its hematocrit is 40% and # RBC/μL = 5.0 million.
4. The Hb of a patient is 15 g/dL and the RBC is $5.7 \times 10^6/\mu L$. Find the MCH.
5. The Hb of a patient is 14 g/dL and the RBC is $5.2 \times 10^6/\mu L$. Find the MCH.
6. The Hb of a patient is 13 g/dL and the RBC is $5.1 \times 10^6/\mu L$. Find the MCH.
7. The Hb of a patient is 14 g/dL with an Hct of 45%. Find the MCHC.
8. The Hb of a patient is 16 g/dL with an Hct of 50%. Find the MCHC.
9. The Hb of a patient is 15 g/dL with an Hct of 55%. Find the MCHC.

8.3 – TRANSFUSION MEDICINE

One pint of whole blood is called a **unit** of blood. When this whole blood is placed into a centrifuge, and the plasma is removed, the RBCs left over constitute a *unit* of packed RBCs. The hemoglobin concentration in this unit of packed RBCs will be about $1.0 \, \text{g}/_{100 \, \text{mL}}$. Thus, if 1 unit of these packed RBCs is transfused into a "normal" patient, we would expect the patient's hemoglobin level to rise by about $1.0 \, \text{g}/_{100 \, \text{mL}}$. Likewise, for each unit of packed RBCs administered to a patient, the patient's hematocrit should rise between 2% and 3%.

EXAMPLE 8-9: A patient had a hematocrit of 25% and his hemoglobin was $5.7 \, \text{g}/_{100 \, \text{mL}}$; therefore, 3 units of packed RBCs were transfused into this patient. What would be his anticipated hemoglobin concentration? In what percentage range would we expect his hematocrit to fall after he is administered the 3 units of packed RBCs?

Because 3 units of packed RBCs were given, his hemoglobin level would be anticipated to rise by 3. Therefore, after the transfusion the patient would be expected to have a hemoglobin level of $5.7 \, \text{g}/_{100 \, \text{mL}} + 3 \, \text{g}/_{100 \, \text{mL}}$, which is $8.7 \, \text{g}/_{100 \, \text{mL}}$.

The hematocrit rises 2% to 3% for every unit of packed RBCs. Because 3 units were given, we would expect an increase of somewhere between 6% and 9%. Therefore, we would expect his overall hematocrit to be between 25% + 6% and 25% + 9% or between 31% and 34%.

Just as RBCs can be transfused, platelets can be transfused as well. A unit of platelets is a concentrate separated from a single unit of whole blood and suspended in a small amount of the original plasma. There are usually at least 5.5×10^9 platelets in 40 mL to 70 mL of plasma. Platelets are typically given to prevent bleeding when platelet levels fall below 10,000 per microliter. Platelets are also given to patients with cancer or who have undergone chemotherapy. When 1 unit of platelets is transfused into a 70 kg adult, a platelet increase of 5,000 to 10,000 per microliter would be expected. Likewise, when 1 unit of platelets is transfused into an 18 kg child, a platelet increase of about 20,000 per microliter would be expected. A common dose is 4 to 8 units. A more precise method for measuring response to the transfusion of platelets is the **corrected count index**, or CCI. The formula for the CCI is

$$\text{CCI} = \frac{\text{Posttransfusion count} - \text{Pretransfusion count}}{\text{Number of platelets transfused} (\times 10^{11})} \times (\text{Body surface area in m}^2)$$

A CCI of at least 5,000 is expected, and a posttransfusion count should be done within 60 minutes. This number will usually decrease with time. Therefore, another dose may need to be administered after one to three days.

EXAMPLE 8-10: A cancer patient with a body surface area of 1.5 m² has a pretransfusion platelet count of 2,500 per microliter. Twenty minutes after being transfused with a platelet dose of 5.0×10^{11}, this patient had a posttransfusion count of 28,000 per microliter. Find the CCI.

Substituting these values into the CCI formula, we obtain

$$\text{CCI} = \frac{28,000 - 2,500}{5.0} \times 1.5 = 7,650.$$

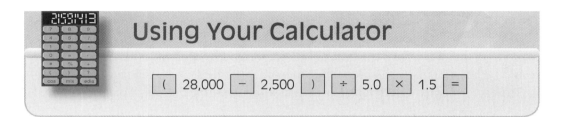

Using Your Calculator

(28,000 − 2,500) ÷ 5.0 × 1.5 =

PRACTICE PROBLEMS: Section 8.3

1. A patient with leukemia has a body surface area of 1.4 m². His pretransfusion platelet count was 2,200 per microliter. Fifteen minutes after being transfused with a platelet dose of 6.5×10^{11}, this patient had a posttransfusion count of 30,000 per microliter. Find the CCI.

2. A cancer patient with a body surface area of 1.6 m² has a pretransfusion platelet count of 2,000 per microliter. Thirty minutes after being transfused with a platelet dose of 5.5×10^{11}, this patient had a posttransfusion count of 25,000 per microliter. Find the CCI.

3. A cancer patient with a body surface area of 1.7 m² has a pretransfusion platelet count of 2,400 per microliter. Twenty minutes after being transfused with a platelet dose of 5.5×10^{11}, this patient had a posttransfusion count of 27,000 per microliter. Find the CCI.

4. A cancer patient with a body surface area of 1.8 m² has a pretransfusion platelet count of 2,700 per microliter. Twenty minutes after being transfused with a platelet dose of 6.0×10^{11}, this patient had a posttransfusion count of 31,000 per microliter. Find the CCI.

5. A patient had a hematocrit of 24% and her hemoglobin was 5.6 $^g/_{100\ mL}$. If this patient was given 3 units of packed RBCs, what would be her anticipated hemoglobin concentration? In what percentage range would we expect her hematocrit to fall after she is administered the 3 units of packed RBCs?

6. A patient in the emergency room was found to be anemic. His hematocrit was 25% and his hemoglobin was 5.7 $^g/_{100\ mL}$. If this patient is not bleeding and he was given 3 units of packed RBCs, what would be his expected hemoglobin concentration? In what percentage range would his hematocrit be expected to fall after he is administered the 3 units of packed RBCs?

7. A patient in the emergency room was found to be anemic. Her hematocrit was 20% and her hemoglobin was 5.5 %/100 mL. If this patient is not bleeding and she was given 3 units of packed RBCs, what would be her expected hemoglobin concentration? In what percentage range would her hematocrit be expected to fall after she is administered the 3 units of packed RBCs?

8. A patient was found to be anemic and was thus admitted to the hospital. His hematocrit was 22% and his hemoglobin was 5.3 %/100 mL. If this patient is not bleeding and he was given 2 units of packed RBCs, what would be his expected hemoglobin concentration? In what percentage range would his hematocrit be expected to fall after he is administered the 2 units of packed RBCs?

CHAPTER SUMMARY

- In the laboratory we often count cells using a microscope together with a hemacytometer. The Neubauer hemacytometer is a common type used in the clinical laboratory.

- $$\frac{\text{Number of cells}}{\text{mm}^3} = \text{No. of cells counted} \times \frac{\text{Depth factor} \times \text{Dilution factor}}{\text{Total area counted (in mm}^2)}$$

- The mean corpuscular volume (MCV) is calculated using the formula

$$\text{MCV} = \frac{\text{Hct (\%)}}{\text{\# RBCs (in millions per microliter)}} \times 10.$$

- The mean corpuscular hemoglobin (MCH) is calculated using the formula

$$\frac{\text{Hb (g/dL)}}{\text{\# RBCs (in millions/}\mu\text{L)}} \times 10.$$

- The mean corpuscular hemoglobin concentration (MCHC) is calculated using the formula

$$\frac{\text{Hb (g/dL)}}{\text{Hct (\%)}} \times 100.$$

- The corrected count index (CCI) is calculated using the formula

$$\text{CCI} = \frac{\text{Posttransfusion count} - \text{Pretransfusion count}}{\text{Number of platelets transfused } (\times 10^{11})} \times (\text{Body surface area in m}^2).$$

CHAPTER TEST

1. A laboratorian is asked to find the WBC count for a blood specimen with a low level of WBCs. A $\frac{1}{10}$ dilution was carried out and 70 WBCs were counted in each of the four corners in each of the two chambers of the hemacytometer. Determine the total WBC count and assume the depth is 0.1 mm.

2. Three hundred platelets were counted in the entire middle square of one of the chambers and a $\frac{1}{100}$ dilution was carried out on the original blood sample. Assume the depth is $\frac{1}{10}$ mm. Calculate the number of platelets in the original blood sample per cubic millimeter.

3. Find the MCV of a blood sample if its Hct is 45% and the RBC count is 5.0 million per microliter.

4. Find the MCV of a blood sample if its Hct is 50% and the RBC count is 5.2 million per microliter.

5. The Hb of a patient is 14 g/dL and the RBC is $5.5 \times 10^6/\mu\text{L}$. Find the MCH.

6. The Hb of a patient is 15 g/dL and the RBC is $5.6 \times 10^6/\mu\text{L}$. Find the MCH.

7. The Hb of a patient is 16 g/dL with an Hct of 45%. Find the MCHC.

8. The Hb of a patient is 15 g/dL with an Hct of 40%. Find the MCHC.

9. A cancer patient with a body surface area of 1.5 m² has a pretransfusion platelet count of 1,800 per microliter. Thirty minutes after being transfused with a platelet dose of 5.2×10^{11}, this patient had a posttransfusion count of 24,000 per microliter. Find the CCI.

10. A patient in the emergency room was found to be anemic. Her hematocrit was 23% and her hemoglobin was 5.4 g/100 mL. If this patient is not bleeding and she was given 3 units of packed RBCs, what would be her expected hemoglobin concentration? In what percentage range would her hematocrit be expected to fall after she is administered the 3 units of packed RBCs?

Urinalysis and Renal Clearance

INTRODUCTION

Urinalysis is the inspection of urine. A urinalysis can be performed to help detect diseases of the organs. A urinalysis is also frequently performed to detect urinary tract infections.

Recall that the renal artery is the artery that supplies the kidneys with blood. *Renal clearance* refers to how fast the kidneys clear the blood of a material. It is usually measured in milliliters of blood cleared per minute. Thus, the units associated with renal clearance are usually $\frac{mL}{min}$ or $mL \cdot min^{-1}$. **Creatinine** is a protein produced by the body that enters the bloodstream. The amount produced by a "normal" person is constant and continuous. Therefore, the rate at which the kidney clears the plasma of creatinine is often used to measure renal clearance. This is referred to as creatinine clearance.

9.1 – URINE PRODUCTION

Usually urine is collected over some period of time such as 24 hours. The average amount of urine output is 1 milliliter per minute. In other words, in a 24-hour period of collecting urine, we would expect to have a total volume of about

$$\frac{1\,mL}{min}\left(\frac{60\,min}{1\,hour}\right)(24\,hours) = 1{,}440\,mL.$$

EXAMPLE 9-1: A 24-hour urine sample contained 1,800 mL and had a creatinine concentration of 75 $\frac{mg}{dL}$. Find the total amount of creatinine this patient excreted and express the result in terms of grams per day ($\frac{g}{day}$ is usually how these results are reported). Also find the number of milliliters of urine excreted per minute.

To find the amount of creatinine in the sample, solve using proportions.

$$\frac{75 \text{ mg}}{1 \text{ dL}} = \frac{x \text{ mg}}{1{,}800 \text{ mL}}$$

Note we cannot yet solve this because the units are not the same in both denominators. However, we know that 100 mL = 1 dL. Substituting this we have

$$\frac{75 \text{ mg}}{100 \text{ mL}} = \frac{x \text{ mg}}{1{,}800 \text{ mL}}.$$

Cross multiplying we get

$$100x = 135{,}000.$$

Dividing both sides by 100, we find

$$x = 1{,}350.$$

Therefore, there are 1,350 mg of creatinine in the entire 1,800 mL sample of urine.

To find how much creatinine was excreted in 24 hours, simply use dimensional analysis. From our previous calculations, we know the creatinine value of this sample is 1,350 mg/24 hours.

The denominator is 24 hours because the urine collection occurred over 24 hours. Now we just convert this to $\frac{\text{g}}{\text{day}}$ as we learned in Chapter 3.

$$\left(\frac{1350 \text{ mg}}{24 \text{ hours}}\right)\left(\frac{24 \text{ hours}}{1 \text{ day}}\right)\left(\frac{10^{-3}\text{g}}{1 \text{ mg}}\right) = 1.35 \frac{\text{g}}{\text{day}}$$

To find the number of milliliters excreted per minute, we again use dimensional analysis. Because there was a total of 1,800 mL collected in 24 hours, we set up our conversion as follows.

$$\frac{1{,}800 \text{ mL}}{24 \text{ hr}}\left(\frac{1 \text{ hr}}{60 \text{ min}}\right) = \frac{1{,}800 \text{ mL}}{(24)(60) \text{ min}} = \frac{1.25 \text{ mL}}{\text{min}}$$

EXAMPLE 9-2: Beginning at 6 a.m. and ending at 6 p.m., a health care professional collected 800 mL of urine from a patient. A laboratorian then analyzed the sample and found a protein concentration of 40 $\frac{\text{mg}}{\text{dL}}$. Find the total amount of protein excreted by this patient and then find the number of milligrams per day. (Protein is often reported in units of $\frac{\text{mg}}{\text{day}}$.)

We begin by setting up a proportion, keeping in mind that 1 dL = 100 mL.

$$\frac{40 \text{ mg}}{100 \text{ mL}} = \frac{x \text{ mg}}{800 \text{ mL}}$$

Cross multiplying we get

$$100x = 32{,}000.$$

Dividing by 100 we find

$$x = 320.$$

Therefore, there is 320 mg of protein in the entire 800 mL sample.

To find milligrams of protein per day, we use dimensional analysis. From our previous calculations, we know the protein value of this sample is

$$\frac{800 \text{ mg}}{12 \text{ hours}}.$$

Converting we have

$$\left(\frac{800 \text{ mg}}{12 \text{ hours}} \right) \left(\frac{24 \text{ hours}}{1 \text{ day}} \right) = 1,600 \text{ }^{mg}/_{day}.$$

PRACTICE PROBLEMS: Section 9.1

1. A 24-hour urine sample contained 1,600 mL of urine and had a creatinine concentration of 80 $^{mg}/_{dL}$. Find the total amount of creatinine excreted by this patient. How many grams of creatinine did this patient excrete in one day? Find the number of milliliters of urine excreted per minute.

2. A 12-hour urine sample contained 750 mL of urine and had a creatinine concentration of 85 $^{mg}/_{dL}$. Find the total amount of creatinine excreted by this patient. How many grams of creatinine did this patient excrete in one day?

3. A 24-hour urine specimen contained 1,700 mL of urine and had a creatinine concentration of 85 $^{mg}/_{dL}$. Find the total amount of creatinine in this entire sample. How many grams of creatinine did this patient excrete in one day?

4. A 12-hour urine specimen contained 700 mL of urine and had a creatinine concentration of 75 $^{mg}/_{dL}$. Find the total amount of creatinine in this entire sample. What is the 24-hour creatinine value?

5. A 12-hour urine collection contained 900 mL of urine. It was found to have a protein concentration of 45 $^{mg}/_{dL}$. Find the total amount of protein excreted by this patient and find the number of milligrams excreted per day.

6. In an 8-hour period 500 mL of urine was collected from a patient. It was found to have a protein concentration of 35 $^{mg}/_{dL}$. Find the total amount of protein excreted and find the 24-hour protein value in terms of milligrams per day.

7. In a 24-hour period a total volume of 1,900 mL of urine was collected. It was found to have 70 $^{mg}/_{dL}$ of creatinine. Find the total amount of creatinine in this entire sample. What is the creatinine value in terms of grams per day?

Continues

PRACTICE PROBLEMS: Section 9.1 (continued)

8. In an 8-hour period a total volume of 600 mL of urine was collected. It was found to have 50 $\frac{mg}{dL}$ of creatinine. Find the total amount of creatinine in this entire sample. Find the creatinine value in terms of grams per day.

9. In a 6-hour period a total volume of 400 mL of urine was collected. It was found to have a creatinine concentration of 48 $\frac{mg}{dL}$. Find the total amount of creatinine excreted. Find the 24-hour creatinine value.

10. In an 8-hour period a total volume of 550 mL of urine was collected. It was found to have a creatinine concentration of 43 $\frac{mg}{dL}$. Find the total amount of creatinine excreted. What is the 24-hour creatinine value?

9.2 – RENAL CLEARANCE

If the kidneys do not rid the blood of creatinine at a rate comparable to the rate at which creatinine is secreted into the urine, blood creatinine concentrations will be out of balance. In general, **renal clearance** values give us information about the rate at which the kidneys rid a material from the blood. The mathematical formula used to calculate the renal clearance for an adult of average size and weight is

$$\text{Clearance} = \frac{\text{Concentration of substance in urine} \times \text{Flow rate of the urine}}{\text{Concentration of substance in plasma}}$$

In shorthand notation we write this formula as

$$Cl = \frac{U \times V}{P}$$

where Cl is the clearance, U is the substance concentration in the urine, V is the rate at which the urine flows (usually in milliliters per minute), and P is the substance concentration in the plasma.

EXAMPLE 9-3: A laboratorian analyzed a sample of blood and found the creatinine concentration to be 12 $\frac{mg}{100\,mL}$. This specialist analyzed additional laboratory data and found that creatinine was secreted into the urine at the rate of 6 $\frac{mg}{min}$. Find the creatinine clearance.

Creatinine clearance is the rate at which creatinine is cleared from the blood and is usually given in units of mL/min. We are given that the blood concentration is $12\ ^{mg}/_{100\ mL}$. But we are also given that 6 mg are passed into the urine every minute. Thus, to find the quantity passed into the urine in terms of milliliters, we simply use proportions.

$$\frac{12\ mg}{100\ mL} = \frac{6\ mg}{x\ mL}$$

Cross multiplying and solving, we find

$$x = 50\ mL.$$

Therefore, 50 mL of blood are cleared of 6 mg of creatinine each minute. In other words, the creatinine clearance is $50\ ^{mL}/_{min}$.

EXAMPLE 9-4: A health care professional collected a total volume of 1,600 mL of urine in 24 hours from a patient. A laboratorian then ran tests to determine the patient's urine and plasma creatinine concentrations. They were found to be $175\ ^{mg}/_{dL}$ and $1.7\ ^{mg}/_{dL}$, respectively. Find the creatinine clearance.

First, convert 1,600 mL per 24 hours to milliliters per minute. To do this all we have to do is divide 1,600 by 1,440. This is because of the conversion involved.

$$\frac{1{,}600\ mL}{24\ hr}\left(\frac{1\ hr}{60\ min}\right) = \frac{1{,}600\ mL}{1{,}440\ min} = 1.1\overline{1}\ ^{mL}/_{min} \approx 1.11\ ^{mL}/_{min}$$

Therefore, the flow rate of urine, V, is $1.11\ ^{mL}/_{min}$.

The concentration of creatinine in the plasma, P, is $1.7\ ^{mg}/_{dL}$, and the concentration of creatinine in the urine, U, is $175\ ^{mg}/_{dL}$. Plugging these into the clearance formula, we find

$$Cl = \frac{175\ ^{mg}/_{dL} \times 1.11\ ^{mL}/_{min}}{1.7\ ^{mg}/_{dL}} = 114.3\ ^{mL}/_{min}.$$

Notice the $^{mg}/_{dL}$ in the numerator cancels with the $^{mg}/_{dL}$ in the denominator and we are left with units of $^{mL}/_{min}$. When using this formula, be careful that the units associated with U are the same as the units associated with P (so they cancel).

EXAMPLE 9-5: A health care professional collected a total volume of 0.45 L of urine in 8 hours from a patient. A laboratorian then ran tests to determine the patient's urine and plasma creatinine concentrations. They were found to be $180\ ^{mg}/_{dL}$ and $1.3\ ^{mg}/_{dL}$, respectively. Find the creatinine clearance.

First, convert 0.45 L to mL: $0.45\ L\left(\dfrac{10^3\ mL}{1\ L}\right) = 450\ mL.$

Next, convert 450 mL per 8 hours to milliliters per minute.

$$\left(\frac{450\ mL}{8\ hr}\right)\left(\frac{1\ hr}{60\ min}\right) = 0.94\ ^{mL}/_{min}$$

The units for the urine concentration and the plasma concentration are the same, so there is no work to be done here. Next, plug everything into the clearance formula, yielding

$$Cl = \frac{180 \; ^{mg}\!/_{dL} \times 0.94 \; ^{mL}\!/_{min}}{1.3 \; ^{mg}\!/_{dL}} = 130.2 \; ^{mL}\!/_{min} \, .$$

As mentioned at the beginning of this section, the clearance formula we have just been using is for adults of average size, where, statistically speaking, average size is 1.73 m^2 (this is the total amount of surface area of the skin). If the patient is not of average size, we must multiply the clearance formula by a *size factor*. The size factor is

$$\frac{1.73 \text{ m}^2}{\text{Size of adult}} \, ,$$

and the corrected clearance formula would then become

$$Cl_c = \frac{U \times V}{P} \times \frac{1.73 \text{ m}^2}{\text{Size of person (in square meters)}} \, .$$

EXAMPLE 9-6: A health care professional was given the following data for a patient. Find the creatinine clearance for this patient.

• Body size: 2.45 m^2

• 24-hour urine volume: 2,000 mL

• Creatinine urine concentration: $130 \; ^{mg}\!/_{dL}$

• Creatinine plasma concentration: $4.9 \; ^{mg}\!/_{dL}$

First, convert 2,000 mL per 24 hours to milliliters per minute by dividing by 1,440.

$$\frac{2,000}{1,440} = 1.39 \; ^{mL}\!/_{min}$$

Next, substitute everything into the corrected clearance formula, yielding

$$Cl_c = \frac{130 \; ^{mg}\!/_{dL} \times 1.39 \; ^{mL}\!/_{min}}{4.9 \; ^{mg}\!/_{dL}} \times \frac{1.73 \text{ m}^2}{2.45 \text{ m}^2} = 26.0 \; ^{mL}\!/_{min} \, .$$

Topics Related to Urine Concentration

Glomerular Filtration

The **glomerular filtration rate (GFR)** measures how well the kidneys remove and filter substances. The GFR for males is typically between 100 and 130 milliliters per minute per 1.73 square meters of body surface area. For women the GFR is typically between

90 and 125 milliliters per minute per 1.73 square meters of body surface area. To calculate the GFR, the bloodstream is typically injected with a fluid that is then measured in a 24-hour urine collection. Inulin is a substance commonly used to measure GFR.

The National Kidney Foundation says that an accurate estimate of the GFR is defined as

$$\text{GFR} = \frac{\text{Urine inulin concentration} \times \text{Urine flow rate}}{\text{Plasma inulin concentration}} = \frac{U_{\text{in}} \times V}{P_{\text{in}}}.$$

GFR can be estimated using blood creatinine levels and a formula combining this with age, race, and gender. The National Kidney Foundation also says that GFR estimates are the best indicators of the level of kidney function and that when clinical laboratories report serum creatinine levels, they should also report GFR estimates ("K/DOQI Clinical Practice," 2002).

Specific Gravity

Recall that specific gravity is the ratio of the density of a liquid to the density of pure water. Urine specific gravity can be used to measure solute concentration in urine and can help in the determination of how well the renal tubules are diluting or concentrating glomerular filtrates. Though "normal" ranges vary from lab to lab, typical urine specific gravity measurements will be between 1.005 and 1.030. If a urine specimen has a relatively high specific gravity, then its solute concentration is relatively high (such as a high protein concentration). Likewise, if the urine specific gravity is relatively low, then its solute concentration is also relatively low (such as a low glucose concentration). Therefore, if the urine specific gravity is relatively low or high, further tests may need to be performed to correctly diagnose what the exact problem is.

PRACTICE PROBLEMS: Section 9.2

1. A health care professional collected a total volume of 1,400 mL of urine in 24 hours from a patient. A specialist then ran tests to determine the patient's urine and plasma creatinine concentrations. They were found to be 185 $\frac{mg}{dL}$ and 1.5 $\frac{mg}{dL}$, respectively. Find the creatinine clearance.

2. A health care professional collected a total volume of 1,550 mL of urine in 24 hours from a patient. A specialist then ran tests to determine the patient's urine and plasma creatinine concentrations. They were found to be 170 $\frac{mg}{dL}$ and 1.2 $\frac{mg}{dL}$, respectively. Find the creatinine clearance.

3. A health care professional collected a total volume of 1,500 mL of urine in 24 hours from a patient. A laboratorian then ran tests to determine the patient's urine and plasma creatinine concentrations. They were found to be 175 $\frac{mg}{dL}$ and 1.6 $\frac{mg}{dL}$, respectively. Find the creatinine clearance.

Continues

PRACTICE PROBLEMS: Section 9.2 *(continued)*

4. In a 12-hour period a total volume of 750 mL of urine was collected. The creatinine concentration in the urine was 170 $\frac{mg}{dL}$ and the concentration of creatinine in the plasma was found to be 1.7 $\frac{mg}{dL}$. Find the creatinine clearance.

5. In an 8-hour period a total volume of 0.6 L of urine was collected. The creatinine concentration in the urine was 190 $\frac{mg}{dL}$ and the concentration of creatinine in the plasma was found to be 1.6 $\frac{mg}{dL}$. Find the creatinine clearance.

6. A health care professional collected a total volume of 0.45 L of urine in 6 hours from a patient. A laboratorian then ran tests to determine the patient's urine and plasma creatinine concentrations. They were found to be 160 $\frac{mg}{dL}$ and 1.1 $\frac{mg}{dL}$, respectively. Find the creatinine clearance.

7. A health care professional collected a total volume of 800 mL of urine in 12 hours from a patient. A laboratorian then ran tests to determine the patient's urine and plasma creatinine concentrations. They were found to be 165 $\frac{mg}{dL}$ and 1.4 $\frac{mg}{dL}$, respectively. Find the creatinine clearance.

8. A health care professional was given the following information. Find the creatinine clearance.
   - Urine volume: 0.75 L in an 8-hour period
   - Creatinine concentration in the urine: 175 $\frac{mg}{dL}$
   - Concentration of creatinine in the plasma: 1.6 $\frac{mg}{dL}$

9. A health care professional was given the following data for a patient. Find the creatinine clearance for this patient.
   - Body size: 2.35 m^2
   - 24-hour urine volume: 1,900 mL
   - Creatinine urine concentration: 135 $\frac{mg}{dL}$
   - Creatinine plasma concentration: 6.7 $\frac{mg}{dL}$

10. A health care professional was given the following data for a patient. Find the creatinine clearance for this patient.
   - Body size: 1.41 m^2
   - 8-hour urine volume: 450 mL
   - Creatinine urine concentration: 140 $\frac{mg}{dL}$
   - Creatinine plasma concentration: 3.1 $\frac{mg}{dL}$

11. A health care professional was given the following data for a patient. Find the creatinine clearance for this patient.
   - Body size: 2.40 m^2
   - 12-hour urine volume: 950 mL
   - Creatinine urine concentration: 130 $\frac{mg}{dL}$
   - Creatinine plasma concentration: 4.2 $\frac{mg}{dL}$

12. A very small patient had a body size of 1.35 square meters. Her 8-hour urine sample had a volume of 500 mL. Her creatinine urine concentration was 145 $\frac{mg}{dL}$ and her creatinine plasma concentration was 3.3 $\frac{mg}{dL}$. Find this patient's creatinine clearance.

13. An obese patient had a body size of 2.60 square meters. His 12-hour urine sample had a volume of 1,000 mL. His creatinine urine and plasma concentrations were 120 $\frac{mg}{dL}$ and 3.9 $\frac{mg}{dL}$, respectively. Find this patient's creatinine clearance.

14. A very small patient had a body size of 1.32 square meters. Her 8-hour urine sample had a volume of 400 mL. Her creatinine urine concentration was 150 $\frac{mg}{dL}$ and her creatinine plasma concentration was 3.3 $\frac{mg}{dL}$. Find this patient's creatinine clearance.

CHAPTER SUMMARY

- The rate at which the kidney clears the plasma of creatinine is often used to measure renal clearance.
- The renal clearance for an adult of average size and weight is calculated by using the following formula where Cl is the clearance, U is the substance concentration in the urine, V is the rate at which the urine flows (usually in milliliters per minute), and P is the substance concentration in the plasma.

$$Cl = \frac{U \times V}{P}$$

- The corrected clearance formula to be used for patients who are not of average size is

$$Cl_c = \frac{U \times V}{P} \times \frac{1.73 \, m^2}{\text{Size of person (in square meters)}}$$

CHAPTER TEST

1. A 12-hour urine sample contained 700 mL and had a protein concentration of 35 $\frac{mg}{dL}$. Find the total amount of protein this patient excreted. How many milligrams of protein did this patient excrete in one day?

2. A health care professional collected a total volume of 850 mL of urine in 12 hours from a patient. A laboratorian then ran tests to determine the patient's urine and plasma creatinine concentrations. They were found to be 160 $\frac{mg}{dL}$ and 1.8 $\frac{mg}{dL}$, respectively. Find the creatinine clearance.

3. An 8-hour urine sample contained 575 mL and had a creatinine concentration of 48 $\frac{mg}{dL}$. Find the total amount of creatinine this patient excreted. How many milligrams of protein did this patient excrete in one day?

4. A health care professional was given the following data for a patient. Find the creatinine clearance for this patient.
   - Body size: 2.20 m^2
   - 24-hour urine volume: 1,700 mL
   - Creatinine urine concentration: 120 mg/dL
   - Creatinine plasma concentration: 4.7 mg/dL

5. A health care professional was given the following data for a patient. Find the creatinine clearance for this patient.
   - Body size: 1.44 m^2
   - 12-hour urine volume: 625 mL
   - Creatinine urine concentration: 136 mg/dL
   - Creatinine plasma concentration: 3.6 mg/dL

6. In a 12-hour period a total volume of 750 mL of urine was collected. It was found to have 70 mg/dL of creatinine. Find the total amount of creatinine in this entire sample. How many grams of creatinine did this patient excrete in one day?

10 Charting Data

INTRODUCTION

In the laboratory and health sciences, we often need to gather data. For example, we might want to determine the average cholesterol level for a group of patients. To do this we would find and record the cholesterol level for each patient. This collected data is referred to as **raw data**. Raw data is usually not very useful because it is not organized. Therefore, once we have all the raw data, our next step is to organize it so we can draw conclusions or make conjectures. One common means of organizing data is to create a frequency distribution. From a **frequency distribution**, we can see how often or how *frequent* certain data appears by subdividing the raw data into classes, where each **class** includes the data values that fall within an established range. We can then create graphs and charts from the frequency distribution to better understand the data.

10.1 – ORGANIZING DATA

The Frequency Distribution Table

A **frequency distribution table** organizes data to show how often certain data values appear within a particular range. Let's look at an example.

EXAMPLE 10-1: Twenty patients had their cholesterol levels tested and their results follow, each in units of milligrams per deciliter.

$$142 \quad 156 \quad 240 \quad 143 \quad 179 \quad 233 \quad 220 \quad 195 \quad 168 \quad 200$$

$$248 \quad 258 \quad 205 \quad 177 \quad 150 \quad 181 \quad 215 \quad 198 \quad 166 \quad 192$$

After the information is gathered (i.e., the cholesterol levels of the 20 patients), it needs to be organized so the results make sense. One way to do this is to create a frequency distribution table.

Steps in Creating a Frequency Distribution Table

1) *Determine the class width.*

$$\text{Class width} = \frac{\text{Largest data value} - \text{Smallest data value}}{\text{Desired number of classes}}$$

If the result is a decimal, round up to the nearest whole number.

2) *Create distinct classes.* The number of classes chosen is usually 5 to 20; however, fewer than 5 or more than 20 is acceptable.

The **lower class limit** of the first class will be the smallest data value (or sometimes a value slightly less; however, in this case caution must be used). Add the class width *less 1* to this number to get the upper class limit of this class. The **upper class limit** of each class is the highest value that can be included in that class. Continue until the last class includes the largest data value contained in the raw data.

3) *Count the number of data values that lie in each class.*

We now organize the raw data into a frequency distribution table by following the process just laid out.

For this example, let's say we want six classes. Then the class width will be

$$\text{Class width} = \frac{258 - 142}{6} = \frac{116}{6} = 20 \text{ (rounded up to the nearest whole number)}.$$

We will pick the lower limit of the first class to be 140 (140 is a nice convenient number that is slightly less than the lowest data value, which is 142). Therefore, the upper class limit for the first class will be $140 + (20 - 1) = 140 + 19 = 159$. The second class will range from 160 to 179 since $160 + 19 = 179$. The third class will range from 180 to 199 and so forth until the last class includes the largest data value, which is 258. Thus, our table will look as follows:

CLASS	FREQUENCY
140–159	
160–179	
180–199	
200–219	
220–239	
240–259	

To get the frequencies, simply count the number of data values that fall within each class limit. There are four data values that fall between 140 and 159, four between 160 and 179, four between 180 and 199, three between 200 and 219, two between 220 and 239, and three between 240 and 259. Placing these tallies into the table, our completed frequency distribution table will look like the following:

CLASS	FREQUENCY
140–159	4
160–179	4
180–199	4
200–219	3
220–239	2
240–259	3
Total	20

Now that the data is organized, we can make observations such as the majority (12 out of 20, or 60%) of these patients have a cholesterol level between 140 and 199.

NOTE

The frequencies should always be totaled to ensure all the data values were included and none were inadvertently left out.

EXAMPLE 10-2: The protein concentrations in milligrams per day of 30 24-hour urine samples were gathered and the raw data for this study follows. Construct a frequency distribution table containing five classes.

70 62 69 74 80 75 91 72 63 87 55 67 85 71 58

71 89 51 64 75 68 92 83 72 65 81 97 65 74 70

Class width $= \dfrac{97-51}{5} = 9.2$, which rounds up to 10.

We will pick 50 to be the lower limit for the first class. Therefore, the first class will range from 50 to 59 since $50 + (10 - 1) = 50 + 9 = 59$. The second class will be 60 to 69 and so forth. Thus, our table will look as follows:

CLASS	FREQUENCY
50–59	
60–69	
70–79	
80–89	
90–99	

After the frequencies for each class have been counted and placed into the table, our completed frequency distribution table will look like the following:

CLASS	FREQUENCY
50–59	3
60–69	8
70–79	10
80–89	6
90–99	3
Total	30

PRACTICE PROBLEMS: Section 10.1

1. Construct a frequency distribution table using six classes for the following data set:

6	13	48	10	3	16	20	17	40	4
8	7	25	8	21	19	15	3	17	14
10	12	45	1	8	4	16	11	18	23
11	6	2	14	13	7	15	46	12	9
12	34	13	41	28	36	17	24	27	29
18	14	26	10	24	37	31	8	16	12

2. Following are systolic blood pressure measurements of 20 women. Construct a frequency distribution table using five classes.

112	91	134	122	124	138	128	113	111	99
115	131	108	102	125	136	117	110	119	130

3. Thirty people were asked how many cups of coffee they consume per day. The results follow. Construct a frequency distribution table using four classes.

0	1	3	1	2	4	5	2	3	1	6	2	3	7	0
4	5	2	1	1	0	2	7	4	5	1	0	6	0	1

4. Forty patients were asked how many minutes they had to wait in an emergency room before they were seen by a doctor. The results follow. Construct a frequency distribution table using five classes.

32	40	66	51	28	35	30	45	49	33
37	41	56	43	59	60	32	48	56	55
50	29	44	54	64	65	49	34	39	30
36	34	47	52	43	47	58	31	61	29

5. Forty-five people were solicited to see how long they could hold their breath. The results are as follows, in seconds. Construct a frequency distribution table using classes 0 to 19, 20 to 39, 40 to 59, and so forth.

12	98	71	20	55	14	62	88	19	39	50	90	81	17	26
75	10	67	53	11	99	19	30	56	61	76	15	45	65	32
22	16	40	37	97	29	49	18	80	54	44	31	72	9	48

6. Twenty-four patients had their cholesterol level checked. Following are the results. Construct a frequency distribution table using five classes.

| 130 | 210 | 153 | 197 | 276 | 184 | 148 | 292 | 281 | 131 | 152 | 178 |
| 200 | 245 | 262 | 159 | 201 | 157 | 188 | 217 | 180 | 233 | 270 | 160 |

7. Thirty people were observed as to how many ounces of meat they ate at an all-you-can-eat buffet. Construct a frequency distribution table using four classes.

| 3 | 18 | 14 | 9 | 18 | 6 | 1 | 7 | 9 | 16 | 2 | 10 | 3 | 12 | 16 |
| 8 | 4 | 16 | 11 | 6 | 15 | 5 | 2 | 8 | 0 | 9 | 17 | 18 | 13 | 7 |

10.2 – GRAPHING DATA

Once a frequency distribution table is developed, we often want to create a graphical representation of these results. There are several types of graphs (or charts) that can be constructed from tables. They include histograms, frequency polygons, bar graphs, and pie graphs. Let's begin with the histogram.

Histograms

A **histogram** is a graph that presents data by using vertical bars with the height of each bar equivalent to the frequency of the class. Before you can create a histogram, you must first know what class boundaries are. To find the **class boundaries**, first add 0.5 to the upper class limit and subtract 0.5 from the lower class limit.

Class boundaries = (Lower class limit − 0.5) to (Upper class limit + 0.5)

For example, for the class 40 to 59, the class boundaries would be

$$(40 - 0.5) \text{ to } (59 + 0.5)$$

or

$$39.5 \text{ to } 59.5.$$

EXAMPLE 10-3: Construct a histogram that corresponds with the frequency distribution table in Example 10-2.

To begin, first determine the boundaries for each class.

CLASS	CLASS BOUNDARIES
50–59	49.5–59.5
60–69	59.5–69.5
70–79	69.5–79.5
80–89	79.5–89.5
90–99	89.5–99.5

Next, draw the first quadrant of the coordinate plane with the class boundaries on the x-axis and frequency on the y-axis.

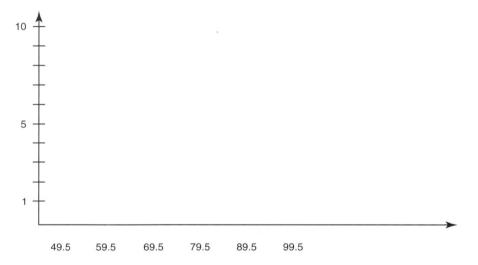

Last, draw vertical bars for each class, with the height of each bar corresponding to its class frequency.

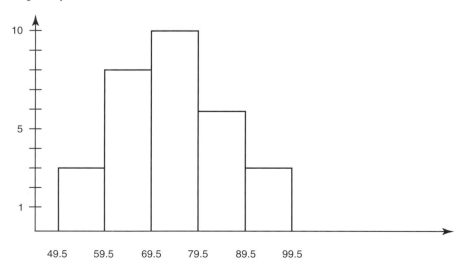

Frequency Polygons

To create a frequency polygon, connect the frequencies at the midpoints of each class. For example, to create a frequency polygon for the frequency distribution table in Example 10-2, begin by placing points at the middle of the top of each vertical bar of the histogram created in Example 10-3.

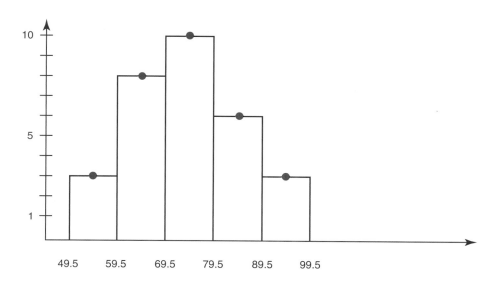

Next, drop the vertical bars but leave the points.

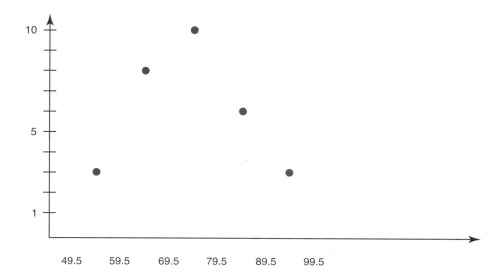

Last, connect each point with a straight line.

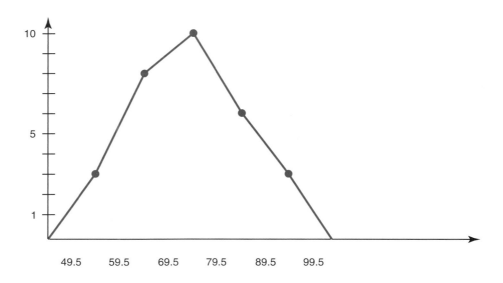

Bar Graphs

Bar graphs (or bar charts) tend to be used when there are specified amounts of specific items.

EXAMPLE 10-4: Following is a bar graph of the average daily calorie intake for four individuals. Determine the average daily intake of calories for Tim.

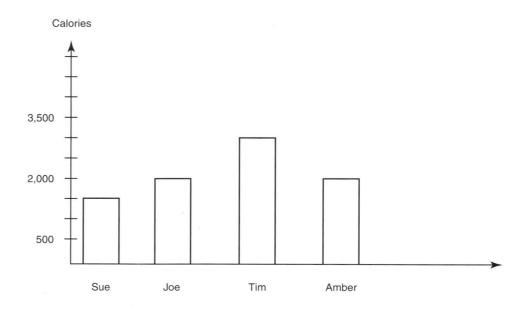

The height of the bar above Tim is 3,000, so Tim's average daily calorie intake is 3,000 calories.

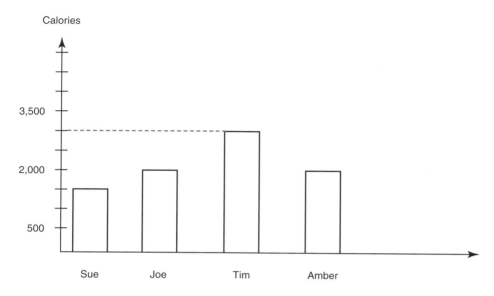

Creating a bar graph is simple using Microsoft Excel.

Using Technology

Creating a Vertical Bar Chart Using Microsoft Excel

1. Enter the word "Sue" in column A, row 1.
2. Enter the word "Joe" in column A, row 2.
3. Enter the word "Tim" in column A, row 3.
4. Enter the word "Amber" in column A, row 4.
5. Enter 1,500 in column B, row 1.
6. Enter 2,000 in column B, row 2.
7. Enter 3,000 in column B, row 3.
8. Enter 2,000 in column B, row 4.
9. Single click on the Chart Wizard icon.
10. Under Chart Type click Column for vertical bars (or bar for horizontal bars).
11. Under Chart sub-type click the first option, which will already be selected by default.
12. Click the Next > button.

Continues

Using Technology *(continued)*

13. On the next pop-up window, click the Next > button.
14. Click the Titles tab.
15. Enter "Calorie Intake" under Chart title.
16. Enter "Person" under Category (X) axis.
17. Enter "Calories" under Value (Y) axis.
18. Click the Next > button.
19. Select: As object in.
20. Click the Finish button.
21. Now select Edit copy and paste into your document.

Following is the bar chart created using Excel.

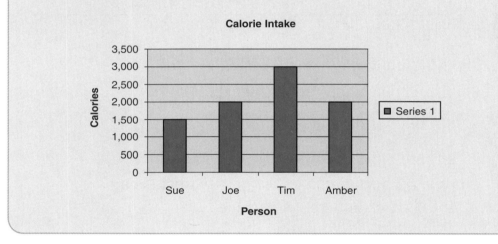

Pie Graphs

Pie graphs (or pie charts) can be used to show the same information as a bar graph. However, pie graphs can be more effective in showing the relationships among different groups.

EXAMPLE 10-5: Construct a pie graph for the information given in the following table.

BLOOD TYPE	FREQUENCY
A	80
B	22
AB	8
O	90
Total	200

To find the number of degrees for each sector, use the formula

$$\text{Degrees} = \frac{\text{Frequency}}{\text{Total}} \times 360°.$$

For type A we have

$$\text{Degrees} = \frac{80}{200} \times 360° = 144°,$$

$$\text{Percentage} = \frac{80}{200} \times 100\% = 40\%.$$

For type B we have

$$\text{Degrees} = \frac{22}{200} \times 360° = 40° \text{ (rounded)},$$

$$\text{Percentage} = \frac{22}{200} \times 100\% = 11\%.$$

For type AB we have

$$\text{Degrees} = \frac{8}{200} \times 360° = 14° \text{ (rounded)},$$

$$\text{Percentage} = \frac{8}{200} \times 100\% = 4\%.$$

For type O we have

$$\text{Degrees} = \frac{90}{200} \times 360° = 162°,$$

$$\text{Percentage} = \frac{90}{200} \times 100\% = 45\%.$$

Now we construct a pie with four sectors, one for type A, one for type B, one for AB, and one for O. The angle within each sector will be the angle we just calculated. A protractor can be used to accurately construct the pie graph.

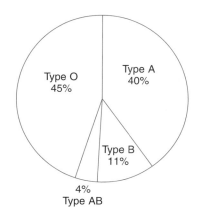

Constructing a pie chart is simple using Microsoft Excel. It is done in almost the same way as creating a bar chart using Excel.

Using Technology

Creating a Pie Chart Using Microsoft Excel

1. Enter the letter "A" in column A, row 1.
2. Enter the letter "B" in column A, row 2.
3. Enter the letters "AB" in column A, row 3.
4. Enter the letter "O" in column A, row 4.
5. Enter 80 in column B, row 1.
6. Enter 22 in column B, row 2.
7. Enter 8 in column B, row 3.
8. Enter 90 in column B, row 4.
9. Single click on the Chart Wizard icon.
10. Under Chart Type click Pie.
11. Under Chart sub-type, click the first option, which will already be selected by default.
12. Click the Next > button.
13. On the next pop-up window, click the Next > button.
14. Click the Titles tab.
15. Enter "Blood Types" under Chart title.
16. Click the Data Labels tab.
17. Select Percentage.
18. Click the Next > button.
19. Select: As object in.
20. Click the Finish button.
21. Now select Edit copy and paste into your document.

Following is the pie chart created using Excel.

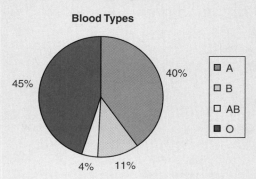

Blood Types

PRACTICE PROBLEMS: Section 10.2

1. One hundred seven hospital employees were sampled and their ages were obtained. Following is a table of the results. Construct a histogram for this table.

CLASS	FREQUENCY
10–19	4
20–29	15
30–39	25
40–49	32
50–59	22
60–69	9
Total	107

2. One hundred students took an exam. Their test results are as follows. Construct a histogram and frequency polygon for this table.

AGE	FREQUENCY
50–59	6
60–69	18
70–79	38
80–89	30
90–99	8
Total	100

3. Construct a bar graph for the following information on transplants.

ORGAN	NUMBER
Liver	3,200
Heart	2,100
Kidney	8,600
Lung	400

4. In an emergency room of a small hospital, the number of life-threatening cases was documented for several months. Following are the results. Construct a bar graph and pie graph.

MONTH	NUMBER
April	12
May	16
June	23
July	20
August	18
September	15

5. Following is the monthly budget of a family whose monthly income is $5,000. Construct a pie chart.

EXPENSE	MONEY SPENT
Rent	$1,000
Utilities	$ 500
Food	$ 600
Insurance and taxes	$1,800
Miscellaneous	$1,100

6. Construct a bar chart and pie chart for the following information on the health status of 5,000 individuals.

STATUS	FREQUENCY
Excellent	2,100
Very good	1,200
Good	800
Fair	600
Poor	300

7. Fifteen people were surveyed and asked how many cups of coffee they drink per day on average. Following are the results. Construct a bar chart for this information.

0   2   1   2   1   2   3   2   3   0   1   0   2   3   3

Continues

PRACTICE PROBLEMS: Section 10.2 *(continued)*

8. Twenty people were asked how many hours on average they watch TV per day. Following are the results. Create a pie chart.

1	2	4	3	5	1	0	2	3	2
4	1	5	2	2	1	2	3	1	2

9. Construct a pie graph for the data in problem 7.
10. Construct a bar graph for the data in problem 8.

CHAPTER SUMMARY

- Frequency distributions are useful in organizing raw data.
- To create a frequency distribution table, first determine the class width using the formula

$$\text{Class width} = \frac{\text{Largest data value} - \text{Smallest data value}}{\text{Desired number of classes}}$$

  Next, create distinct classes and count the number of data values that lie in each class.
- There are several types of graphs that can be used in conjunction with frequency distribution tables. These include histograms, frequency polygons, bar charts, and pie charts.

CHAPTER TEST

1. Name the type of graphs discussed in this chapter.

2. Create a frequency distribution table with five classes for the following raw data. Then construct a histogram and frequency polygon.

25	6	44	61	56	100	84	93	19	32	77	21	72	89	8
9	35	70	36	91	83	59	62	46	24	17	90	29	17	49
88	97	75	82	66	59	21	36	11	8	87	18	51	50	52

3. Create a bar chart and pie chart for the following information.

Category	Frequency
A	28
B	35
C	10
D	27

Basic Statistics and Quality Control

INTRODUCTION

Statistics has two main branches: inferential statistics and descriptive statistics. **Descriptive statistics** involves the collection of data followed by summarizing and describing the characteristics of that data. **Inferential statistics** involves the process of gathering a portion of the data, called a **sample**, from an entire **population** and using the information from the sample to make a general conjecture about some characteristic of the entire population. For example, say we wanted to know how many hours of television the average teenager in the United States watches per week. The only way to get the exact answer is to ask every single teenager in the United States (this would be the population). Obviously, this is not practical and may be almost impossible. So instead we ask a "small" collection of teenagers (this would be our sample) how many hours they watch, and from these results we might draw conclusions about teenagers in general. This is essentially inferential statistics.

For the sample to validate results in the lab, it must represent the population. We call this a representative sample. For example, if we asked 100 teenagers studying in a library how much TV they watch, this sample would not be a representative sample because it would most likely not represent the entire teenage population. When working in the laboratory, we must be careful that our sample is representative of our population. As we will learn in this chapter, the analysis of data will show whether our sample is representative.

When practicing quality control in the laboratory, we often generate descriptive statistics. For example, a typical validation procedure in the laboratory is to analyze a control specimen such as determining the glucose value of a control sample. In this case we usually use an instrument to measure the glucose values. We then summarize and describe the characteristics of the outcomes provided by the instrument and report those results. This chapter gives guidelines for determining whether the results from a procedure are accurate, dependable, and reliable.

11.1 – MEASURES OF CENTRAL TENDENCY

The most common measure of central tendency is the average, also called the mean. The next most common measure of central tendency is the median. Occasionally the mode is also used.

The Mean

The **mean** is found by adding up all the data values and dividing that result by the total number of data values. In statistics x represents data values, and two symbols are used to notate the mean. Those two symbols are μ and $\bar{x}$; μ is the symbol used to notate the mean of the entire population and $\bar{x}$ is used to notate the mean of the sample. To express the mean as a mathematical formula, we must first discuss a few more symbols and what they represent. First, in statistics N usually refers to the number of data values in the *entire population* while n refers to the number of data values in the *sample* of an entire population. The Greek letter $\sum$ means "the sum of." Therefore, $\sum x$ means to sum up, or add up, all of the data values. Now that we are familiar with the notation used, we can present the mathematical formulas for the mean of a population,

$$\mu = \frac{\sum x}{N},$$

and the mean of a sample,

$$\bar{x} = \frac{\sum x}{n}.$$

EXAMPLE 11-1: Find the mean of the following sample.

$$12 \quad 20 \quad 11 \quad 16 \quad 16 \quad 13 \quad 18$$

$$\bar{x} = \frac{\sum x}{n} = \frac{12+20+11+16+16+13+18}{7} = \frac{106}{7} = 15.14 \text{ (rounded to two decimal places)}$$

Using Your Calculator

To find the mean using your calculator, first enter the data values. To enter data values, you must first access STAT 1. STAT 1 is the one-variable stats mode. This is typically done by pressing the 3rd key and then the $\boxed{x><y}$ key. Above the $\boxed{x><y}$ key, you should see STAT 1. Once in one-variable stats mode, enter the data values as follows.

12 $\boxed{\Sigma+}$ 20 $\boxed{\Sigma+}$ 11 $\boxed{\Sigma+}$ 16 $\boxed{\Sigma+}$ 16 $\boxed{\Sigma+}$ 13 $\boxed{\Sigma+}$ 18 $\boxed{\Sigma+}$

To calculate the mean, press the 2nd key and the $\boxed{x^2}$ key. Your calculator should now display 15.14.

NOTE

For computations of the mean in the laboratory, it is desirable to have at least two more significant figures than what is expected in the patient's test result. To be safe, it is always best to carry more significant figures than needed.

The Median

The **median** is another common measure of central tendency. It is the middle value of the entire data set. To find this middle value, first write all the data values in ascending order (from smallest to largest) and then find the middle value by counting inward from both sides. If the data set has an odd amount of data values, there will be only one middle number and this number will be the median. If the data set has an even amount of data values, there will be two middle numbers and the median will be the mean of these two middle numbers.

EXAMPLE 11-2: Find the median of the following data set.

$$12 \quad 20 \quad 11 \quad 16 \quad 16 \quad 13 \quad 18$$

First, rearrange this set in ascending order.

$$11 \quad 12 \quad 13 \quad 16 \quad 16 \quad 18 \quad 20$$
$$\uparrow$$
$$\text{middle}$$

Thus, the median is 16.

NOTE

The data sets in Examples 11-1 and 11-2 are the same. The mean and the median are fairly close to each other. This is because they are both giving us an idea of what the central value for the entire data set is.

EXAMPLE 11-3: Find the median of the following data set.

$$6 \quad 12 \quad 15 \quad 8 \quad 10 \quad 14$$

First, arrange in ascending order. Keep in mind there are six data values, and because this is an even number, the median will be the mean of the two middle numbers.

$$6 \quad 8 \quad \underline{10} \quad \underline{12} \quad 14 \quad 15$$

The two middle numbers are 10 and 12; therefore,

$$\text{Median} = \frac{10+12}{2} = 11.$$

NOTE

When a small data set has an extreme value, the mean is greatly affected, but the median is not. For example, let's modify the data set used in Examples 11-1 and 11-2 by changing just one number, namely 12 to 60. Clearly, 60 is an extreme value relative to the other values in the set. Now let's recalculate the mean and median. Changing 12 to 60 the set would become

$$60 \quad 20 \quad 11 \quad 16 \quad 16 \quad 13 \quad 18$$

The mean is $\bar{x} = \frac{60+20+11+16+16+13+18}{7} = 22$. But the original set had a mean of 15.14, and there is a big difference between 15.14 and 22. However, if we recalculate the median we have

$$11 \quad 13 \quad 16 \quad \underset{\underset{\text{Median}}{\uparrow}}{16} \quad 18 \quad 20 \quad 60$$

and the median is still 16. The lesson here is that when the data set is relatively small, the mean is greatly affected by extreme values, but the median is not.

The Mode

The last measure of central tendency discussed here is the mode. The **mode** is the number in the data set that appears most frequently. In the data set given in Examples 11-1 and 11-2, the mode is 16 because 16 appears twice and all the other numbers appear only once. If all the numbers in a data set appear only once, there is no mode. However, sometimes two numbers appear the same amount of times and more than any of the other numbers. In this case the data set is **bimodal**. Following is an example of a data set that is bimodal.

$$65 \quad 90 \quad 70 \quad 80 \quad 65 \quad 78 \quad 95 \quad 90$$

In this set the numbers 65 and 90 both appear twice and the other numbers appear only once. Therefore, this set has two modes, 65 and 90. It should be mentioned that sets can also have more than two modes.

Note: Practice problems for Sections 11.1 through 11.3 are grouped together in the practice problems in Section 11.3.

11.2 – STANDARD DEVIATION

Before discussing standard deviation, let's analyze two different data sets by calculating their mean, median, and mode.

DATA SET 1

0 4 4 8

$$\bar{x} = \frac{\Sigma x}{n} = \frac{0+4+4+8}{4} = \frac{16}{4} = 4$$

DATA SET 2

2 4 4 6

$$\bar{x} = \frac{\Sigma x}{n} = \frac{2+4+4+6}{4} = \frac{16}{4} = 4$$

The data sets are already in ascending order and the number of data values is even, so the median in each set will be the mean of the two middle values.

$$\text{Median} = \frac{4+4}{2} = 4 \qquad\qquad \text{Median} = \frac{4+4}{2} = 4$$

$$\text{Mode} = 4 \qquad\qquad\qquad \text{Mode} = 4$$

The mean, median, and mode for both sets are the same, namely 4. Yet the two sets are clearly different. Set 1 is more spread out, or dispersed, than set 2 because the values range from 0 to 8 whereas in set 2 the values range from 2 to 6. The **standard deviation** of a data set gives us information about how dispersed, or spread out, a given data set is (Section 11.3 discusses how standard deviation can be used to help determine precision). Thus, the standard deviation of data set 1 will be larger than the standard deviation of data set 2. The following example illustrates this. In statistics the letter s is used to denote standard deviation. There are two mathematical formulas that can be used to calculate the standard deviation. Both formulas are presented here; however, this book uses standard deviation formula 1.

Standard Deviation Formula 1	Standard Deviation Formula 2
$$s = \sqrt{\frac{\sum(x-\bar{x})^2}{n-1}}$$	$$s = \sqrt{\frac{\sum x^2 - \frac{(\sum x)^2}{n}}{n-1}}$$

Before we do some examples, let's examine formula 1 more closely. Remember that x stands for the data values, $\bar{x}$ is the mean of all the data values in the set, and n is the total number of data values. To calculate s using formula 1, proceed one step at a time. Following is a step-by-step procedure for calculating the standard deviation, s.

Procedure for calculating the standard deviation:

1) Calculate $\bar{x}$.

2) Calculate $x - \bar{x}$ for each data value.

3) Square each result in step 2.

4) Add up all the results in step 3.

5) Divide the result in step 4 by $(n-1)$.

6) Take the square root of the result in step 5.

Note: The answer obtained in step 5 is called the **variance**.

EXAMPLE 11-4: Now let's calculate the standard deviation of the two data sets discussed at the beginning of this section. Recall that data set 1 consisted of the numbers 0, 4, 4, and 8, and data set 2 consisted of the numbers 2, 4, 4, and 6.

1) We know from our earlier calculations that $\bar{x}$ is 4 for both sets.

2) Calculate $x - \bar{x}$ for each data value.

Data Set 1	Data Set 2
$0 - 4 = -4$	$2 - 4 = -2$
$4 - 4 = 0$	$4 - 4 = 0$
$4 - 4 = 0$	$4 - 4 = 0$
$8 - 4 = 4$	$6 - 4 = 2$

3) Square each result in step 2.

$(-4)^2 = 16$	$(-2)^2 = 4$
$0^2 = 0$	$0^2 = 0$
$0^2 = 0$	$0^2 = 0$
$4^2 = 16$	$2^2 = 4$

4) Add the results in step 3.

$$16 + 0 + 0 + 16 = 32 \qquad 4 + 0 + 0 + 4 = 8$$

5) Divide the result in step 4 by $(n - 1)$.

The number of data values in each set is 4; therefore, $n - 1 = 3$.

$$\frac{32}{3} = 10.67 \qquad\qquad \frac{8}{3} = 2.67$$

6) Take the square root of the result in step 5. Round to two decimal places.

$$\sqrt{10.67} = 3.27 \qquad\qquad \sqrt{2.67} = 1.63$$

As expected, the standard deviation for set 1 is larger because it is more spread out.

> ### NOTE
>
> For computations of standard deviation in the laboratory, it is desirable to have at least one more significant figure than what is expected in the patient's test result. To be safe it is always best to carry more significant figures than needed. However, in many of the examples that follow, we round to two decimal places. This is only to keep some level of simplicity and consistency for illustration purposes.

EXAMPLE 11-5: A laboratory has received a large shipment of boxes containing glass test tubes. An employee randomly samples eight boxes and finds the following numbers of broken test tubes per box. Find the variance and standard deviation.

$$2 \quad 3 \quad 4 \quad 5 \quad 6 \quad 8 \quad 10 \quad 10$$

To solve, use standard deviation formula 1.

1) Calculate $\bar{x}$.

$$\bar{x} = \frac{\Sigma x}{n} = \frac{2+3+4+5+6+8+10+10}{8} = \frac{48}{8} = 6.00$$

Using Your Calculator

First, be sure the calculator is in the STAT 1 mode. Now enter the following data values.

$$2 \; \boxed{\Sigma +} \; 3 \; \boxed{\Sigma +} \; 4 \; \boxed{\Sigma +} \; 5 \; \boxed{\Sigma +} \; 6 \; \boxed{\Sigma +} \; 8 \; \boxed{\Sigma +} \; 10 \; \boxed{\Sigma +}$$

To calculate the mean, press the 2nd key and the $\boxed{x^2}$ key. Your calculator should now display 6.

2) Calculate $x - \bar{x}$ for each data value.

$2 - 6 = -4$

$3 - 6 = -3$

$4 - 6 = -2$

$5 - 6 = -1$

$6 - 6 = 0$

$8 - 6 = 2$

$10 - 6 = 4$

$10 - 6 = 4$

3) Square each result in step 2.

$(-4)^2 = 16$

$(-3)^2 = 9$

$(-2)^2 = 4$

$(-1)^2 = 1$

$0^2 = 0$

$2^2 = 4$

$4^2 = 16$

$4^2 = 16$

4) Add the results in step 3.

$$16 + 9 + 4 + 1 + 0 + 4 + 16 + 16 = 66$$

5) Divide the result in step 4 by $(n - 1)$.

$$n = 8, \text{which means } n - 1 = 7$$

$$\frac{66}{7} = 9.43$$

Therefore, the variance is 9.43.

6) Take the square root of the result in step 5.

$$s = \sqrt{9.43} = 3.07$$

Therefore, the standard deviation is 3.07.

Using Your Calculator

Because we already entered the data values to find the mean, the data values will still be in the memory of our calculator. To find the standard deviation, press the 2nd key and the $\sqrt{x}$ key and 3.07 should be displayed on your calculator. If we had not yet entered the data values, we would first have to do that as follows. First be sure you are in the STAT 1 mode. To calculate the standard deviation, begin by entering the data values.

2 $\boxed{\Sigma+}$ 3 $\boxed{\Sigma+}$ 4 $\boxed{\Sigma+}$ 5 $\boxed{\Sigma+}$ 6 $\boxed{\Sigma+}$ 8 $\boxed{\Sigma+}$ 10 $\boxed{\Sigma+}$ 10 $\boxed{\Sigma+}$

To find the standard deviation, press the 2nd key and the $\sqrt{x}$ key. Your calculator should now display 3.07.

EXAMPLE 11-6: Consider the following group of six glucose values all having the unit of milligrams per deciliter. Find the variance and standard deviation.

$$87 \quad 91 \quad 85 \quad 89 \quad 82 \quad 83$$

1) Calculate $\bar{x}$.

$$\bar{x} = \frac{\Sigma x}{n} = \frac{87+91+85+89+82+83}{6} = \frac{517}{6} = 86.17$$

2) Calculate $x - \bar{x}$ for each data value.

$87 - 86.17 = 0.83$

$91 - 86.17 = 4.83$

$85 - 86.17 = -1.17$

$89 - 86.17 = 2.83$

$82 - 86.17 = -4.17$

$83 - 86.17 = -3.17$

3) Square each result in step 2.

$(0.83)^2 = 0.69$

$(4.83)^2 = 23.33$

$(-1.17)^2 = 1.37$

$(2.83)^2 = 8.01$

$(-4.17)^2 = 17.39$

$(-3.17)^2 = 10.05$

4)   Add the results in step 3.

$$0.69 + 23.33 + 1.37 + 8.01 + 17.39 + 10.05 = 60.84$$

5)   Divide the result in step 4 by $(n-1)$.

$$n = 6, \text{ which implies } n - 1 = 5$$

$$\frac{60.84}{5} = 12.17$$

Therefore, the variance is 12.17.

6)   Take the square root of the result in step 5.

$$s = \sqrt{12.17} = 3.49$$

Therefore, the standard deviation is 3.49.

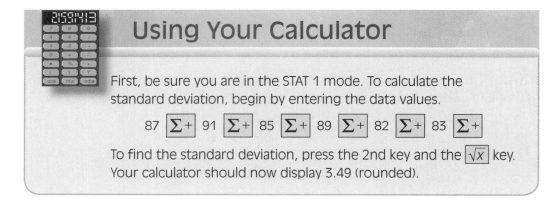

Using Your Calculator

First, be sure you are in the STAT 1 mode. To calculate the standard deviation, begin by entering the data values.

87 $\boxed{\Sigma +}$ 91 $\boxed{\Sigma +}$ 85 $\boxed{\Sigma +}$ 89 $\boxed{\Sigma +}$ 82 $\boxed{\Sigma +}$ 83 $\boxed{\Sigma +}$

To find the standard deviation, press the 2nd key and the $\boxed{\sqrt{x}}$ key. Your calculator should now display 3.49 (rounded).

Note: Practice problems for Sections 11.1 through 11.3 are grouped together in the practice problems in Section 11.3.

11.3 – COEFFICIENT OF VARIATION

The **coefficient of variation (CV)** is used to compare two or more data sets. The numerical value of the CV for each data set can then be used to determine which data set is more precise. The larger the CV, the more variation within the data set. Likewise, the lower the CV, the less dispersed the data set. Therefore, lower CVs imply more precision. For example, in the laboratory we use instruments to measure things such as glucose values in blood samples. However, when we use any type of instrument to measure something, there is inevitably going to be some error involved. When two or more groups of data are compared, the value of the coefficient of variation for each set can tell us which data set is more precise. If several different instruments were used to measure the same specimen, we could then calculate the CV for each set and determine which instrument is most precise. If the instrument used is precise, the measurements should all be fairly close together (i.e., a low s and therefore a low CV). If the instrument is not precise, the measurements will most likely be more spread apart (i.e., a high CV). The mathematical formula for the coefficient of variation is

$$CV = \frac{s}{\bar{x}}$$

The CV is simply the standard deviation divided by the mean of the data set. To express the CV as a percentage, multiply the result by 100%. That is,

$$\%CV = \frac{s}{\bar{x}} \times 100\%.$$

EXAMPLE 11-7: In example 11-6 we found

$$\bar{x} = 86.17 \qquad s = 3.49$$

The coefficient of variation in this case would be

$$CV = \frac{s}{\bar{x}} = \frac{3.49}{86.17} = 0.04.$$

As a percent the coefficient of variation would be

$$\%CV = 0.04 \times 100\% = 4.00\%.$$

EXAMPLE 11-8: A medical technologist in laboratory 1 calculated the cholesterol values of a group of specimens using the instrument provided in that lab. The CV for that instrument was 3.5%. In laboratory 2, using aliquots of the same group of specimens but a different instrument, a technologist found the CV to be 2.9%. Which instrument is more precise?

As previously discussed, the lower the CV, the more precise the data set. Clearly, 2.9% < 3.5%; therefore, instrument 2 is more precise than instrument 1.

NOTE

When using the CV, be careful about drawing conclusions. The CV should not be used to compare the precision of two variables if there are several varying conditions. Also, be sure the units of the two variables are the same. Most clinical laboratories want the CV to be less than 5%.

PRACTICE PROBLEMS: Section 11.3

1. Thirty patients had their glucose level tested and the results follow.

85	100	72	92	76	83	88	96	80	103	70	79	91	82	90
101	92	93	85	74	98	71	87	80	92	85	99	85	68	81

   a) Find the mean.
   b) Find the median.
   c) Find the mode.
   d) Find the variance.
   e) Find the standard deviation.
   f) Find the coefficient of variation.
   g) Find the ±1, ±2, and ±3 SD *range*.

2. Twenty patients had their cholesterol level tested and the results follow.

150	195	184	220	168	241	148	198	177	219
182	265	203	236	162	184	190	215	229	155

   a) Find the mean.
   b) Find the median.
   c) Find the mode.
   d) Find the variance.
   e) Find the standard deviation.
   f) Find the coefficient of variation.
   g) Find the ±1, ±2, and ±3 SD *range*.

3. Ten patients had their cholesterol level tested and the results follow.

130	240	195	166	182	144	320	210	171	150

   a) Find the mean.
   b) Find the median.
   c) Find the mode.
   d) Find the variance.
   e) Find the standard deviation.
   f) Find the coefficient of variation.
   g) Find the ±1, ±2, and ±3 SD *range*.
   h) How many of the actual data values fall within ±1 SD from the mean?

   i) How many of the actual data values fall within ±2 SD from the mean?

   j) How many of the actual data values fall within ±3 SD from the mean?

4. Twenty patients had their protein concentrations measured and the results follow (in grams per liter).

$$52 \quad 98 \quad 68 \quad 85 \quad 110 \quad 60 \quad 50 \quad 89 \quad 84 \quad 57$$
$$102 \quad 77 \quad 91 \quad 59 \quad 70 \quad 62 \quad 86 \quad 88 \quad 70 \quad 51$$

   a) Find the mean.

   b) Find the median.

   c) Find the mode.

   d) Find the variance.

   e) Find the standard deviation.

   f) Find the coefficient of variation.

   g) Find the ±1, ±2, and ±3 SD *range*.

   h) How many of the actual data values fall within ±1 SD from the mean?

   i) How many of the actual data values fall within ±2 SD from the mean?

   j) How many of the actual data values fall within ±3 SD from the mean?

5. Following are the results of measuring six items using two different methods. Answer parts a through g for each data set.

SET 1	SET 2
60 61 59 62 61 63	58 55 60 66 67 63

   a) Find the mean.

   b) Find the median.

   c) Find the mode.

   d) Find the variance.

   e) Find the standard deviation.

   f) Find the coefficient of variation.

   g) Which set is more precise? Explain your answer.

6. A sample is tested using two different methods. The resulting data is as follows:

METHOD A	METHOD B
77 68 65 77 66 74 73 67 77 71	85 54 58 62 100 42 77 93 67 77

   a) Find the mean.

   b) Find the median.

   c) Find the mode.

   d) Find the variance.

   e) Find the standard deviation.

Continues

PRACTICE PROBLEMS: Section 11.3 (continued)

  f) Find the coefficient of variation.

  g) Which method is more precise? Explain your answer.

7. A sample is tested using two different methods. The resulting data is as follows:

SET 1	SET 2
12 20 16 12 15 12 17 19	13 10 15 12 13 19 22 16

  a) Find the mean.

  b) Find the median.

  c) Find the mode.

  d) Find the variance.

  e) Find the standard deviation.

  f) Find the coefficient of variation.

  g) Which method is more precise? Explain your answer.

8. A sample is tested using two different methods. The resulting data is as follows:

METHOD A	METHOD B
2 9 4 11 9 3 12 1	5 10 7 8 9 6 8 8

  a) Find the mean.

  b) Find the median.

  c) Find the mode.

  d) Find the variance.

  e) Find the standard deviation.

  f) Find the coefficient of variation.

  g) Which method is more precise? Explain your answer.

9. A sample is tested using two different methods. The resulting data is as follows:

METHOD A	METHOD B
150 162 154 145 154	142 168 150 138 152

  a) Find the mean.

  b) Find the median.

  c) Find the mode.

  d) Find the variance.

  e) Find the standard deviation.

  f) Find the coefficient of variation.

  g) Which method is more precise? Explain your answer.

10. A sample is tested using two different methods. The resulting data is as follows:

METHOD A	METHOD B
250 235 230 225 220 240 233	268 251 245 232 222 245 240

   a) Find the mean.

   b) Find the median.

   c) Find the mode.

   d) Find the variance.

   e) Find the standard deviation.

   f) Find the coefficient of variation.

   g) Which method is more precise? Explain your answer.

11.4 – NORMAL DISTRIBUTION

Many populations and samples are dispersed in such a way that graphing the distribution of the population or sample results in a bell-shaped curve. This bell-shaped curve is referred to as a **normal distribution** or a **Gaussian distribution**. This type of curve has a graph that looks similar to the graph in Figure 11–1.

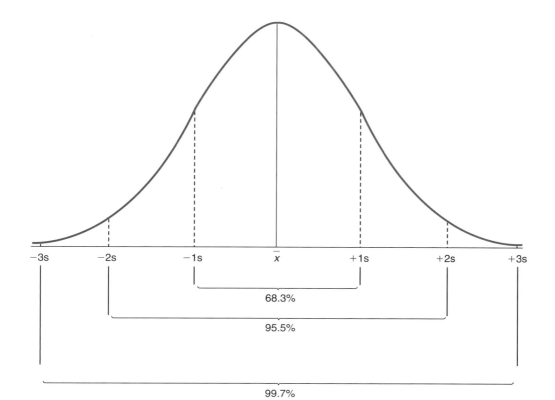

FIGURE 11–1 The Normal Distribution

The mean is located at 0 in Figure 11–1, and $-3s$ represents 3 standard deviations *below* the mean, $-2s$ represents 2 standard deviations *below* the mean, $+1s$ is 1 standard deviation *above* the mean, and so on. It turns out that for populations (or samples) whose distribution is approximately normal, about 68.3% of all the data values in that population will fall within ±1 standard deviation from the mean, about 95.5% will fall within ±2 standard deviations from the mean, and about 99.7% (almost all of the data values) will fall within ±3 standard deviations from the mean. This is all summarized in the empirical rule, which is given next.

The Empirical Rule

The **empirical rule** states that if a set of measurements has a normal distribution, then the following is true:

- Approximately 68.3% of all values fall within 1 standard deviation of the mean (i.e., between $\bar{x} - s$ and $\bar{x} + s$).

- Approximately 95.5% of all values fall within 2 standard deviations of the mean (i.e., between $\bar{x} - 2s$ and $\bar{x} + 2s$).

- Approximately 99.7% of all values fall within 3 standard deviations of the mean (i.e., between $\bar{x} - 3s$ and $\bar{x} + 3s$).

EXAMPLE 11-9: A glucose assay was performed on 400 specimens of urine collected in a 24-hour period. They were found to have a mean of 1.0 $\frac{g}{day}$ and a standard deviation of 0.2 grams. Assuming the distribution is approximately bell shaped, use the empirical rule to determine about how many of the 400 specimens fall within

a)   1 standard deviation from the mean.

b)   2 standard deviations from the mean.

c)   3 standard deviations from the mean.

a)   By the empirical rule, we know approximately 68.3% of the specimens have values falling within 1 standard deviation from the mean. Mathematically that is

$1.0 \pm 1(0.2) = 1.0 \pm 0.2$

$1.0 + 0.2 = \underline{\mathbf{1.2}}$ and $1.0 - 0.2 = \underline{\mathbf{0.8}}$.

So approximately 68.3% of the 400 specimens, or $(0.683)(400) = 273$, of the specimens will have values between 0.8 and 1.2 $\frac{g}{day}$.

b)   By the empirical rule, we know approximately 95.5% of the specimens have values falling within 2 standard deviations from the mean. Mathematically that is

$1.0 \pm 2(0.2) = 1.0 \pm 0.4$

$1.0 + 0.4 = \underline{\mathbf{1.4}}$ and $1.0 - 0.4 = \underline{\mathbf{0.6}}$.

So approximately 95.5% of the 400 specimens, or $(0.955)(400) = 382$, of the specimens will have values between 0.6 and 1.4 $\frac{g}{day}$.

c) By the empirical rule, we know approximately 99.7% of the specimens have values falling within 3 standard deviations from the mean. Mathematically that is

$1.0 \pm 3(0.2) = 1.0 \pm 0.6$

$1.0 + 0.6 = \underline{\textbf{1.6}}$ and $1.0 - 0.6 = \underline{\textbf{0.4}}$.

So approximately 99.7% of the 400 specimens, or $(0.997)(400) \oplus 399$, of the specimens will have values between 0.4 and 1.6 $\frac{g}{day}$.

EXAMPLE 11-10: By the empirical rule, approximately what percentage of data values having a normal distribution will fall

a) outside ± 1 standard deviation from the mean?

b) outside ± 2 standard deviations from the mean?

c) outside ± 3 standard deviations from the mean?

a) We know about 68.3% fall within ± 1 SD; therefore, about $100\% - 68.3\% = \underline{\textbf{31.7}}\%$ will fall outside ± 1 SD from $\bar{x}$.

b) We know approximately 95.5% fall within ± 2 SD; therefore, approximately $100\% - 95.5\% = \underline{\textbf{4.5}}\%$ will fall outside ± 2 SD from $\bar{x}$.

c) We know about 99.7% fall within ± 3 SD; thus, about $100\% - 99.7\% = \underline{\textbf{0.3}}\%$ will fall outside ± 3 SD from $\bar{x}$.

PRACTICE PROBLEMS: Section 11.4

1. Assume the data set is approximately normally distributed (bell shaped). List the percentage associated with each of the following events.

   a) A control result falls *within* ± 1 SD from the mean.

   b) A control result falls *within* ± 2 SD from the mean.

   c) A control result falls *within* ± 3 SD from the mean.

   d) A control result falls *outside* ± 2 SD from the mean.

   e) A control result falls *outside* ± 3 SD from the mean.

   f) A control result falls *outside* ± 1 SD from the mean.

Continues

PRACTICE PROBLEMS: Section 11.4 (continued)

2. A set of approximately normally distributed data has a standard deviation of 5 and a mean of 80.

   a) Calculate the ±1, ±2, and ±3 standard deviation *ranges* for the data.

   b) Approximately what percent of the data values could be expected to fall within each of the standard deviation ranges calculated in part a?

   c) Approximately what percent of the data values could be expected to fall outside each of the standard deviation ranges calculated in part a?

3. A group of approximately normally distributed data has a standard deviation of 12.5 and a mean of 225.

   a) Calculate the ±1, ±2, and ±3 standard deviation *ranges* for the data.

   b) Approximately what percent of the data values could be expected to fall within each of the standard deviation ranges calculated in part a?

   c) Approximately what percent of the data values could be expected to fall outside each of the standard deviation ranges calculated in part a?

4. A group of approximately normally distributed data has a standard deviation of 1.7 and a mean of 28.3.

   a) Calculate the ±1, ±2, and ±3 standard deviation *ranges* for the data.

   b) Approximately what percent of the data values could be expected to fall within each of the standard deviation ranges calculated in part a?

   c) Approximately what percent of the data values could be expected to fall outside each of the standard deviation ranges calculated in part a?

5. A group of approximately normally distributed data has a standard deviation of 5.8 and a mean of 80.

   a) Calculate the ±1, ±2, and ±3 standard deviation *ranges* for the data.

   b) Approximately what percent of the data values could be expected to fall within each of the standard deviation ranges calculated in part a?

   c) Approximately what percent of the data values could be expected to fall outside each of the standard deviation ranges calculated in part a?

6. A group of approximately normally distributed data has a standard deviation of 6 and a mean of 160.

   a) Calculate the ±1, ±2, and ±3 standard deviation *ranges* for the data.

   b) Approximately what percent of the data values could be expected to fall within each of the standard deviation ranges calculated in part a?

   c) Approximately what percent of the data values could be expected to fall outside each of the standard deviation ranges calculated in part a?

11.5 – QUALITY CONTROL

One process used to make sure laboratory results are precise and dependable is called **quality control**. How do we know whether the numbers obtained are of good quality? To be confident, we compare our results with previous measurements we know are accurate. We can get these accurate measurements from commercial control products, or we can generate them in the lab ourselves. Measurements we know are accurate are called **controls**. When measuring these controls, we must be sure the materials and conditions simulate the materials we are analyzing and conditions in which they are analyzed. Therefore the control material must have the same chemical and physical characteristics as the material we are examining.

We always try to use at least two if not three control materials for each method to be sure the results of the patient's specimen are reliable. For instance, an instrument can typically measure at least three levels of a sample: low, medium, and high. Therefore, instead of just checking the precision and reliability of the instrument at the low level, we would also test at the medium and/or high levels. This gives us more reliable and dependable results. If we check the instrument at two levels, we will need two different control materials, and, likewise, if we check at three levels, we will need three different control materials.

If the results of a specimen do not fall within an established range of the controls, we can assume something has gone wrong, and we must inspect our work process for errors. The established range of acceptable values varies from laboratory to laboratory, but either way the $\pm 1s$, $\pm 2s$, and $\pm 3s$ standard deviation (SD) ranges are used. For example, if the ± 2 SD range is determined to be acceptable, this means we would expect at least 95.5% of the control values to fall within the ± 2 SD range. Keep in mind that the expectation of 95.5% falling within ± 2 SD is the same as 4.5% falling outside the ± 2 SD range. Also remember that 4.5% means $\frac{4.5}{100}$, which is approximately $\frac{1}{22}$. Therefore, we could expect about 1 in 22 of our control values to fall outside the ± 2 SD range. If about 1 in 22 of the control values falls outside this range, we usually consider our work process to be reliable and we say the test run is **in control**. If more than 1 in 22 fall outside this range, we assume there are errors, check our work process to detect and correct those errors, and say the test run is **out of control**. However, if we have a relatively small sample (fewer than 22), we would expect none of the control values to fall outside the ± 2 SD range. Likewise, if the established range of acceptable values is ± 3 SD, we would expect 99.7% of the sample values to fall within the ± 3 SD range of the control values and 0.3% to fall outside. Because 0.3% is such a small number, we would not expect any control values to fall outside the ± 3 SD range. To help us visually see whether a test procedure is in or out of control, we usually construct a control chart. The Levey-Jennings control chart is typically used in the laboratory to record control results.

Note: Practice problems for Section 11.5 are contained in the practice problems in Section 11.6.

11.6 – LEVEY-JENNINGS CHARTS
AND WESTGARD MULTIRULES

Levey-Jennings control charts are useful in helping laboratory scientists to be sure their instruments are working well and the results are precise and dependable. In other words, the Levey-Jennings chart is commonly used in the medical laboratory for quality control. The process behind this method of quality control is the following:

1) Gather data.

2) Calculate the mean, standard deviation, and $+1s, +2s, +3s, -1s, -2s, -3s$.

3) Prepare the chart, indicating with a line where the mean and $\pm1s, +2s, +3s, -1s, -2s, -3s$ are located.

4) Plot the data set and inspect for outliers, trends, and shifts (we will discuss these shortly—daily control values).

Once you have completed this chart, you then need to analyze it and determine whether the test run is in control or out of control. When analyzing the chart, you are looking for control values that fall outside the established range of acceptable values determined by the laboratory. Any values that lie outside this established range are called outliers. In general, **outliers** are values that deviate from the mean by an extreme amount.

In addition to looking for outliers, we also look for a condition referred to as a trend. A **trend** is when six or more consecutive plots all fall in one direction, specifically upward or downward. If we observe a trend, the assay procedure should be examined to detect and correct problems, and depending on the problem, we may or may not report the results. This will be explained in more detail shortly.

Another situation that arises when analyzing a Levey-Jennings chart is a condition referred to as a shift. A **shift** is when six or more consecutive plots all fall on/above or on/below the mean line. If they all fall on/above the mean line, we call this a *positive* shift, and if they are all on/below, we call this a *negative* shift. If we observe a shift, the assay procedure should be examined to detect and correct problems. Depending on the problem discovered, we may or may not report the results.

Sometimes, however, a shift and/or trend can happen by chance. Because the probability of this happening by chance is quite small, whenever a shift or trend is observed, the procedure should always be examined for problems.

NOTE

In the examples that follow, the number of days is relatively small. We are using a small number for illustration purposes. When using the Levey-Jennings chart in the lab, it is suggested to collect at least 20 measurements over a four-week period.

EXAMPLE 11-11: A laboratory control for iron levels has a mean for the level of 18 $\mu mol/L$ with a standard deviation of 2 $\mu mol/L$. New control values were collected throughout an eight-day period as a part of routine work. Those values follow. Construct a Levey-Jennings chart for the eight control results and determine whether there are any trends and/or shifts.

Day 1: 16 $\mu mol/L$

Day 2: 21 $\mu mol/L$

Day 3: 19 $\mu mol/L$

Day 4: 20 $\mu mol/L$

Day 5: 19 $\mu mol/L$

Day 6: 21 $\mu mol/L$

Day 7: 20 $\mu mol/L$

Day 8: 17 $\mu mol/L$

We are given the mean and standard deviation. From these we will calculate the $+1s$, $+2s$, $+3s$, $-1s$, $-2s$, $-3s$ ranges.

$$\bar{x} + 1s = 18 + 1(2) = 20$$
$$\bar{x} + 2s = 18 + 2(2) = 22$$
$$\bar{x} + 3s = 18 + 3(2) = 24$$
$$\bar{x} - 1s = 18 - 1(2) = 16$$
$$\bar{x} - 2s = 18 - 2(2) = 14$$
$$\bar{x} - 3s = 18 - 3(2) = 12$$

Next we plot the mean and $\pm 1s$, $\pm 2s$, and $\pm 3s$ lines on the Levey-Jennings chart.

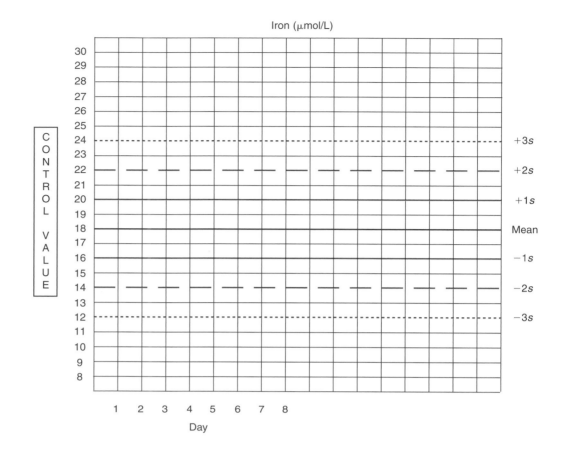

NOTE

The use of the dotted lines is strictly for visual purposes so we can better see and distinguish between the ±1, ±2, and ±3 standard deviation lines.

Next we plot the control values for each of the eight days on the chart.

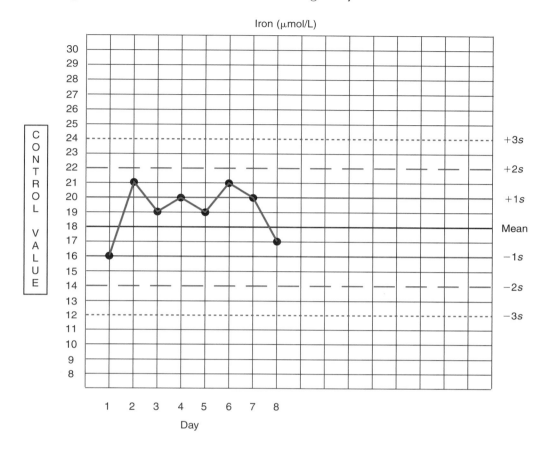

By inspection we see there is a positive shift from days 2 to 7 because all these data points lie above the mean. Therefore, the assay procedure should be examined to detect and correct problems. It should be noted that the results could still be reported depending on the outcome of the investigation. For example, the instrument might just need to be recalibrated. In either case, the laboratory procedure manual should be followed.

EXAMPLE 11-12: Two different commercial control products were selected for a cholesterol method, one for the low level and one for the middle level. These two materials were analyzed for 20 runs, and from the results, the mean and standard deviation of each control were calculated and found to be

Control 1: $\bar{x} = 150$ $^{mg}\!/_{dL}$ and $s = 3$ $^{mg}\!/_{dL}$,

Control 2: $\bar{x} = 200$ $^{mg}\!/_{dL}$ and $s = 4$ $^{mg}\!/_{dL}$.

Later, for 10 consecutive days, controls were analyzed as a part of routine lab work. That data follows.

DAY	CONTROL 1	CONTROL 2
1	152	195
2	151	206
3	155	209
4	155	205
5	154	196
6	152	200
7	145	198
8	150	199
9	146	202
10	143	204

Construct a Levey-Jennings chart and determine whether the assay procedure should be examined. Assume the ±2 SD range is the established range of acceptable values.

Solution:

We are given the mean and standard deviation for each control, so we continue by calculating the $+1s, +2s, +3s, -1s, -2s, -3s$ ranges.

Control 1: $\bar{x} + 1s = 150 + 1(3) = 153$ Control 2: $\bar{x} + 1s = 200 + 1(4) = 204$
$\qquad \bar{x} + 2s = 150 + 2(3) = 156$ $\qquad \bar{x} + 2s = 200 + 2(4) = 208$
$\qquad \bar{x} + 3s = 150 + 3(3) = 159$ $\qquad \bar{x} + 3s = 200 + 3(4) = 212$
$\qquad \bar{x} - 1s = 150 - 1(3) = 147$ $\qquad \bar{x} - 1s = 200 - 1(4) = 196$
$\qquad \bar{x} - 2s = 150 - 2(3) = 144$ $\qquad \bar{x} - 2s = 200 - 2(4) = 192$
$\qquad \bar{x} - 3s = 150 - 3(3) = 141$ $\qquad \bar{x} - 3s = 200 - 3(4) = 188$

We now prepare the charts. In this case we need two charts because we have two controls. These charts are found in Figures 11–2 and 11–3.

Next we plot the control results from our routine runs on the Levey-Jennings charts we just constructed (Figure 11–2 and Figure 11–3). These results are found in Figure 11–4 and Figure 11–5.

By inspection of the charts in Figures 11–2 through 11–5, we can see there is a shift in control 1 from day 1 to day 6 that warrants our attention. The established range of acceptable values is ±2 SD, so the method or run would be considered out of control on day 10 in control 1 because the data value falls below −2 SD. For control 2 on day 3 the data value is above +2 SD and again this warrants the conclusion that the assay procedure needs to be analyzed to correct any problems.

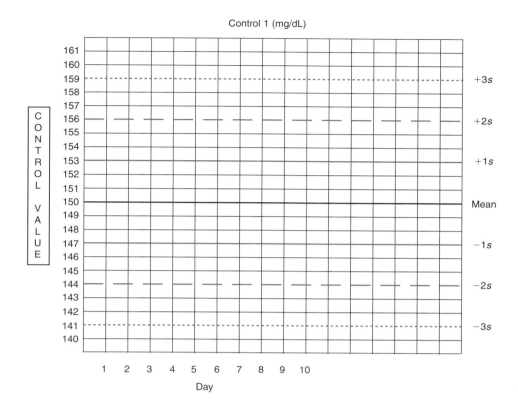

FIGURE 11–2
Control 1 (mg/dL).

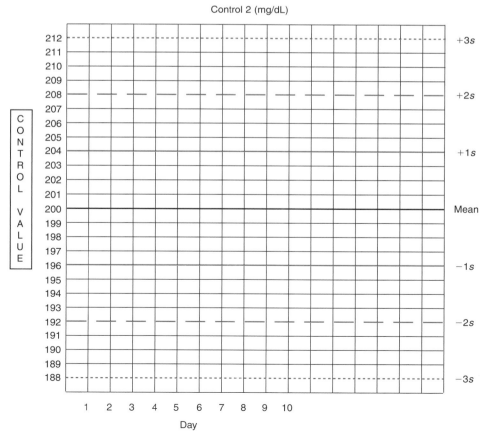

FIGURE 11–3
Control 2 (mg/dL).

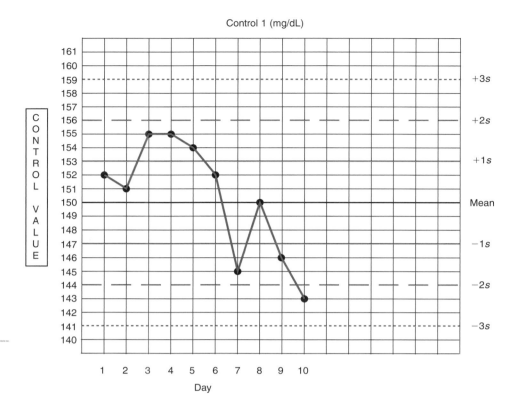

FIGURE 11–4 Test results for control 1 (mg/dL).

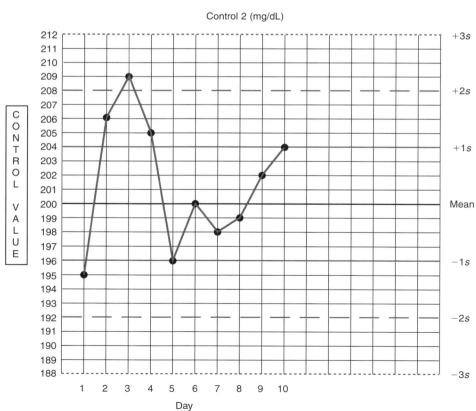

FIGURE 11–5 Test results for control 2 (mg/dL).

NOTE

In this next example we are rounding to the nearest whole number. However, this is solely for the sake of simplicity to illustrate the concept. As mentioned before, when computing the standard deviation in the lab, we want at least one more significant figure than what is expected in the patient's test result and two more significant figures for the mean. It is always best to carry more significant figures than needed.

EXAMPLE 11-13: For a protein method, a new control product was purchased and eight consecutive measurements were taken. Following are the results.

Measurement #:	1	2	3	4	5	6	7	8
Measurement (mg/day)	80	85	78	82	84	80	79	77

Later, for eight consecutive days, new control values were collected as a part of routine lab work. That data follows.

Day:	1	2	3	4	5	6	7	8
Measurement (mg/day)	77	82	76	84	86	79	81	79

Construct a Levey-Jennings chart and determine whether the assay procedure should be examined. Assume the ±2 SD range is the established range of acceptable values.

First, calculate the mean and standard deviation for the control product.

$$\bar{x} = \frac{80+85+78+82+84+80+79+77}{8} = 81$$

Using Your Calculator

First be sure the calculator is in the STAT 1 mode. Now enter the data values.

80 $\boxed{\Sigma +}$ 85 $\boxed{\Sigma +}$ 78 $\boxed{\Sigma +}$ 82 $\boxed{\Sigma +}$ 84

$\boxed{\Sigma +}$ 80 $\boxed{\Sigma +}$ 79 $\boxed{\Sigma +}$ 77 $\boxed{\Sigma +}$

To calculate the mean, press the 2nd key and the $\boxed{x^2}$ key. Your calculator should now display 80.625. We will round to 81 for illustration purposes.

Next calculate the SD.

$$(80 - 81)^2 = 1$$
$$(85 - 81)^2 = 16$$
$$(78 - 81)^2 = 9$$
$$(82 - 81)^2 = 1$$
$$(84 - 81)^2 = 9$$
$$(80 - 81)^2 = 1$$
$$(79 - 81)^2 = 4$$
$$(77 - 81)^2 = 16$$

Adding these results we get $1 + 16 + 9 + 1 + 9 + 1 + 4 + 16 = 57$.

Divide by $n - 1 = 7$ to get $\dfrac{57}{7} = 8$.

Take the square root to get $s = \sqrt{8} = 3$ (again, we are rounding to the nearest whole number for illustration purposes).

 ## Using Your Calculator

We already entered the data values to find the mean, so we can immediately move to finding the standard deviation. Press the 2nd key and then the $\boxed{\sqrt{x}}$ key. Your calculator should now display 2.83 (rounded), but we will round to 3 for the sake of illustration purposes.

Now we calculate the $\pm 1, \pm 2,$ and ± 3 SD locations.

$$\overline{x} + 1s = 81 + 1(3) = 84$$
$$\overline{x} + 2s = 81 + 2(3) = 87$$
$$\overline{x} + 3s = 81 + 3(3) = 90$$
$$\overline{x} - 1s = 81 - 1(3) = 78$$
$$\overline{x} - 2s = 81 - 2(3) = 75$$
$$\overline{x} - 3s = 81 - 3(3) = 72$$

Now we plot these lines on the Levey-Jennings chart. See Figure 11-6.

Next we plot the test results from our routine run on the Levey-Jennings chart we just constructed. See Figure 11-7.

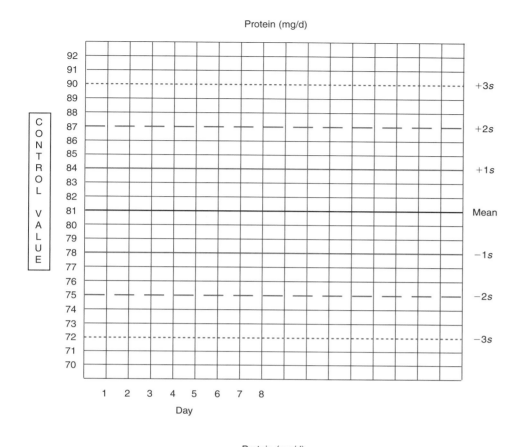

FIGURE 11–6
Calculations plotted on Levey-Jennings chart.

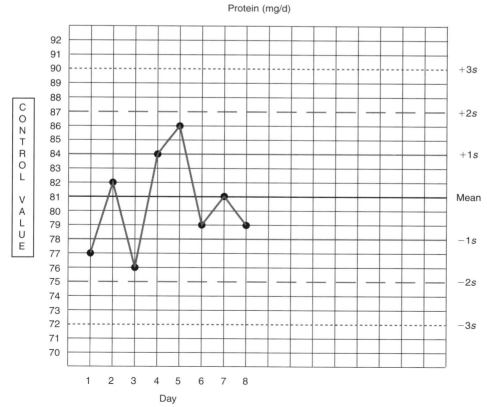

FIGURE 11–7
Test results.

By inspection of this chart, we see there is no trend, no shift, and none of these measurements falls above $+2s$ or below $-2s$. We conclude the method is in control for those days and shows acceptable results. Therefore, the control is satisfactory for continued patient work.

Westgard Multirules

Up to this point, if the established range of acceptable values is $\pm 2s$ and any of the measurements falls above or below these two lines, we must investigate the assay procedure to detect problems. However, this rule is often too stringent for many labs. As a result, an individual by the name of Westgard, together with his colleagues, came up with a multiple rule design to determine whether a method is in or out of control. When applying the **Westgard multirules**, a run outside $\pm 2s$ does not necessarily mean we do not report the results. It is just a warning. Also, when applying these rules, we must be sure to use two or three levels of control. After each rule is presented, there is a single chart illustrating the concept. The Westgard multirules are as follows:

Rule 1_{3s}: The results are not reported whenever a *single* control measure lies above $+3s$ or below $-3s$.

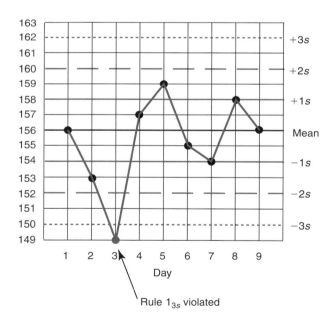

EXAMPLE 11-14: For a cholesterol method, two different materials for two levels of control are each plotted on a Levey-Jennings chart. Determine whether a Westgard rule has been violated.

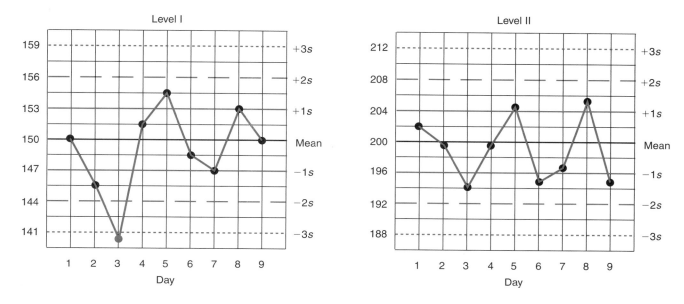

In level II all of the control results are between +2s and −2s; however, in level I, on day 3 rule 1_{3s} is violated, so we do not report the results and the assay procedure needs to be analyzed to correct the problem.

Rule 1_{2s}: This rule is typically used when the established range of acceptable values is ±2s. This rule says if a *single* control measure in either level falls above +2s or below −2s, a warning goes up and we must look at the other Westgard rules. If *any* of the other rules are violated, we do not report the results. Therefore, whenever we see any control value that falls above +2s or below −2s, it does not necessarily mean we reject the run. We must check to see whether other rules are violated first before we reject the run.

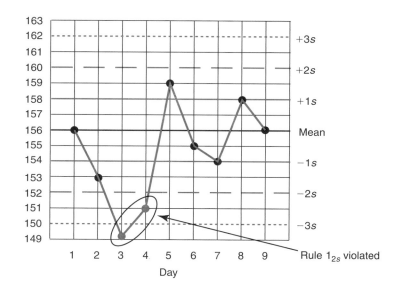

Rule 2₂ₛ: If *two consecutive* control values fall above $+2s$ or below $-2s$, corrective action must be taken. This rule is also violated if corresponding runs across two different materials (or levels) both satisfy this condition.

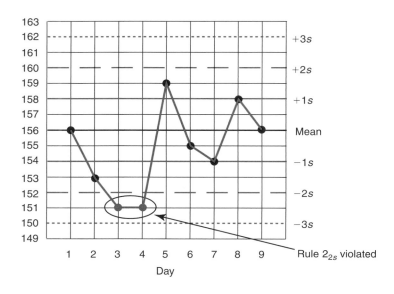

EXAMPLE 11-15: For a cholesterol method, two different materials for two levels of control are each plotted on a Levey-Jennings chart. Determine whether a Westgard rule has been violated.

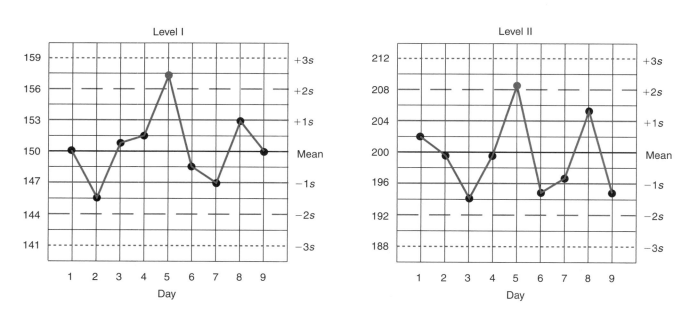

Rule 2_{2s} is violated across materials on day 5; therefore, the assay procedure needs to be analyzed to correct the problem.

EXAMPLE 11-16: For a cholesterol method, two levels of control are each plotted on a Levey-Jennings chart. Determine whether a Westgard rule has been violated.

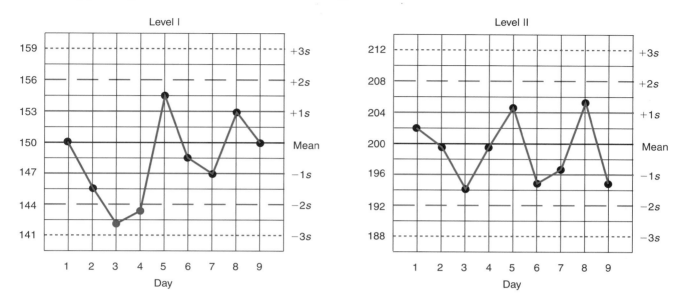

We see rule 2_{2s} is violated within the level I material on days 3 and 4; therefore, the work process needs to be analyzed to correct the problem.

Rule R_{4s}: If one control measure falls above $+2s$ and another falls below $-2s$, we reject the run. This rule is also violated if corresponding runs across two different materials both satisfy this condition.

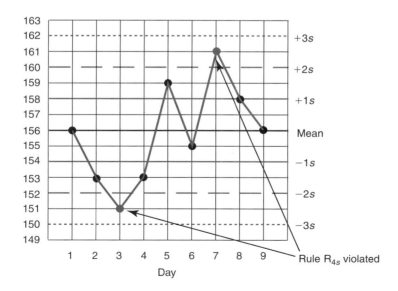

EXAMPLE 11-17: For a cholesterol method, two levels of control are each plotted on a Levey-Jennings chart. Determine whether a Westgard rule has been violated.

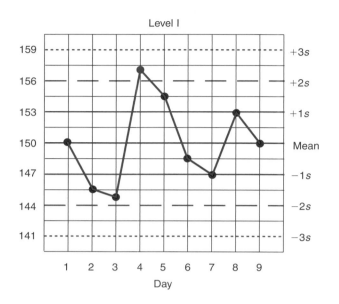

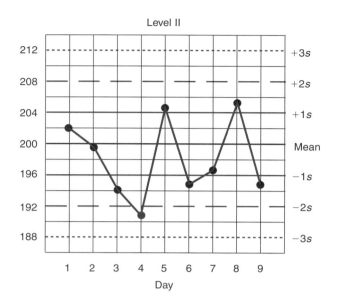

Rule R$_{4s}$ is violated across materials on day 4; therefore, the assay procedure needs to be analyzed to correct the problem.

Rule 4$_{1s}$: If *four consecutive* controls all fall above or below ±1s of that level's mean, we reject the run. Note that to initiate a 4$_{1s}$ violation, there must also be a run falling outside the ±2s range. This rule can also be violated if two consecutive corresponding runs across two different materials satisfy the same conditions.

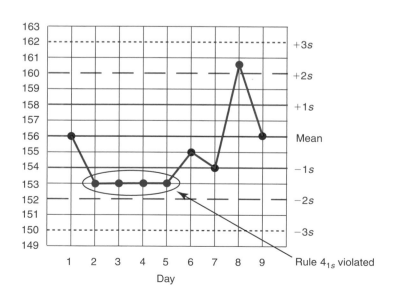

EXAMPLE 11-18: For a cholesterol method, two levels of control are each plotted on a Levey-Jennings chart. Determine whether a Westgard rule has been violated.

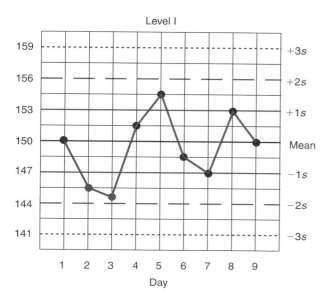

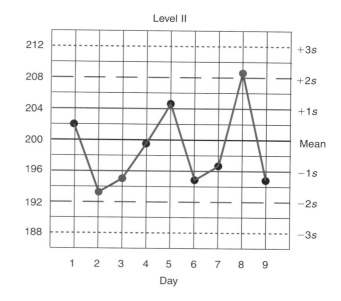

First note there is a run falling outside ±2s in level II, day 8. We also see on days 2 and 3 rule 4_{1s} is violated across materials; therefore, corrective action must be taken.

Rule 10_X: If the last *10 consecutive* control results, within one level of control, all fall on one side of the mean, we reject the run. This rule can also be violated if we have two control levels and the last five runs all fall on one side of the mean for both levels of control.

EXAMPLE 11-19: For a cholesterol method, two different materials for two levels of control are each plotted on a Levey-Jennings chart. Determine whether a Westgard rule has been violated.

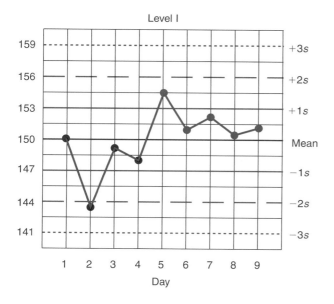

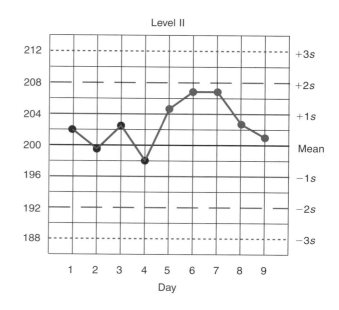

We see rule 10_x is violated across materials on days 5 through 9; therefore, the work process needs to be analyzed to correct the problem.

> Following is the protocol for determining whether a Westgard rule has been violated given two levels of control.
>
> - If all the results of both controls fall within $+2s$ and $-2s$ from the mean, we report the results.
>
> - If any one control result falls above $+2s$ or below $-2s$, there is a warning and we need to check whether other rules are violated as follows:
>   - If the 1_{3s} rule is violated in either material, we do not report the results.
>   - If any of the remaining rules are violated within one of the materials, we do not report the results.
>   - If any of the remaining rules are violated across materials, we do not report the results.
>   - If none of the remaining rules is violated within one of the materials or across materials, we report the results.

EXAMPLE 11-20: For a cholesterol method, two different materials for two levels of control are each plotted on a Levey-Jennings chart. Determine whether a Westgard rule has been violated.

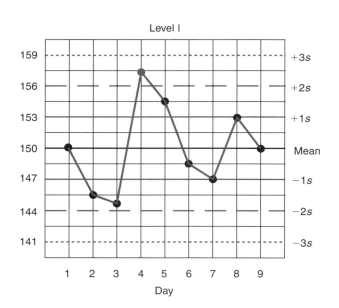

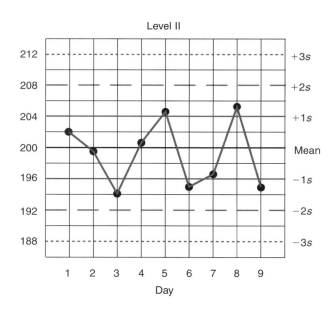

A rule 1_{2s} warning goes up because of the day 4 run in level I. However, none of the other rules is violated; therefore, we can report the results.

PRACTICE PROBLEMS: Section 11.6

For problems 1 through 5, do the following. Do *not* use the Westgard rules.

a) Construct a Levey-Jennings chart using the control results/values.

b) Is there a shift? Answer yes or no, and if the answer is yes, determine whether it is positive or negative.

c) Is there a trend? Answer yes or no, and if the answer is yes, determine whether it is upward or downward.

d) Assume the acceptable range of values for the laboratory is the $\pm 2s$ range.

e) Explain whether the test procedure is in control or out of control and whether the test procedure should be used for patient diagnosis.

1. A control product was selected for test interpretation. This material was analyzed once each day for 25 days, and from the results the mean and standard deviation were calculated and found to be

   Control: $\overline{x} = 84\ ^{mg}\!/_{dL}$ and $s = 6.0\ ^{mg}\!/_{dL}$.

   Later, for 7 consecutive days new control values were collected as a part of routine lab work. That data follows.

Day:	1	2	3	4	5	6	7
Measurement (mg/dL):	94	90	85	83	81	80	75

2. A control product was selected for test interpretation. This material was analyzed once each day for 20 days, and from the results the mean and standard deviation were calculated and found to be

   Control: $\overline{x} = 86\ ^{mg}\!/_{dL}$ and $s = 5.0\ ^{mg}\!/_{dL}$.

   Later, for 10 consecutive days new control values were collected as a part of routine lab work. That data follows.

Day:	1	2	3	4	5	6	7	8	9	10
Measurement (mg/dL):	83	98	94	92	97	80	85	82	81	81

3. A control product was selected for glucose test interpretation. This material was analyzed once each day for 30 days, and from the results the mean and standard deviation were calculated and found to be

   Control: $\overline{x} = 110\ ^{mg}\!/_{dL}$ and $s = 6.0\ ^{mg}\!/_{dL}$.

   Later, for 10 consecutive days new glucose control values were collected as a part of routine lab work. That data follows.

Day:	1	2	3	4	5	6	7	8	9	10
Measurement (mg/dL):	107	114	90	93	105	110	115	120	112	107

Continues

PRACTICE PROBLEMS: Section 11.6 *(continued)*

4. A control product was selected for glucose test interpretation. This material was analyzed once each day for 30 days, and from the results the mean and standard deviation were calculated and found to be

    Control: $\bar{x} = 100$ $^{mg}/_{dL}$ and $s = 5.0$ $^{mg}/_{dL}$.

    Later, for 10 consecutive days new glucose control values were collected as a part of routine lab work. That data follows.

Day:	1	2	3	4	5	6	7	8	9	10
Measurement (mg/dL):	102	110	93	99	95	100	108	105	112	90

5. A control product was selected for test interpretation. This material was analyzed once each day for 20 days, and from the results the mean and standard deviation were calculated and found to be

    Control: $\bar{x} = 90$ $^{mg}/_{dL}$ and $s = 4.0$ $^{mg}/_{dL}$.

    Later, for 10 consecutive days new control values were collected as a part of routine lab work. That data follows.

Day:	1	2	3	4	5	6	7	8	9	10
Measurement (mg/dL):	87	90	95	100	85	104	84	81	81	94

6. For a protein method, a control product was purchased and for eight consecutive days measurements were taken. Those results were

Day:	1	2	3	4	5	6	7	8
Measurement (mg/day):	75	80	77	76	72	73	79	76

    Later, for eight consecutive days new control values were collected as a part of routine lab work. That data follows.

Day:	1	2	3	4	5	6	7	8
Measurement (mg/day):	77	79	79	74	73	75	68	79

    Construct a Levey-Jennings chart and determine whether the run should be rejected. Assume the ±2 SD range is the established range of acceptable values.

7. For a urine urea method, a control product was purchased and for eight consecutive days measurements were taken. Those results follow.

Day:	1	2	3	4	5	6	7	8
Measurement (mg/dL):	30	32	28	26	25	29	31	28

Later, for eight consecutive days new control values were collected as a part of routine lab work. That data follows.

Day:	1	2	3	4	5	6	7	8
Measurement (mg/dL):	25	24	28	30	26	24	27	25

Construct a Levey-Jennings chart and determine whether the run should be rejected. Assume the ±2 SD range is the established range of acceptable values.

8. The means of two different quality control products for cholesterol levels are 200 $\frac{mg}{dL}$ and 250 $\frac{mg}{dL}$ with standard deviations of 4.0 $\frac{mg}{dL}$ and 5.0 $\frac{mg}{dL}$ for control 1 and control 2, respectively. For 10 consecutive days new cholesterol control values were collected as a part of routine lab work. That data follows.

Day:	1	2	3	4	5	6	7	8	9	10
Control 1 (mg/dL):	202	204	205	196	203	190	198	195	204	200
Control 2 (mg/dL):	250	245	248	254	252	246	247	253	263	250

By applying the Westgard multiple rules, determine whether these results should be reported. If they should not, determine which Westgard rule or rules have been violated.

9. The means of two different levels of quality control groups are 100 $\frac{mg}{dL}$ for the middle range and 120 $\frac{mg}{dL}$ for the high range. Their standard deviations are 3.0 $\frac{mg}{dL}$ for the middle range and 3.5 $\frac{mg}{dL}$ for the high range. For 10 consecutive days new control values were collected as a part of routine lab work. That data follows.

Day:	1	2	3	4	5	6	7	8	9	10
Control 1 (mg/dL):	98	104	105	101	102	103	95	100	96	97
Control 2 (mg/dL):	115	121	125	126	123	122	117	116	118	121

By applying the Westgard multiple rules, determine whether these results should be reported. If they should not, determine which Westgard rule or rules have been violated.

For problems 10, 11, and 12, apply the Westgard multiple rules to determine whether the results should be reported. If they should not, determine which Westgard rule or rules have been violated.

10. The means of two different levels of quality control groups are 150 $\frac{mg}{dL}$ for the middle range and 180 $\frac{mg}{dL}$ for the high range. Their standard deviations are 3.0 $\frac{mg}{dL}$ for the middle range and 4.0 $\frac{mg}{dL}$ for the high range. For 10 consecutive days new control values were collected as a part of routine lab work. That data follows.

Day:	1	2	3	4	5	6	7	8	9	10
Control 1 (mg/dL):	155	151	148	157	152	145	149	143	150	152
Control 2 (mg/dL):	186	179	174	181	189	190	177	175	178	180

Continues

PRACTICE PROBLEMS: Section 11.6 *(continued)*

11. The means of two different levels of quality control groups are 90 $^{mg}/_{dL}$ for the middle range and 150 $^{mg}/_{dL}$ for the high range. Their standard deviations are 2.0 $^{mg}/_{dL}$ for the middle range and 3.0 $^{mg}/_{dL}$ for the high range. For 10 consecutive days new control values were collected as a part of routine lab work. That data follows.

Day:	1	2	3	4	5	6	7	8	9	10
Control 1 (mg/dL):	89	92	87	89	93	95	90	85	88	93
Control 2 (mg/dL):	148	151	147	150	154	157	148	145	149	155

12. The means of two different levels of quality control groups are 150 $^{mg}/_{dL}$ for the middle range and 200 $^{mg}/_{dL}$ for the high range. Their standard deviations are 4.0 $^{mg}/_{dL}$ for the middle range and 5.0 $^{mg}/_{dL}$ for the high range. For 10 consecutive days new control values were collected as a part of routine lab work. That data follows.

Day:	1	2	3	4	5	6	7	8	9	10
Control 1 (mg/dL):	151	157	156	146	147	148	143	150	159	151
Control 2 (mg/dL):	196	208	207	197	199	198	195	202	206	203

13. Following are Levey-Jennings charts for a cholesterol method using two materials at two different levels. By applying the Westgard multiple rules, determine whether these results should be reported. If they should not, determine which Westgard rule or rules have been violated.

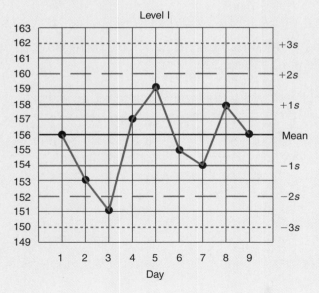

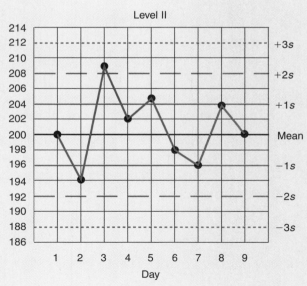

14. Following are Levey-Jennings charts for a cholesterol method using two materials at two different levels. By applying the Westgard multiple rules, determine whether these results should be reported. If they should not, determine which Westgard rule or rules have been violated.

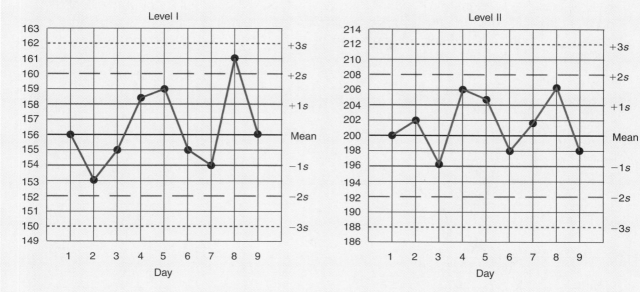

15. Following are Levey-Jennings charts for a protein method using two different materials at two different levels. By applying the Westgard multiple rules, determine whether these results should be reported. If they should not, determine which Westgard rule or rules have been violated.

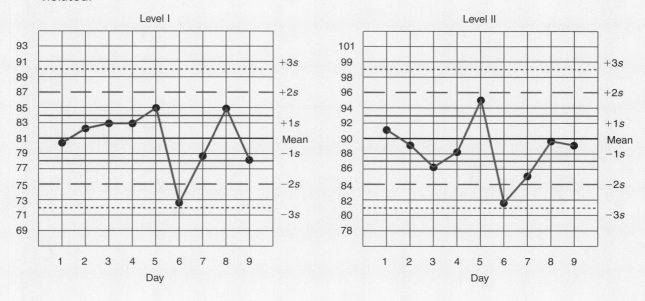

Continues

PRACTICE PROBLEMS: Section 11.6 (continued)

16. Following are Levey-Jennings charts for a protein method using two different materials at two different levels. By applying the Westgard multiple rules, determine whether these results should be reported. If they should not, determine which Westgard rule or rules have been violated.

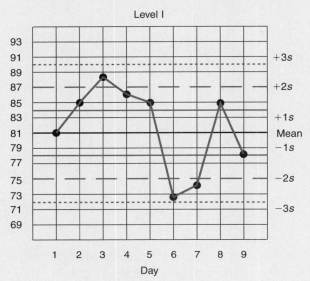

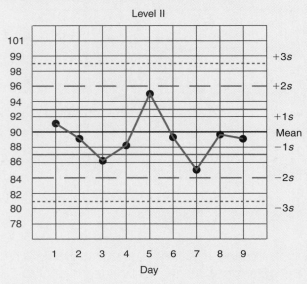

17. Following are Levey-Jennings charts for a protein method using two different materials at two different levels. By applying the Westgard multiple rules, determine whether these results should be reported. If they should not, determine which Westgard rule or rules have been violated.

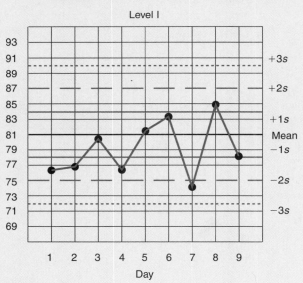

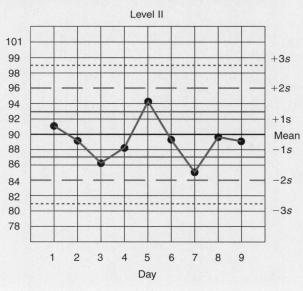

18. Following are Levey-Jennings charts for a protein method using two different materials at two different levels. By applying the Westgard multiple rules, determine whether these results should be reported. If they should not, determine which Westgard rule or rules have been violated.

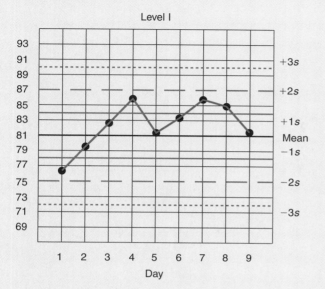

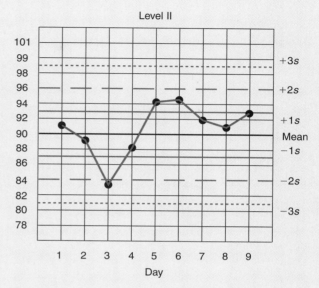

19. Following are Levey-Jennings charts for a cholesterol method using two materials at two different levels. By applying the Westgard multiple rules, determine whether these results should be reported. If they should not, determine which Westgard rule or rules have been violated.

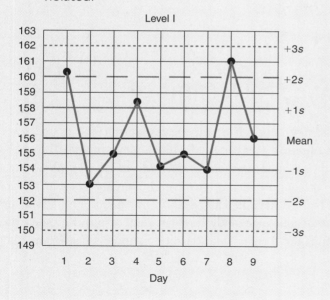

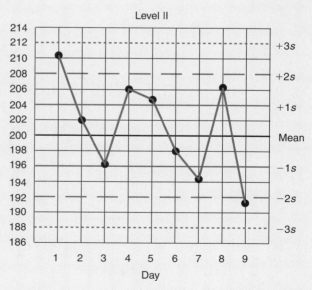

Continues

PRACTICE PROBLEMS: Section 11.6 (continued)

20. Following are Levey-Jennings charts for a cholesterol method using two materials at two different levels. By applying the Westgard multiple rules, determine whether these results should be reported. If they should not, determine which Westgard rule or rules have been violated.

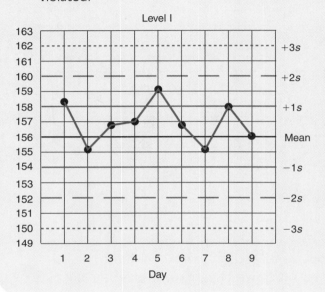

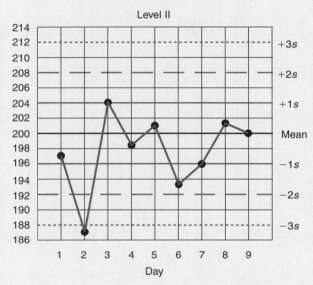

11.7 – THE Z-SCORE AND APPLYING THE CV

The *z-score* tells us how far a measurement is from the mean in terms of standard deviations. For example, if a set of cholesterol measurements had a mean of 240 $\frac{mg}{dL}$ with a standard deviation of 5 $\frac{mg}{dL}$, then a measurement of 245 would be +1 SD from the mean while 235 would be −1 SD from the mean. However, how many standard deviations is 248 from the mean? This is a little harder to do in our head. There is a very simple formula for the z-score that tells us exactly how far, plus or minus, a measurement is away from the sample mean in terms of standard deviations. That formula is

$$z = \frac{x - \bar{x}}{s}.$$

EXAMPLE 11-21: For a set of cholesterol measurements, the mean was found to be 240 $\frac{mg}{dL}$ with a standard deviation of 5 $\frac{mg}{dL}$. How many standard deviations is a measurement of 248 $\frac{mg}{dL}$ away from the mean?

We are given that $\bar{x} = 240$, $x = 248$, and $s = 5$. Substituting these values into the z-score formula, we find

$$z = \frac{248-240}{5} = \frac{8}{5} = 1.6.$$

Therefore, 248 is 1.6 standard deviations above the mean (above because it is positive).

EXAMPLE 11-22: For a set of cholesterol measurements, the mean was found to be 240 $\frac{mg}{dL}$ with a standard deviation of 5 $\frac{mg}{dL}$. How many standard deviations is a measurement of 237 $\frac{mg}{dL}$ away from the mean?

$$z = \frac{237-240}{5} = \frac{-3}{5} = -0.6$$

Therefore, 237 is 0.6 standard deviations below the mean (below because of the negative sign).

Finding the z-score can be very useful when inspecting control results from different materials. We can compute the z-score and immediately see whether the measurement is above $+3s$ or below $-3s$, if there are any trends, and so on.

EXAMPLE 11-23: The behavior of five consecutive measurements from a cholesterol method using two different materials appeared to be odd. For the level I control, $\bar{x} = 190$ $\frac{mg}{dL}$ and $s = 3$ $\frac{mg}{dL}$. For the level II control, $\bar{x} = 230$ $\frac{mg}{dL}$ and $s = 4$ $\frac{mg}{dL}$. Can we conclude there has been a Westgard rule violated by just inspecting the following five measurements?

Day	Level I Measurement	Level II Measurement
2	194	228
3	197	240
4	198	239
5	189	231
6	194	229

First calculate the z-score for each measurement.

	Level I	Level II

Day 2: $z = \dfrac{194-190}{3} = \dfrac{4}{3} = 1.3$ $z = \dfrac{228-230}{4} = \dfrac{-2}{4} = -0.5$

Day 3: $z = \dfrac{197-190}{3} = \dfrac{7}{3} = 2.3$ $z = \dfrac{240-230}{4} = \dfrac{10}{4} = 2.5$

Day 4: $z = \dfrac{198-190}{3} = \dfrac{8}{3} = 2.7$ $z = \dfrac{239-230}{4} = \dfrac{9}{4} = 2.3$

Day 5: $z = \dfrac{189-190}{3} = \dfrac{-1}{3} = -0.3$ $z = \dfrac{231-230}{4} = \dfrac{1}{4} = 0.3$

Day 6: $z = \dfrac{194-190}{3} = \dfrac{4}{3} = 1.3$ $z = \dfrac{229-230}{4} = \dfrac{-1}{4} = -0.3$

By inspection we can see that on days 3 and 4, for both levels, the standard deviation is greater than +2. Therefore, rule 4_{1s} was violated and the assay procedure needs to be analyzed to correct the problem.

EXAMPLE 11-24: The behavior of one particular measurement from the level III material of a cholesterol method appeared to be extreme. For the level III material, $\bar{x} = 250$ $^{mg}\!/_{dL}$ and $s = 4$ $^{mg}\!/_{dL}$. Can we conclude there has been a Westgard rule violated by just inspecting the fact that the measurement had a value of 237?

First calculate the z-score for this measurement.

$$z = \frac{237-250}{4} = \frac{-13}{4} = -3.3$$

Clearly, this value is more than 3 standard deviations away from the mean. Therefore, rule 1_{3s} was violated and the work process needs to be analyzed to correct the problem.

Applying the Coefficient of Variation

The coefficient of variation can be used to evaluate method performance over the span of concentrations within the different levels. For example, in example 11-12, control 1 had a mean and SD of $\bar{x} = 150$ $^{mg}\!/_{dL}$ and $s = 3$ $^{mg}\!/_{dL}$ while control 2 had a mean and SD of $\bar{x} = 200$ $^{mg}\!/_{dL}$ and $s = 4$ $^{mg}\!/_{dL}$. If we calculate the CV for both controls, we find

$$\%CV_1 = \frac{3}{150} \times 100\% = 2\% \text{ and } \%CV_2 = \frac{4}{200} \times 100\% = 2\%.$$

Because they have the same values, they have the same amount of variation.

EXAMPLE 11-25: A commercial control product for glucose has a mean of 90.0 $^{U}\!/_{L}$ with a standard deviation of 2.0 $^{U}\!/_{L}$. However, all the laboratory has at its disposal is a control product whose mean is 85.0 $^U/_L$. From observed results with the 85.0 $^U/_L$ level, it was found the standard deviation was 1.9 $^U/_L$. Calculate the CV for each and compare the results.

$$\%CV_1 = \frac{2.0}{90.0} \times 100\% = 2.2\%$$

$$\%CV_2 = \frac{1.9}{85.0} \times 100\% = 2.2\%$$

The control product available to the laboratory, to one significant figure, is just as variable as the commercial control product and should therefore be very reliable.

PRACTICE PROBLEMS: Section 11.7

1. The behavior of five consecutive measurements from a cholesterol method using two different materials appeared to be strange. For the level I control, $\bar{x} = 190$ $^{mg}/_{dL}$ and $s = 3$ $^{mg}/_{dL}$. For the level II control, $\bar{x} = 230$ $^{mg}/_{dL}$ and $s = 4$ $^{mg}/_{dL}$. Can we conclude there has been a Westgard rule violated by just inspecting the following five measurements?

DAY	LEVEL I MEASUREMENT	LEVEL II MEASUREMENT
12	190	232
13	186	227
14	195	236
15	183	220
16	182	221

2. The behavior of a measurement from a glucose method using two different materials appeared to be strange for one particular day. For the level I control, $\bar{x} = 100$ $^{mg}/_{dL}$ and $s = 2$ $^{mg}/_{dL}$. For the level II control, $\bar{x} = 120$ $^{mg}/_{dL}$ and $s = 3$ $^{mg}/_{dL}$. Can we conclude there has been a Westgard rule violated by just inspecting the following measurement of each material for that day?

DAY	LEVEL I MEASUREMENT	LEVEL II MEASUREMENT
17	93	130

3. The behavior of a measurement from a glucose method using two different materials appeared to be strange for one particular day. For the level I control, $\bar{x} = 100$ $^{mg}/_{dL}$ and $s = 2$ $^{mg}/_{dL}$. For the level II control, $\bar{x} = 120$ $^{mg}/_{dL}$ and $s = 3$ $^{mg}/_{dL}$. Can we conclude there has been a Westgard rule violated by just inspecting the following measurement of each material for that day?

DAY	LEVEL I MEASUREMENT	LEVEL II MEASUREMENT
3	107	128

Continues

PRACTICE PROBLEMS: Section 11.7 (continued)

4. A commercial control product had a mean of 250.0 $^{mg}\!/_{dL}$ with a standard deviation of 5.0 $^{mg}\!/_{dL}$. However, all the laboratory has at its disposal is a control product whose mean is 230.0 $^{mg}\!/_{dL}$. From the observed results at the 230.0 $^{mg}\!/_{dL}$ level, it was found the standard deviation was 4.9 $^{mg}\!/_{dL}$. Calculate the CV for each and compare the results.

5. The behavior of a measurement from a glucose method using two different materials appeared to be strange for one particular day. For the level I control, $\bar{x} = 110$ $^{mg}\!/_{dL}$ and $s = 2$ $^{mg}\!/_{dL}$. For the level II control, $\bar{x} = 120$ $^{mg}\!/_{dL}$ and $s = 3$ $^{mg}\!/_{dL}$. Can we conclude there has been a Westgard rule violated by just inspecting the following measurement of each material for that day?

DAY	LEVEL I MEASUREMENT	LEVEL II MEASUREMENT
17	102	110

6. A commercial control product had a mean of 150.0 $^{mg}\!/_{dL}$ with a standard deviation of 3.0 $^{mg}\!/_{dL}$. However, all the laboratory has at its disposal is a control product whose mean is 200.0 $^{mg}\!/_{dL}$. From the observed results at the 200.0 $^{mg}\!/_{dL}$ level, it was found the standard deviation was 5.0 $^{mg}\!/_{dL}$. Calculate the CV for each and compare the results.

CHAPTER SUMMARY

- Samples must be representative of the population.
- The mean is calculated using the formula $\bar{x} = \dfrac{\Sigma x}{n}$.
- The median is the middle value of the entire data set.
- The mode is the number in the data set that appears most frequently.
- The standard deviation is calculated using the formula $s = \sqrt{\dfrac{\Sigma (x-\bar{x})^2}{n-1}}$.
- The coefficient of variation is calculated using the formula $CV = \dfrac{s}{\bar{x}}$.
- The bell-shaped curve is usually referred to as a normal distribution or a Gaussian distribution.
- For a normal distribution, approximately 68.3% of all values fall within 1 standard deviation of the mean, approximately 95.5% of all values fall within 2 standard deviations of the mean, and approximately 99.7% of all values fall within 3 standard deviations of the mean.
- Levey-Jennings control charts and Westgard multirules are useful in quality control.

- The Westgard multirules are as follows:
  - **Rule 1$_{3s}$**: The results are not reported whenever a *single* control measure lies above $+3s$ or below $-3s$.
  - **Rule 1$_{2s}$**: This rule is typically used when the established range of acceptable values is $\pm 2s$. This rule says if a *single* control measure in either level falls above $+2s$ or below $-2s$, a warning goes up and we must look at the other Westgard rules. If *any* of the other rules are violated, we do not report the results. Therefore, whenever any control value falls above $+2s$ or below $-2s$, a warning goes up. It does not necessarily mean we reject the run. We must check to see whether other rules are violated first before we reject the run.
  - **Rule 2$_{2s}$**: If *two consecutive* control values fall above $+2s$ or below $-2s$, corrective action must be taken. This rule is also violated if corresponding runs across two different materials (or levels) both satisfy this condition.
  - **Rule R$_{4s}$**: If one control measure falls above $+2s$ and another falls below $-2s$, we reject the run. This rule is also violated if corresponding runs across two different materials both satisfy this condition.
  - **Rule 4$_{1s}$**: If *four consecutive* controls all fall above or below $\pm 1s$ of that level's mean, we reject the run. Note that to initiate a 4_{1s} violation, there must also be a run falling outside the $\pm 2s$ range. This rule can also be violated if two consecutive corresponding runs across two different materials satisfy the same conditions.
  - **Rule 10$_x$**: If the last *10 consecutive* control results, within one level of control, all fall on one side of the mean, we reject the run. This rule can also be violated if we have two control levels and the last five runs all fall on one side of the mean for both levels of control.
- The number of standard deviations a data value lies from its mean is calculated using the formula $z = \dfrac{x - \bar{x}}{s}$. This can be useful in determining whether a Westgard rule has been violated.

CHAPTER TEST

1. A sample is tested using two different methods. The resulting data is as follows:

METHOD A	METHOD B
2 5 3 12 6 8 10 2	7 13 9 11 9 9 12 10

   a) Find the mean.
   b) Find the median.
   c) Find the mode.
   d) Find the standard deviation.
   e) Find the coefficient of variation.
   f) Which method is more precise? Explain your answer.

2. A control product was selected for test interpretation. This material was analyzed once each day for 20 days, and from the results the mean and standard deviation were calculated and found to be

Control: $\bar{x} = 7.6 \ \text{mg}/\text{dL}$ and $s = 0.2 \ \text{mg}/\text{dL}$.

Later, for 10 consecutive days new control values were collected as a part of routine lab work. That data follows.

Day:	1	2	3	4	5	6	7	8	9	10
Measurement (mg/dL):	7.4	7.5	7.7	7.4	7.3	7.6	7.5	7.8	7.9	7.9

Do not use the Westgard multirules.

a) Construct a Levey-Jennings chart using the control measures.
b) Is there a shift? Answer yes or no, and if the answer is yes, determine whether it is positive or negative.
c) Is there a trend? Answer yes or no, and if the answer is yes, determine whether it is upward or downward.
d) Assume the acceptable range of values for the laboratory is the $\pm 2s$ range.
e) Explain whether the test procedure is in control or out of control and whether the test procedure should be used for patient diagnosis.

3. Assuming a data set is approximately normally distributed, what percentage of the data values will approximately fall within ± 2 standard deviations from the mean?

4. For a urine urea method, a control product was purchased and for eight consecutive days measurements were taken. Those results follow.

Day:	1	2	3	4	5	6	7	8
Measurement (mg/dL):	30	32	28	26	25	29	31	28

Later, for eight consecutive days new control values were collected as a part of routine lab work. That data follows.

Day:	1	2	3	4	5	6	7	8
Measurement (mg/dL):	25	24	28	29	26	22	27	25

Construct a Levey-Jennings chart and determine whether the run should be rejected. Assume the ± 2 SD range is the established range of acceptable values.

5. For a set of cholesterol measurements, the mean was found to be $200 \ \text{mg}/\text{dL}$ with a standard deviation of $4 \ \text{mg}/\text{dL}$. During routine lab work on day 17, the measurement was $186 \ \text{mg}/\text{dL}$. How many standard deviations is a measurement of $186 \ \text{mg}/\text{dL}$ away from the mean? Has a Westgard multirule been violated on this day?

6. Explain each of the Westgard multirules.

7. For a cholesterol method, two different materials for two levels of control are
    each plotted on a Levey-Jennings chart. Determine whether a Westgard rule has
    been violated.

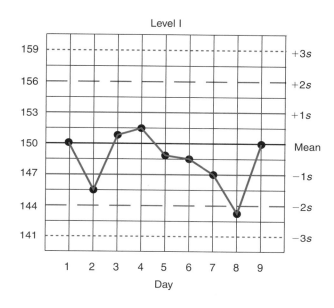

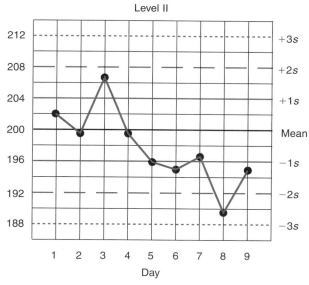

12 Statistics for Laboratory Medicine

$$y = -\frac{2}{5}x + 8$$

INTRODUCTION

As discussed in Chapter 11, instruments are used frequently in the laboratory to obtain measurements and control reliability. However, in many situations we have results from two different instruments or two different methods and the relationships between the two results must be compared. Though results from two different instruments (or two different methods) may be different, they may still be reliable. So how do we determine whether results from two instruments or two different methods are reliable? In Chapter 11 we did so by using Levey-Jennings charts. This chapter presents another approach that provides information beyond knowing whether a method is reliable. To understand this let's take a deeper look into applications of the normal distribution. We first look at some diagnostic probabilities.

12.1 – DIAGNOSTIC PROBABILITIES

One error we certainly want to avoid is reporting that a patient is infected with a disease when that is not the case or reporting that a patient is not infected with a disease when the patient actually is. The probability that all patients who are infected will test positive is called **diagnostic sensitivity**. The probability that all patients who are not infected will not test positive is called **diagnostic specificity**.

When you see the word *probability*, think of percentage. Probabilities are always between 0 and 1. In other words, probabilities can be thought of as percentages between 0% and 100%. A probability of 0.25 can be thought of as 25%. Before we give the formulas for the two diagnostic scenarios, we must first familiarize ourselves with the notation used.

tp: **True positives** are the number of patients who are infected and test positive.

fp: **False positives** are the number of patients who are not infected but test positive.

tn: **True negatives** are the number of patients who are not infected and also test negative.

fn: **False negatives** are the number of patients who are infected but test negative.

Following are the formulas for these probabilities.

$$\text{Diagnostic sensitivity} = \frac{tp}{tp + fn}$$

$$\text{Diagnostic specificity} = \frac{tn}{tn + fp}$$

EXAMPLE 12-1:   Six hundred patients who all showed symptoms of having mononucleosis were tested using a new test; 425 tested positive. Of these 425 patients, 25 were verified by culture to actually be negative. Of the patients who tested negative, 10 actually had mono. Find the diagnostic sensitivity and specificity for this new test.

By reading this information, we see that

$tp = 425 - 25 = 400,$

$fp = 25,$

$tn = 175 - 10 = 165$ (note that 175 comes from the fact that $600 - 425 = 175$),

$fn = 10.$

Substitute these values into the appropriate formulas.

$$\text{Diagnostic sensitivity} = \frac{tp}{tp + fn} = \frac{400}{400 + 10} = \frac{400}{410} = 0.976$$

$$\text{Diagnostic specificity} = \frac{tn}{tn + fp} = \frac{165}{165 + 25} = \frac{165}{190} = 0.868$$

Because sensitivity and specificity do not depend on the underlying probability of disease, test sensitivity and specificity can be applied in a variety of settings in which the disease prevalence is more or less common. Two values that are predictive are the positive predictive value (PPV) and the negative predictive value (NPV). The formulas for these are

$$PPV = \frac{tp}{\text{All positive tests}} = \frac{tp}{tp + fp},$$

$$NPV = \frac{tn}{\text{All negative tests}} = \frac{tn}{tn + fn}.$$

NOTE

To determine PPV and NPV, we must know something about the disease prevalence in the population.

EXAMPLE 12-2: Twenty thousand patients were tested last year for lyme disease using a new assay; 12,000 tested positive. Of these 12,000 that tested positive, 600 did not have lyme disease. Of the 8,000 that tested negative, 40 actually had lyme disease. Find the PPV and the NPV.

$tp = 12,000 - 600 = 11,400$

$fp = 600$

$tn = 8,000 - 40 = 7,960$

$fn = 40$

$$PPV = \frac{11,400}{11,400 + 600} = \frac{11,400}{12,000} = 0.950$$

$$NPV = \frac{7,960}{7,960 + 40} = \frac{7,960}{8,000} = 0.995$$

PRACTICE PROBLEMS: Section 12.1

1. Seven hundred patients who all showed symptoms of having hepatitis A were tested using a new test; 500 tested positive. Of these 500 patients, 50 were verified by culture to actually be negative. Of the patients who tested negative, 25 actually had hepatitis. Find the diagnostic sensitivity and specificity for this new test.

2. Six hundred and fifty patients who all showed symptoms of having mononucleosis were tested using a new test; 400 tested positive. Of these 400 patients, 35 were verified by culture to actually be negative. Of the patients who tested negative, 65 actually had mono. Find the diagnostic sensitivity and specificity for this new test.

3. Four hundred patients who all showed symptoms of having lyme disease were tested using a new test; 200 tested positive. Of these 200 patients, 50 were verified to actually be negative. Of the patients who tested negative, 40 actually had the disease. Find the diagnostic sensitivity and specificity for this new test.

4. Fifteen thousand patients were tested for lyme disease using a new assay; 11,000 tested positive. Of these 11,000 that tested positive, 500 did not have lyme disease. Of the 4,000 that tested negative, 60 actually had lyme disease. Find the PPV and the NPV.

5. One hundred twenty thousand patients were tested for mononucleosis using a new assay; 80,000 tested positive. Of these 80,000 that tested positive, 1,800 did not have mono. Of the 40,000 that tested negative, 800 actually had mono. Find the PPV and the NPV.

6. Ninety thousand patients were tested for hepatitis C using a new assay; 60,000 tested positive. Of these 60,000 that tested positive, 1,000 did not have the disease. Of the 30,000 that tested negative, 400 actually had hepatitis C. Find the PPV and the NPV.

12.2 – CONFIDENCE INTERVALS

A **confidence interval** is an interval of values that comes from sample information and gives us a percentage that measures our level of confidence. In the 95% confidence interval, we are 95% confident our hypothesis is correct. Keep in mind this means there is a 5% chance we are wrong. This 5% chance of being wrong is called the **significance level** and is denoted by $\alpha = 0.05$. Likewise, using a 99% confidence interval, we will be 99% confident our hypothesis is correct with only a 1% chance we are wrong; therefore, the significance level in this case is $\alpha = 0.01$. It logically follows to ask why we would ever use a 95% interval if we can use a 99% instead. To answer this we will first give the formulas for each confidence interval and then follow up with an example.

The formula for a 95% confidence interval for a single sample whose standard deviation is s and size, n, is 30 or greater is

$$\bar{x} \pm 1.96\frac{s}{\sqrt{n}}.$$

The formula for a 99% confidence interval for a single sample whose size, n, is 30 or greater is

$$\bar{x} \pm 2.58\frac{s}{\sqrt{n}}.$$

EXAMPLE 12-3: Each of 30 specimens in a sample was measured using an instrument to determine glucose levels. This sample was found to have a mean glucose level of 90 $^{mg}/_{dL}$ with a standard deviation of 5.0 $^{mg}/_{dL}$. Find the 95% and 99% confidence intervals for this sample.

The 95% confidence interval is $\bar{x} \pm 1.96\frac{s}{\sqrt{n}}$. We are given that $\bar{x} = 90$, $s = 5.0$, and $n = 30$. Substituting these into the formula, we get

$$90 \pm 1.96\frac{5.0}{\sqrt{30}} = 90 \pm 1.8.$$

Now $90 - 1.8 = 88.2$ and $90 + 1.8 = 91.8$.

Therefore, the 95% confidence interval is 88.2 to 91.8.

The 99% confidence interval is $\bar{x} \pm 2.58\frac{s}{\sqrt{n}}$.

Substituting the given values into this formula, we get

$$90 \pm 2.58\frac{5.0}{\sqrt{30}} = 90 \pm 2.4.$$

Now $90 - 2.4 = 87.6$ and $90 + 2.4 = 92.4$.

Therefore, the 99% confidence interval is 87.6 to 92.4.

Looking at these two results, we see the 95% interval is smaller than the 99% interval. We must realize that the more confident we are, the larger our interval. The larger the interval, the more likely a data value will fall within that range. There is a give and take between confidence and the interval size associated with that confidence.

PRACTICE PROBLEMS: Section 12.2

1. Each of 20 specimens in a sample was measured using an instrument to determine glucose levels. This sample was found to have a mean glucose level of 95 $\frac{mg}{dL}$ with a standard deviation of 4.5 $\frac{mg}{dL}$. Find the 95% and 99% confidence intervals for this sample.

2. Each of 25 specimens in a sample was measured using an instrument to determine cholesterol levels. This sample was found to have a mean cholesterol level of 240 $\frac{mg}{dL}$ with a standard deviation of 5.5 $\frac{mg}{dL}$. Find the 95% and 99% confidence intervals for this sample.

3. Each of 30 specimens in a sample was measured using an instrument to determine fibrinogen levels. This sample was found to have a mean fibrinogen level of 300 $\frac{mg}{dL}$ with a standard deviation of 3.2 $\frac{mg}{dL}$. Find the 95% and 99% confidence intervals for this sample.

4. Each of 30 specimens in a sample was measured using an instrument to determine glucose levels. This sample was found to have a mean glucose level of 100 $\frac{mg}{dL}$ with a standard deviation of 5.5 $\frac{mg}{dL}$. Find the 95% confidence interval for this sample. If the sample size were 10, find the 95% confidence interval. What observation is seen between the two sample sizes?

12.3 – TESTING THE DIFFERENCE BETWEEN TWO MEANS

In Example 12-3 we had only one sample. However, often we are comparing two instruments (or methods). When two instruments are compared, one is the *reference* instrument (known to be reliable), and the other is the *test* instrument. To analyze the two, we formulate hypotheses. These hypotheses involve the mean of the two instruments. The null hypothesis, H_0, is a statement about the relationship between the means of the two instruments, and the alternative hypothesis, H_1, is a statement about how the relationship stated in H_0 is not true. The alternative hypothesis in usually in one of the following forms:

a) The mean of instrument A is statistically less than the mean of instrument B.

b) The mean of instrument A is statistically greater than the mean of instrument B.

c) The statistical mean of instrument A is significantly different from the statistical mean of instrument B.

In the case of a or b when there is an inequality involved, we have a situation called a one-tailed test. The graph involving a *greater than* inequality would look like the diagram in Figure 12–1. The shaded region is called the **rejection region**, and we discuss this further in Example 12-4.

The graph involving a *less than* inequality would look like the diagram in Figure 12–2.

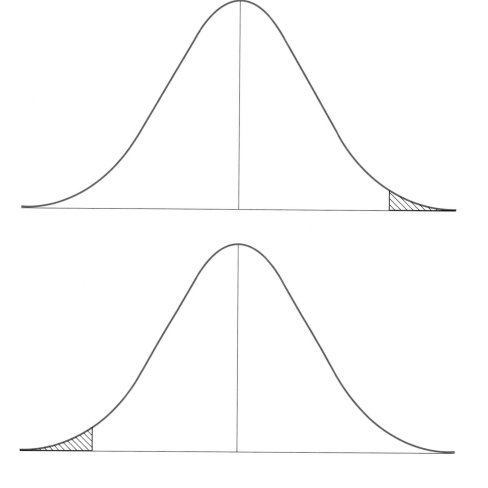

FIGURE 12–1
Rejection Region for
Greater than Inequality

FIGURE 12–2
Rejection Region for
Less than Inequality

When we are looking to see whether the results from instrument A are significantly *different* from those of instrument B, we have a situation called a two-tailed test, and the corresponding graph would look like the diagram in Figure 12–3.

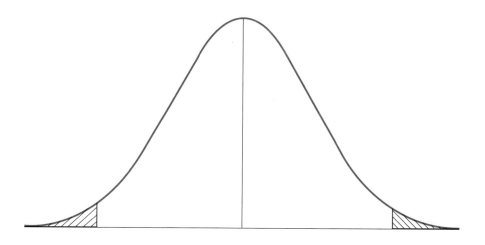

FIGURE 12–3
Rejection Region for
Significantly Different

To compare two normally distributed, grouped sets of data (two methods or two instruments), the paired *t*-test or paired *z*-test is used to determine whether there is a significant difference between the two sets. If the set contains more than 30 data values, the *z*-test is used, and if the sample size is less than or equal to 30, the *t*-test is used. In this section we concentrate on samples with 30 or fewer data values because, as mentioned before, 20 measurements (1 measurement each working day for four weeks) is commonly worked with in the laboratory. When using these tests, we are comparing the means of the two sets. For either test there are five steps to follow.

1) State hypotheses.

2) State the significance level.

3) Perform calculations and state the test.

4) Determine the rejection region.

5) Draw conclusions.

One last comment, the **degrees of freedom**, or **d.f.**, is defined as being 1 less than the number of data values, or aliquots, in a sample. Thus, $d.f. = n - 1$.

The formula for testing the null hypothesis, H_0, with a small sample (≤ 30) is

$$t = \frac{\bar{x} - \mu}{\frac{s}{\sqrt{n}}} \qquad \text{where } d.f. = n - 1.$$

EXAMPLE 12-4: A distributor of laboratory control products makes a claim that the average price for all its controls is $75 per control. Twenty controls were randomly sampled, and it was found that the mean price was $84 and the standard deviation was $14. Is there sufficient evidence that the distributor is falsely advertising? Test at the 1% level of significance.

Step 1: Assume the distributor's claim is correct (the null hypothesis) and try to prove it is incorrect by showing the alternative hypothesis is truthful. To prove false advertising, you must show that the mean cost μ of all the controls is more than $75. The burden of proof lies on the claim that the mean cost is actually more than $75. Thus,

$$H_0 : \mu = 75$$
$$H_1 : \mu > 75$$

Step 2: $\alpha = 0.01$ because we are testing at the 1% significance level.

Step 3: Because $n \leq 30$, we use the *t*-test where $n = 20, \bar{x} = 84, s = 14$.

$$t = \frac{\bar{x} - \mu}{\frac{s}{\sqrt{n}}} = \frac{84 - 75}{\frac{14}{\sqrt{20}}} = 2.875$$

NOTE

We rounded to three decimal places because the numbers in Table 12–1 contain three decimal places.

Step 4: Because H_1 involves the *greater than* relationship, the rejection region is the right-hand tail.

Refer to Table 12–1, where $d.f. = n - 1 = 19$, and we have one tail, $\alpha = 0.01$. Now find 19 under the *d.f.* column and $\alpha = 0.01$ in the one-tail row. The number associated with 19 in the *d.f.* column *and* the $\alpha = 0.01$ row is 2.539. Therefore, the one-tailed graph in this case would look like the following:

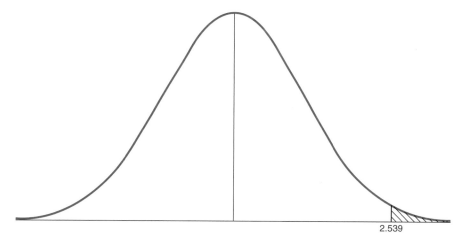

Step 5: From step 3 we know $t = 2.875$. The location of this value on the curve lies in the shaded rejection region (see the following diagram). Therefore, $H_0: \mu = 75$ is rejected, and we conclude that the mean price charged by this distributor is greater than \$75. But remember, we are 99% confident that our conclusion is correct, which means there is a 1% chance we could be wrong.

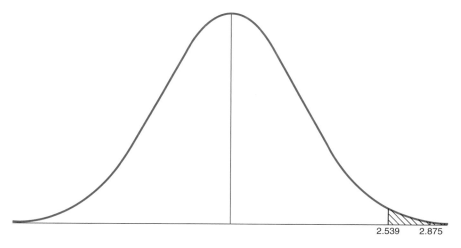

TABLE 12-1 The *t*-Table

d.f.	CONFIDENCE INTERVALS ONE TAIL, α TWO TAILS, α	50% 0.25 0.50	80% 0.10 0.20	90% 0.05 0.10	95% 0.025 0.05	98% 0.01 0.02	99% 0.005 0.01
1		1.000	3.078	6.314	12.706	31.821	63.657
2		.816	1.886	2.920	4.303	6.965	9.925
3		.765	1.638	2.353	3.182	4.541	5.841
4		.741	1.533	2.132	2.776	3.747	4.604
5		.727	1.476	2.015	2.571	3.365	4.032
6		.718	1.440	1.943	2.447	3.143	3.707
7		.711	1.415	1.895	2.365	2.998	3.499
8		.706	1.397	1.860	2.306	2.896	3.355
9		.703	1.383	1.833	2.262	2.821	3.250
10		.700	1.372	1.812	2.228	2.764	3.169
11		.697	1.363	1.796	2.201	2.718	3.106
12		.695	1.356	1.782	2.179	2.681	3.055
13		.694	1.350	1.771	2.160	2.650	3.012
14		.692	1.345	1.761	2.145	2.624	2.977
15		.691	1.341	1.753	2.131	2.602	2.947
16		.690	1.337	1.746	2.120	2.583	2.921
17		.689	1.333	1.740	2.110	2.567	2.898
18		.688	1.330	1.734	2.101	2.552	2.878
19		.688	1.328	1.729	2.093	2.539	2.861
20		.687	1.325	1.725	2.086	2.528	2.845
21		.686	1.323	1.721	2.080	2.518	2.831
22		.686	1.321	1.717	2.074	2.508	2.819
23		.685	1.319	1.714	2.069	2.500	2.807
24		.685	1.318	1.711	2.064	2.492	2.797
25		.684	1.316	1.708	2.060	2.485	2.787
26		.684	1.315	1.706	2.056	2.479	2.779
27		.684	1.314	1.703	2.052	2.473	2.771
28		.683	1.313	1.701	2.048	2.467	2.763
(z) ∞		.674	1.282	1.645	1.960	2.326	2.576

Source: From Beyer, W. H. (1986). *Handbook of Tables for Probability and Statistics* (2nd ed.). Boca Raton, FL: CRC Press. Reprinted with permission.

Shortly we will give the formula for the paired *t*-test, but first we need to be familiar with the notation contained in this formula.

Let *A* represent the sample values from instrument 1 and *B* represent the sample values from instrument 2. Let *n* represent the number of aliquots, let μ_A be the mean of the values obtained from instrument 1, and let μ_B be the mean of the values obtained from instrument 2. The formula for the *t*-statistic is then

$$t = \frac{\sum(A-B)/n - \mu}{\sqrt{\dfrac{\sum(A-B)^2 - \dfrac{(\sum(A-B))^2}{n}}{n-1}}} \times \sqrt{n}.$$

We now explain in more detail the meaning of the notation in this formula.

$\sum(A-B)$ means subtract each value of instrument 2 from each corresponding value of instrument 1 and then add up each of these resulting differences.

$\sum(A-B)^2$ means subtract each value of instrument 2 from each corresponding value of instrument 1, square each of the resulting differences, and then add up those results.

$\left(\sum(A-B)\right)^2$ means take the result of $\sum(A-B)$ and square it.

If we let $D=A-B$ and $\overline{D}=\sum(A-B)=\sum D$, we can express the t-statistic formula in the following way.

$$t = \frac{\overline{D}/n-\mu}{\sqrt{\dfrac{\sum D^2-(\overline{D})^2/n}{(n-1)}}} \times \sqrt{n}$$

EXAMPLE 12-5: Two different laboratories are often asked to analyze aliquots from the same specimen. The medical company sending the samples to the two labs wants to know whether there is a statistically significant difference between the instruments used at each lab at the 99% confidence level. To determine whether there is a significant difference, 10 patient samples were divided into two aliquots and then each aliquot was analyzed on the two instruments in each lab for protein. Following are the results in grams per deciliter.

ALIQUOT	INSTRUMENT A	B
1.	6	8
2.	7	8
3.	5	7
4.	7	8
5.	8	6
6.	5	4
7.	7	6
8.	5	6
9.	6	5
10.	7	9

Because we want to know whether there is a statistically significant difference between the two, we will let $\mu = \mu_A - \mu_B$. If there is no significant difference between the two instruments, $\mu_A = \mu_B$ and thus $\mu = \mu_A - \mu_B = 0$. Therefore, we will let H_0 be $\mu = 0$ and H_1 be $\mu \neq 0$.

Step 1: $H_0 : \mu = 0$

$H_1 : \mu \neq 0$

Step 2: The confidence level is 99%, so $\alpha = 0.01$.

Step 3: Because $n = 10$, we must use the t-test. To calculate the values of D and $\overline{D}$, begin by setting up a table from the given data.

A	B	D = A − B	D²
6	8	−2	4
7	8	−1	1
5	7	−2	4
7	8	−1	1
8	6	2	4
5	4	1	1
7	6	1	1
5	6	−1	1
6	5	1	1
7	9	−2	4

$$\overline{D} = \sum D = -4 \qquad \sum D^2 = 22$$

Substituting these results into

$$t = \frac{\overline{D}/n - \mu}{\sqrt{\frac{\sum D^2 - \left(\overline{D}\right)^2 / n}{(n-1)}}} \times \sqrt{n},$$

we get

$$t = \frac{-4/10 - 0}{\sqrt{\frac{22 - (-4)^2/10}{9}}} \times \sqrt{10}.$$

Simplifying some we get

$$t = \frac{-0.400}{\sqrt{\frac{22 - 16/10}{9}}} \times 3.162$$

$$= \frac{-0.400}{\sqrt{2.267}} \times 3.162.$$

Finally we find

$$t = \frac{-0.400}{1.506} \times 3.162 = -0.840.$$

Step 4: The number of aliquots is 10, so $d.f. = 10 - 1 = 9$. Last, we compare this t value with the value obtained from the t distribution chart given in Table 12–1. When looking at this chart, keep in mind that $\alpha = 0.01$, $d.f. = 9$, and we have a two-tailed test (because we are determining whether the two instruments are different). Next we find 9 under the $d.f.$ column and $\alpha = 0.01$ in the two-tails row. The number associated with 9 in the $d.f.$ column *and* the $\alpha = 0.01$ row is 3.250. Therefore, the two-tailed graph in this case would look like the following diagram. The location of $+3.250$ and -3.250 should be more to the right and left, respectively, but they are positioned in this manner so we can easily see the shaded area.

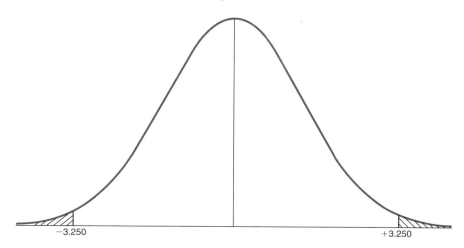

Step 5: Our t value is -0.840, whose position is labeled on the following graph. We can see this t value does not lie in the shaded rejection region, so this means we accept the null hypothesis, which says $\mu = \mu_A - \mu_B = 0$. That there is not a significant statistical difference between their means implies that there is not a significant statistical difference between the two protein values of the two instruments.

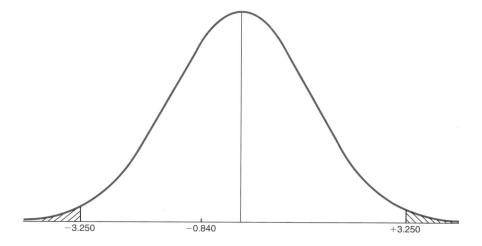

EXAMPLE 12-6: Twelve patient samples were each divided into two aliquots and then one aliquot was analyzed on the "home" instrument for glucose values. The other aliquot was shipped to another lab to be tested. Following are the results in

milligrams per deciliter. Determine at the 95% confidence level whether there is a statistically significant difference between the two instruments used.

ALIQUOT	INSTRUMENT A	B
1.	121	130
2.	104	108
3.	70	85
4.	120	144
5.	100	109
6.	140	155
7.	112	125
8.	95	100
9.	130	124
10.	140	152
11.	98	110
12.	94	103

We want to know whether there is a statistically significant difference between the two, so we will let $\mu = \mu_A - \mu_B$. If there is no difference between the two means, then $\mu = \mu_A - \mu_B = 0$. Thus, we will let H_0 be $\mu = 0$ and H_1 be $\mu \neq 0$.

Step 1: $H_0 : \mu = 0$

$\quad\quad H_1 : \mu \neq 0$

Step 2: The confidence level is 95%, so $\alpha = 0.05$.

Step 3: Because $n = 12$, we must use the t-test. To calculate the values of D and $\overline{D}$, we begin by setting up a table from the given data.

A	B	D = A − B	D²
121	130	−9	81
104	108	−4	16
70	80	−10	100
120	118	2	4
100	109	−9	81
140	145	−5	25
112	125	−13	169
95	100	−5	25
130	124	6	36
140	152	−12	144
98	110	−12	144
94	91	3	9

$$\overline{D} = \sum D = -68 \qquad \sum D^2 = 834$$

Substituting these results into

$$t = \frac{\overline{D}/n-\mu}{\sqrt{\dfrac{\sum D^2 - \left(\overline{D}\right)^2/n}{(n-1)}}} \times \sqrt{n}$$

we get

$$t = \frac{-68/12-0}{\sqrt{\dfrac{834-(-68)^2/12}{11}}} \times \sqrt{12}.$$

Simplifying some we get

$$t = \frac{-5.667}{\sqrt{\dfrac{834-4{,}624/12}{11}}} \times 3.464$$

$$= \frac{-5.667}{\sqrt{40.788}} \times 3.464.$$

Finally we find

$$t = \frac{-5.667}{6.387} \times 3.464 = -3.074.$$

Step 4: The number of aliquots is 12, so $d.f. = 12 - 1 = 11$. Finally, we compare this t value with the value obtained from the t distribution chart given in Table 12–1. When looking at this chart, keep in mind that $\alpha = 0.05$, $d.f. = 11$, and we have a two-tailed test (because we are determining whether the two instruments are different). Next, find the number 11 under the $d.f.$ column and $\alpha = 0.05$ in the two-tails row. The number associated with the $d.f.$ column *and* the $\alpha = 0.05$ row is 2.201. Therefore, the two-tailed graph, including the location of our calculated value for t, would look like the following:

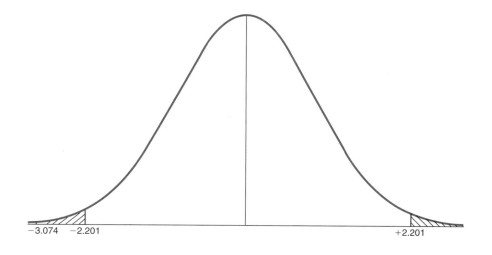

Step 5: Our t value is -3.074, whose position is labeled on the graph; note that this t value does lie in the shaded rejection region, so this means we reject the null hypothesis, which says $\mu = \mu_A - \mu_B = 0$. This implies there is a significant statistical difference between their means, or in other words, there is a significant statistical difference between the two protein values of the two instruments.

PRACTICE PROBLEMS: Section 12.3

1. Find the t value for $\alpha = 0.01$ with $d.f. = 22$ for a right-tailed test.

2. Find the t value for $\alpha = 0.05$ with $d.f. = 17$ for a left-tailed test.

3. Find the t value for $\alpha = 0.01$ with $d.f. = 25$ for a two-tailed test.

4. Find the t value for $\alpha = 0.05$ with $d.f. = 20$ for a two-tailed test.

5. A laboratory claims that the average salary for its technicians is $50,000. A random sample of 10 technicians from this lab had a mean salary of $49,500 with a standard deviation of $500. Is there enough evidence to reject the laboratory's claim at the $\alpha = 0.01$ level?

6. A supervisor claims the average amount of time to measure glucose values for a set amount of specimens is 45 minutes. A random sample of 12 employees had a mean time of 50 minutes per set with a standard deviation of 3 minutes. Is there enough evidence to reject the supervisor's claim at the $\alpha = 0.05$ level?

7. A supervisor claims that the average amount of time needed to count the number of RBCs for a specimen is 25 minutes. A random sample of 15 employees had a mean time of 27 minutes with a standard deviation of 2 minutes. Is there enough evidence to reject the supervisor's claim at the $\alpha = 0.01$ level?

8. A laboratory just purchased a new instrument, and it wants to determine whether there is a statistically significant difference between its older instrument and the new one at the 95% confidence level. To determine whether there is a significant difference, 12 patient samples were divided into two aliquots and then each aliquot was analyzed on both instruments for protein. Following are the results in grams per deciliter. Is there a significant difference?

| | INSTRUMENT | |
ALIQUOT	A	B
1.	8	7
2.	7	6
3.	6	5
4.	7	6
5.	8	8
6.	5	4
7.	7	6
8.	5	4
9.	6	7
10.	7	7
11.	8	7
12.	6	6

9. A laboratory just purchased a new instrument, and it wants to determine whether there is a statistically significant difference between its older instrument and the new one at the 99% confidence level. To determine whether there is a significant difference, 10 patient samples

were divided into two aliquots and then each aliquot was analyzed on both instruments for protein. Following are the results in grams per deciliter. Is there a significant difference?

	INSTRUMENT	
ALIQUOT	A	B
1.	5	6
2.	7	6
3.	5	7
4.	7	6
5.	8	9
6.	5	5
7.	7	8
8.	5	4
9.	6	5
10.	7	8

10. Twenty patient samples were each divided into two aliquots and then one aliquot was analyzed on the "home" instrument for glucose values. The other aliquot was shipped to another lab to be tested. Following are the results in milligrams per deciliter. Determine whether there is a statistically significant difference between the two instruments used at the 95% confidence level.

	INSTRUMENT	
ALIQUOT	A	B
1.	109	121
2.	115	123
3.	70	78
4.	120	129
5.	100	110
6.	130	145
7.	102	115
8.	97	103
9.	120	131
10.	131	143
11.	93	100
12.	99	105
13.	107	118
14.	106	103
15.	128	132
16.	136	148
17.	124	129
18.	107	105
19.	115	122
20.	104	111

11. Twelve patient samples were each divided into two aliquots and then one aliquot was analyzed on the "home" instrument for glucose values. The other aliquot was shipped to another lab to be tested. Following are the results in milligrams per deciliter. Determine whether there is a statistically significant difference between the two instruments used at the 99% confidence level.

	INSTRUMENT	
ALIQUOT	A	B
1.	120	122
2.	112	110
3.	80	83
4.	130	127
5.	120	119
6.	132	130
7.	115	118
8.	105	104
9.	110	110
10.	138	136
11.	100	102
12.	97	100

12. Fifteen patient samples were each divided into two aliquots and then one aliquot was analyzed on the one instrument for glucose values. The other aliquot was shipped to another lab to be tested. Following are the results in milligrams per deciliter. Determine whether there is a statistically significant difference between the two instruments used at the 95% confidence level.

	INSTRUMENT	
ALIQUOT	A	B
1.	119	120
2.	115	118
3.	110	102
4.	110	104
5.	120	124
6.	130	131
7.	132	136
8.	99	108
9.	120	118
10.	100	103
11.	98	98
12.	104	103
13.	106	110
14.	118	112
15.	128	134

12.4 – CORRELATION

The next section covers linear regression analysis. However, applying a linear regression analysis is not always appropriate. To determine whether this type of analysis should be applied, we first need to determine whether there is a correlation between the variables involved in the analysis. As an everyday example, if x is the temperature on some summer day and y is the number of ice creams sold at an ice cream shop, then there is probably a correlation between x and y. Two variables will either have no linear relationship, a positive linear relationship, a negative linear relationship, or a nonlinear relationship. Following is an example of each scenario.

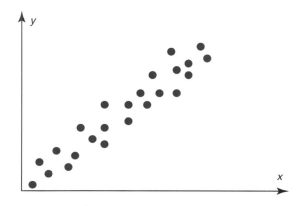

Positive linear correlation (as x increases y tends to increase).

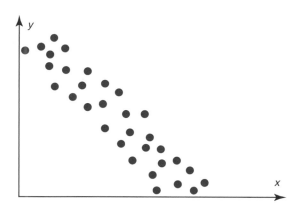

Negative linear correlation (as x increases y tends to decrease).

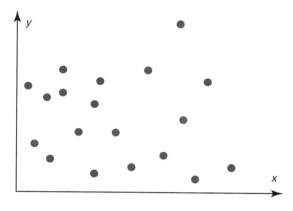

No correlation.

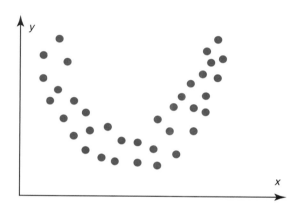

Nonlinear correlation.

To determine whether there is a linear correlation between two variables, we must calculate the **correlation coefficient**, r. The formula for r is

$$r = \frac{n\sum xy - (\sum x)(\sum y)}{\sqrt{n(\sum x^2) - (\sum x)^2}\sqrt{n(\sum y^2) - (\sum y)^2}}$$

where n is the number of pairs of data. The numerical value of r will always be between -1 and $+1$. If r is close to 0, then there is no linear correlation between x and y. If r is close to -1, there is a strong negative linear correlation, and if r is close to $+1$ there is a strong positive linear correlation. If there is no linear correlation (r is close to 0) between the variables, then there is no point in trying to do a linear regression analysis.

EXAMPLE 12-7: The following table lists values obtained from measuring 12 citrate levels using two different instruments. Each number is in milligrams per deciliter. Calculate the correlation coefficient and determine whether it would be wise to do a linear regression analysis.

Measurement	1	2	3	4	5	6	7	8	9	10	11	12
Reference instrument x	2.0	1.8	2.1	2.2	2.3	2.0	1.9	2.4	2.0	2.3	2.2	2.0
Test instrument y	2.1	1.9	2.2	2.3	2.4	2.0	2.1	2.4	2.1	2.4	2.3	2.2

To use the correlation coefficient formula, first calculate each piece within the formula by constructing a table:

MEASUREMENT	x	y	x^2	y^2
1	2.0	2.1	4.0	4.41
2	1.8	1.9	3.24	3.61
3	2.1	2.2	4.41	4.84
4	2.2	2.3	4.84	5.29
5	2.3	2.4	5.29	5.76
6	2.0	2.0	4.00	4.00
7	1.9	2.1	3.61	4.41
8	2.4	2.4	5.76	5.76
9	2.0	2.1	4.00	4.41
10	2.3	2.4	5.29	5.76
11	2.2	2.3	4.84	5.29
12	2.0	2.2	4.00	4.84
	$\sum x = 25.2$	$\sum y = 26.4$	$\sum x^2 = 53.28$	$\sum y^2 = 58.38$

Adding the product of each x with each corresponding y, we get $\sum xy = 55.75$.

$$\left(\sum x\right)^2 = (25.2)^2 = 635.0$$

$$\left(\sum y\right)^2 = (26.4)^2 = 697.0$$

Plugging all this into the formula $r = \dfrac{n\sum xy - \left(\sum x\right)\left(\sum y\right)}{\sqrt{n\left(\sum x^2\right) - \left(\sum x\right)^2}\sqrt{n\left(\sum y^2\right) - \left(\sum y\right)^2}}$,

we get

$$r = \frac{12(55.75) - (25.2)(26.4)}{\sqrt{12(53.28) - (25.2)^2}\sqrt{12(58.38) - (26.4)^2}}.$$

Simplifying some we get

$$r = \frac{669-665.28}{\sqrt{639.36-635.04}\sqrt{700.56-696.96}}$$

$$= \frac{3.72}{\sqrt{4.32}\sqrt{3.6}}$$

$$= \frac{3.72}{3.94} = 0.944.$$

Clearly, 0.944 is very close to +1; therefore, there is a strong positive relationship between the two instruments, and it would be appropriate to proceed with a linear regression analysis.

EXAMPLE 12-8: The correlation coefficient was calculated for a set of data gathered from two instruments measuring creatinine levels. The value of the correlation coefficient was found to be $r = 0.215$. Would it be appropriate to use a linear regression analysis to make predictions based on this sample?

Because r is close to zero, there is not a significant correlation and it would not be appropriate to do a linear regression analysis.

Note: Practice problems for Section 12.4 are grouped with the practice problems for Section 12.5.

12.5 – LINEAR REGRESSION ANALYSIS

As discussed in Section 12-3, the *t*-test can tell us whether there is a significant difference between two instruments, but that is all it tells us. A linear regression analysis, on the other hand, can help us understand why there is a significant difference. In this section we do linear regression analyses using the method of least squares. Before discussing this further, let's refresh our memories with the basic format of any linear equation, which is

$$y = mx + b.$$

When we are applying linear regression, the formula $y = mx + b$ is often written as $y_c = mx + b$ where y_c stands for the *calculated* value, m is the slope, b is the y-intercept, and x is a value from the reference instrument. Once we have the values for m, b, and x, we can then substitute those values into the equation to predict the value of y_c. Remember, the calculated values of y are estimates. When we see the notation y_m, this denotes a *measured* value of y obtained by using the test instrument. When applying linear

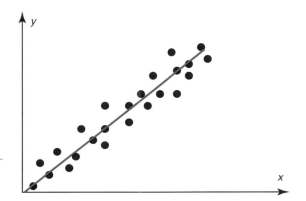

FIGURE 12–4
Line of Best Fit

regression analysis in the lab, we must be sure the reference instrument/method is precise and reliable; we should not use old data because it may not be valid; when using the equation to predict values, we must stay within the scope of the sample; each instrument/method must be functioning properly; and random error must be at a minimum.

Following are the formulas for m and b.

$$m = \frac{n(\sum xy)-(\sum x)(\sum y)}{n(\sum x^2)-(\sum x)^2} \qquad b = \frac{(\sum y)(\sum x^2)-(\sum x)(\sum xy)}{n(\sum x^2)-(\sum x)^2}$$

The line in Figure 12–4 is a line calculated by using linear regression analysis. This line is also called the **line of best fit**. We can see when we calculate values using the equation for this line that those values will be close but not exact because all the data points do not lie on the line.

CLSI standards should be referenced when doing linear regression analyses. The examples in this book contain samples that are relatively small, but this is just to illustrate the concepts being taught. Typically there will more data values as suggested by CLSI standards and guidelines, not just 12 to 15.

EXAMPLE 12-9: As we determined, the data set in Example 12-7 had a strong positive relationship because $r = 0.944$; thus, it makes sense to continue with a linear regression analysis to find the line of best fit.

As we found in Example 12-7:

$$\sum xy = 55.75 \qquad \sum x = 25.2 \qquad \sum y = 26.4$$

$$\sum x^2 = 53.28 \qquad (\sum x)^2 = (25.2)^2 = 635.0$$

Substituting these into the formula for the slope, we get

$$m = \frac{n(\sum xy)-(\sum x)(\sum y)}{n(\sum x^2)-(\sum x)^2} = \frac{12(55.75)-(25.2)(26.4)}{12(53.28)-635.0}$$

$$= \frac{669-665.28}{639.36-635.0},$$

which simplifies to

$$m = \frac{3.72}{4.36} = 0.853.$$

NOTE

The closer m is to 1.000, the stronger the correlation between the two instruments.

Now we will calculate b:

$$b = \frac{(\sum y)(\sum x^2)-(\sum x)(\sum xy)}{n(\sum x^2)-(\sum x)^2}.$$

Substituting the values we get

$$b = \frac{(26.4)(53.28)-(25.2)(55.75)}{12(53.28)-(25.2)^2}$$

$$= \frac{1,406.592-1,404.9}{639.36-635.04},$$

which simplifies to

$$b = \frac{1,406.592-1,404.9}{639.36-635.04} = \frac{1.692}{4.32} = 0.392.$$

Substituting the values we just calculated for m and b into the equation $y_c = mx + b$, we get

$$y_c = 0.853x + 0.392.$$

Now we can use this formula to calculate (estimated) values of y given some value for x. For example, if the value of x is 2.4 mg/dL, the calculated value of y would be

$$y_c = 0.853(2.4) + 0.392 = 2.439.$$

However, this is an estimate and there is a certain amount of error involved. If we graph the line $y_c = 0.853x + 0.392$, the points from our data set would not all fall exactly on this line. Some will deviate from this line (see Figure 12–4). In order to get a better understanding of how many data points deviate from this line, and by how much, we need to calculate the **standard error estimate** (SEE). The closer this value is to zero, the better. This is because in order for the SEE to be zero, all the calculated values of y_c would have to be the same as all the measured values of y_m as seen in the following formula for the SEE.

$$SEE = \sqrt{\frac{\sum(y_m - y_c)^2}{n-2}}$$

In this formula y_m is the measured value of y obtained from the test instrument and y_c is the calculated value of y obtained by using the measured value x from the reference instrument. If we look at the data given in Example 12-7, we can compute $y_m - y_c$ and $(y_m - y_c)^2$ for each set of corresponding measurements as shown in the following table. The values of $(y_m - y_c)^2$ are rounded to four decimal places so that we can get a more precise value for the SEE. Five or six decimal places would be even better.

MEASUREMENT	x		y_c	y_m	$y_m - y_c$	$(y_m - y_c)^2$
1	2.0	$y_c = 0.853(2.0) + 0.392 = 2.1$	2.098	2.1	0.002	0.0000
2	1.8	$y_c = 0.853(1.8) + 0.392 = 1.9$	1.927	1.9	−0.027	0.0007
3	2.1	$y_c = 0.853(2.1) + 0.392 = 2.2$	2.183	2.2	0.017	0.0003
4	2.2		2.269	2.3	0.031	0.0010
5	2.3		2.354	2.4	0.046	0.0021
6	2.0		2.098	2.0	−0.098	0.0096
7	1.9		2.013	2.1	0.087	0.0076
8	2.4		2.439	2.4	−0.039	0.0015
9	2.0		2.098	2.1	0.002	0.0000
10	2.3		2.354	2.4	0.046	0.0021
11	2.2		2.269	2.3	0.031	0.0010
12	2.0		2.098	2.2	0.102	0.0104

To compute the value of SEE, we first need to add up all of the $(y_m - y_c)^2$ values.

$$\sum(y_m - y_c)^2 = 0.0363$$

Substituting this value along with the fact that $n = 12$ into the SEE formula, we get

$$SEE = \sqrt{\frac{\sum(y_m - y_c)^2}{n-2}} = \sqrt{\frac{0.0363}{10}} = 0.0602.$$

This value of 0.0602 is telling us that the standard deviation of the measured values y_m about the predicted values y_c is 0.0602. Therefore, the measured values will deviate by no more than 0.0602 from the calculated values about 68.3% of the time. If we double this value, we get 0.1204, which gives us information about how often and by how much the measured values will deviate from the predicted values by 2 standard deviations. The value of 0.1204 is telling us the measured values will deviate by no more than 0.1204 from the calculated values about 95.5% of the time.

EXAMPLE 12-10: A new instrument was used to measure iron levels. Following are the results of 15 measurements done using the new instrument (instrument B) and 15 corresponding measurements from the reference instrument (instrument A). The units associated with each measurement are micrograms per 100 milliliters. Calculate the correlation coefficient and determine whether it would be sensible to do a regression analysis. If it is sensible, find the line of best fit and also calculate the SEE and interpret its results.

ALIQUOT	INSTRUMENT A	B
1.	68	72
2.	91	94
3.	123	127
4.	70	72
5.	86	89
6.	126	130
7.	122	125
8.	148	153
9.	109	113
10.	89	93
11.	62	65
12.	150	155
13.	102	106
14.	137	142
15.	128	132

From this table the following calculations were computed. (Use the calculator to see whether you obtain the same values.)

$\sum x = 1,611$ $\sum y = 1,668$ $\sum xy = 191,075$ $\sum x^2 = 184,697$

$\sum y^2 = 197,680$ $(\sum x)^2 = 2,595,321$ $(\sum y)^2 = 2,782,224$

Substituting these values into the correlation coefficient formula, we obtain

$$r = \frac{n\sum xy - (\sum x)(\sum y)}{\sqrt{n(\sum x^2) - (\sum x)^2}\sqrt{n(\sum y^2) - (\sum y)^2}}$$

$$= \frac{(15)(191,075) - (1,611)(1,668)}{\sqrt{(15)(184,697) - 2,595,321}\sqrt{(15)(197,680) - 2,782,224}}$$

$$= \frac{178,977}{\sqrt{175,134}\sqrt{182,976}} = 0.999.$$

Because this is very close to 1, there is a very strong correlation between the two instruments. Therefore, it would be appropriate to do a linear regression analysis.

$$m = \frac{n(\Sigma xy)-(\Sigma x)(\Sigma y)}{n(\Sigma x^2)-(\Sigma x)^2} = \frac{(15)(191,075)-(1,611)(1,668)}{(15)(184,697)-2,595,321} = \frac{178,977}{175,134} = 1.022$$

$$b = \frac{(\Sigma y)(\Sigma x^2)-(\Sigma x)(\Sigma xy)}{n(\Sigma x^2)-(\Sigma x)^2} = \frac{(1,668)(184,697)-(1,611)(191,075)}{(15)(184,697)-2,595,321} = \frac{252,771}{175,134} = 1.443$$

Therefore, the line of best fit is $y_c = 1.022x + 1.443$.

Plugging the values of the reference instrument A in for x to find the corresponding calculated values of y_c and then substituting these into the SEE formula, we find

$$\text{SEE} = \sqrt{\frac{\Sigma(y_m-y_c)^2}{n-2}} = 0.6063.$$

Again, use your calculator to do these computations to make sure you get the same value. Your answer may vary a little bit depending upon how many decimal places you round to.

PRACTICE PROBLEMS: Section 12.5

1. The correlation coefficient was calculated for a set of data gathered from two instruments measuring creatinine levels. The value of the correlation coefficient was found to be $r = -0.115$. Would it be appropriate to use a linear regression analysis to make predictions based on this sample?

2. The correlation coefficient was calculated for a set of data gathered from two instruments measuring creatinine levels. The value of the correlation coefficient was found to be $r = -0.815$. Would it be appropriate to use a linear regression analysis to make predictions based on this sample?

3. The correlation coefficient was calculated for a set of data gathered from two instruments measuring creatinine levels. The value of the correlation coefficient was found to be $r = 0.871$. Would it be appropriate to use a linear regression analysis to make predictions based on this sample?

4. The following table lists values obtained from measuring 12 citrate levels using two different instruments. Each number is in milligrams per deciliter. Calculate the correlation coefficient and determine whether it would be wise to do a regression analysis. If it is wise, find the line of best fit and also calculate the SEE and interpret its results.

MEASUREMENT	1	2	3	4	5	6	7	8	9	10	11	12
Reference instrument x	2.3	1.9	2.2	2.1	2.2	1.9	2.0	2.1	2.2	2.0	2.2	2.3
Test instrument y	2.1	1.9	2.3	2.0	2.3	2.0	2.1	2.0	2.3	2.1	2.0	2.2

5. A new instrument was used to measure iron levels. Following are the results of 15 measurements using the new instrument (instrument B) and 15 corresponding measurements from the reference instrument (instrument A). Each measurement is in micrograms per 100 mL. Calculate the correlation coefficient and determine whether it would be wise to do a regression analysis. If it is wise, find the line of best fit and also calculate the SEE and interpret its results.

ALIQUOT	INSTRUMENT A	B
1.	96	100
2.	125	128
3.	80	84
4.	75	80
5.	130	135
6.	141	143
7.	122	127
8.	99	102
9.	110	115
10.	90	92
11.	98	102
12.	104	109
13.	106	110
14.	113	115
15.	138	143

6. A new instrument was used to measure iron levels. Following are the results of 15 measurements using the new instrument (instrument B) and 15 corresponding measurements from the reference instrument (instrument A). Each measurement is in micrograms per 100 mL. Calculate the correlation coefficient and determine whether it would be wise to do a regression analysis. If it is wise, find the line of best fit and also calculate the SEE and interpret its results.

ALIQUOT	INSTRUMENT A	B
1.	112	104
2.	122	130
3.	100	112
4.	83	101
5.	121	111
6.	116	125
7.	122	121
8.	99	100
9.	119	120
10.	97	110
11.	88	75
12.	135	144
13.	112	103
14.	127	130
15.	128	122

7. A new instrument was used to measure nitrogen levels in serum. Following are the results of 15 measurements using the new instrument (instrument B) and 15 corresponding measurements from the reference instrument (instrument A). Each measurement is in milligrams per 100 mL. Calculate the correlation coefficient and determine whether it would be wise to do a regression analysis. If it is wise, find the line of best fit and also calculate the SEE and interpret its results.

ALIQUOT	INSTRUMENT A	B
1.	22	20
2.	28	25
3.	32	31
4.	34	35
5.	20	20
6.	29	28
7.	32	33
8.	30	29
9.	35	34
10.	27	25
11.	26	25
12.	30	28
13.	34	37
14.	29	27
15.	26	25

CHAPTER SUMMARY

- Diagnostic sensitivity $= \dfrac{tp}{tp+fn}$

- Diagnostic specificity $= \dfrac{tn}{tn+fp}$

- The positive predictive value, PPV, is calculated using the formula

$$\text{PPV} = \frac{tp}{\text{All positive tests}} = \frac{tp}{tp+fp}.$$

- The negative predictive value, NPV, is calculated using the formula

$$\text{NPV} = \frac{tn}{\text{All negative tests}} = \frac{tn}{tn+fn}.$$

- The formula for a 95% confidence interval for a single sample whose standard deviation is s and size, n, is 30 or greater is

$$\bar{x} \pm 1.96\frac{s}{\sqrt{n}}.$$

- The formula for a 99% confidence interval for a single sample whose size, n, is 30 or greater is

$$\bar{x} \pm 2.58\frac{s}{\sqrt{n}}.$$

- The t-statistic is calculated by $t = \dfrac{\bar{x}-\mu}{\frac{s}{\sqrt{n}}}$ where $d.f. = n-1$.

- The t-statistic for two samples is $t = \dfrac{\overline{D}/n-\mu}{\sqrt{\dfrac{\sum D^2-\left(\overline{D}\right)^2/n}{(n-1)}}} \times \sqrt{n}$.

- The correlation coefficient is calculated by

$$r = \frac{n\sum xy-\left(\sum x\right)\left(\sum y\right)}{\sqrt{n\left(\sum x^2\right)-\left(\sum x\right)^2}\sqrt{n\left(\sum y^2\right)-\left(\sum y\right)^2}}.$$

- For $y = mx + b$

$$m = \frac{n\left(\sum xy\right)-\left(\sum x\right)\left(\sum y\right)}{n\left(\sum x^2\right)-\left(\sum x\right)^2}, \qquad b = \frac{\left(\sum y\right)\left(\sum x^2\right)-\left(\sum x\right)\left(\sum xy\right)}{n\left(\sum x^2\right)-\left(\sum x\right)^2}.$$

- The standard error estimate is calculated using the formula $\text{SEE} = \sqrt{\dfrac{\sum\left(y_m-y_c\right)^2}{n-2}}$.

CHAPTER TEST

1. Give the formulas for diagnostic sensitivity and diagnostic specificity.

2. Five hundred twenty-five patients who all showed symptoms of having mononucleosis were tested using a new test; 400 tested positive. Of these 400 patients, 30 were verified by culture to actually be negative. Of the patients who tested negative, 20 actually had mono. Find the diagnostic sensitivity and specificity for this new test.

3. Give the formula for a 95% confidence interval for a single sample whose standard deviation is s and size, n, is 30 or greater.

4. Two different laboratories are often asked to analyze aliquots from the same specimen. The medical company sending the samples to the two labs wants to know whether there is a statistically significant difference between the instruments used at each lab at the 95% confidence level. To determine whether there is a significant difference, 10 patient samples were divided into two aliquots and then each aliquot was analyzed on the two instruments in each lab for protein. Following are the results in grams per deciliter.

| | INSTRUMENT | |
ALIQUOT	A	B
1.	7	9
2.	7	8
3.	5	6
4.	7	8
5.	8	7
6.	5	5
7.	7	5
8.	5	7
9.	6	5
10.	7	8

Is there a significant statistical difference between the two instruments?

5. Is there a strong linear correlation between two variables if $r = 0.96$, and would a linear regression analysis be appropriate?

APPENDIX A

Common Greek Symbols Used in Math and Science

UPPERCASE	LOWERCASE	NAME
A	α	Alpha
B	β	Beta
Γ	γ	Gamma
Δ	δ	Delta
E	ϵ	Epsilon
Θ	θ	Theta
Λ	λ	Lambda
M	μ	Mu
X	χ	Xi
Π	π	Pi
P	ρ	Rho
Σ	σ	Sigma
Φ	ϕ	Phi
X	χ	Chi
Ω	ω	Omega

APPENDIX B

Periodic Table of the Elements

Group period	1	2	3	4	5	6	7	8	9	10	11	12	13	14	15	16	17	18
1	1 **H** 1.008																	2 **He** 4.003
2	3 **Li** 6.941	4 **Be** 9.012											5 **B** 10.811	6 **C** 12.011	7 **N** 14.007	8 **O** 15.999	9 **F** 18.998	10 **Ne** 20.180
3	11 **Na** 22.990	12 **Mg** 21.305											13 **Al** 26.982	14 **Si** 28.086	15 **P** 30.974	16 **S** 32.066	17 **Cl** 35.453	18 **Ar** 39.948
4	19 **K** 39.098	20 **Ca** 40.078	21 **Sc** 44.956	22 **Ti** 47.867	23 **V** 50.942	24 **Cr** 51.996	25 **Mn** 54.938	26 **Fe** 55.845	27 **Co** 58.933	28 **Ni** 58.693	29 **Cu** 63.546	30 **Zn** 65.39	31 **Ga** 69.723	32 **Ge** 72.61	33 **As** 74.922	34 **Se** 78.96	35 **Br** 79.904	36 **Kr** 83.8
5	37 **Rb** 85.468	38 **Sr** 87.62	39 **Y** 88.906	40 **Zr** 91.224	41 **Nb** 92.906	42 **Mo** 95.94	43 **Tc** (98)	44 **Ru** 101.07	45 **Rh** 102.905	46 **Pd** 106.42	47 **Ag** 107.868	48 **Cd** 112.411	49 **In** 114.818	50 **Sn** 118.71	51 **Sb** 121.76	52 **Te** 127.6	53 **I** 126.904	54 **Xe** 131.29
6	55 **Cs** 132.905	56 **Ba** 137.327		72 **Hf** 178.49	73 **Ta** 180.948	74 **W** 183.84	75 **Re** 186.207	76 **Os** 190.23	77 **Ir** 192.217	78 **Pt** 195.078	79 **Au** 196.967	80 **Hg** 200.59	81 **Tl** 204.38	82 **Pb** 207.2	83 **Bi** 208.98	84 **Po** (210)	85 **At** (210)	86 **Rn** (222)
7	87 **Fr** (223)	88 **Ra** (226)		104 **Rf** (261)	105 **Db** (262)	106 **Sg** (263)	107 **Bh** (262)	108 **Hs** (264)	109 **Mt** (266)	110 **Uun** (269)	111 **Uuu** (272)	112 **Uub** (277)	113 **Uut**	114 **Uuq** (289)	115 **Uup**	116 **Uuh** (289)	117 **Uus**	118 **Uuo** (293)

Lanthanoids	57 **La** 138.905	58 **Ce** 140.16	59 **Pr** 140.908	60 **Nd** 144.24	61 **Pm** (145)	62 **Sm** 150.36	63 **Eu** 151.964	64 **Gd** 157.25	65 **Tb** 158.925	66 **Dy** 162.5	67 **Ho** 164.930	68 **Er** 167.26	69 **Tm** 168.934	70 **Yb** 173.04	71 **Lu** 174.957
Actinoids	89 **Ac** (227)	90 **Th** (232)	91 **Pa** (231)	92 **U** (238)	93 **Np** (237)	94 **Pu** (244)	95 **Am** (243)	96 **Cm** (247)	97 **Bk** (247)	98 **Cf** (251)	99 **Es** (252)	100 **Fm** (257)	101 **Md** (258)	102 **No** (259)	103 **Lr** (262)

APPENDIX C

Pertinent Formulas

ALGEBRA

- In the proportion $\dfrac{a}{b} = \dfrac{c}{d}$, the cross product equation holds true: $ad = bc$

- Properties of exponents:

  Product rule: $x^A \cdot x^B = x^{A+B}$ **Quotient rule:** $\dfrac{x^A}{x^B} = x^{A-B}$

  Power rule: $\left(x^A\right)^B = x^{A \times B}$ **Negative exponent rule:** $x^{-A} = \dfrac{1}{x^A}$

- Scientific notation: $A \times 10^n$ where $1 \le A < 10$ and n is an integer

- $m = \dfrac{\text{Change in } y}{\text{Change in } x} = \dfrac{\Delta y}{\Delta x} = \dfrac{y_2 - y_1}{x_2 - x_1}$

- The slope-intercept form of a linear equation: $y = mx + b$

- Direct variation: $y = kx$

- Inverse variation: $y = \dfrac{k}{x}$

- $y = \log x$ if and only if $10^y = x$

- $\log(10^y) = y$

CHEMISTRY

- Parts concentrate + Parts diluent = Total volume

- Original concentration $\times$ Dilution = Final concentration

- Dilutions of two concentrations: $V_1 \times C_1 = V_2 \times C_2$

- Percent weight per unit weight:

$$\% \, \text{w/w} = \frac{\text{Unit weights of solute}}{100 \text{ unit weights of solution}} = \frac{\text{Grams of solute}}{100 \text{ grams of solution}}$$

- Percent weight per unit volume:

$$\% \, \text{w/v} = \frac{\text{Grams of solute}}{100 \text{ mL of solution}} = \frac{\text{Grams of solute}}{1 \text{ dL of solution}}$$

- Percent volume per unit volume:

$$\% \, \text{v/v} = \frac{\text{mL of concentrate}}{100 \text{ mL of solution}} = \frac{\text{mL of concentrate}}{1 \text{ dL of solution}}$$

- $\text{Molarity} = \dfrac{\text{Number of moles of solute}}{\text{Unit volume of solution}}$

- $\text{Normality} = \dfrac{\text{Number of equivalent weights}}{\text{Unit volume}}$

- $\text{Specific gravity} = \dfrac{\text{Density of some liquid}}{\text{Density of pure water at some specific temperature}}$

- $\text{pH} = -\log\left(\text{H}^+\right)$

- Absorbance: $A = -\log T$

- Transmittance: $T = 10^{-A}$

HEMATOLOGY

- $\dfrac{\text{Number of cells}}{\text{mm}^3} = \text{Total \# of cells counted} \times \dfrac{\text{Depth factor} \times \text{dilution factor}}{\text{Total area counted (in mm}^2)}$

- Mean corpuscular volume: $\text{MCV} = \dfrac{\text{Hct (\%)}}{\text{\# RBCs (in millions}/\mu\text{L)}} \times 10$

- Mean corpuscular hemoglobin: $\text{MCH} = \dfrac{\text{Hb (g/dL)}}{\text{\# RBCs (in millions}/\mu L)} \times 10$

- Mean corpuscular hemoglobin concentration: $\text{MCHC} = \dfrac{\text{Hb (g/dL)}}{\text{Hct (\%)}} \times 100$

- Corrected count index:

$$\text{CCI} = \frac{\text{Posttransfusion count} - \text{Pretransfusion count}}{\text{Number of platelets transfused}\,(\times 10^{11})} \times (\text{Body surface area in m}^2)$$

RENAL CLEARANCE

- Renal clearance: $Cl = \dfrac{U \times V}{P}$

- Corrected clearance: $Cl_c = \dfrac{U \times V}{P} \times \dfrac{1.73\,\text{m}^2}{\text{Size of person (in square meters)}}$

STATISTICS AND QUALITY CONTROL

- Mean: $\bar{x} = \dfrac{\sum x}{n}$

- Standard deviation: $s = \sqrt{\dfrac{\sum (x - \bar{x})^2}{n-1}}$

- Coefficient of variation: $\text{CV} = \dfrac{s}{\bar{x}}$

- The z-score: $z = \dfrac{x - \bar{x}}{s}$

- Diagnostic sensitivity $= \dfrac{tp}{tp + fn}$

- Diagnostic specificity $= \dfrac{tn}{tn + fp}$

- Positive predictive value: $\text{PPV} = \dfrac{tp}{\text{All positive tests}} = \dfrac{tp}{tp + fp}$

- Negative predictive value: $\text{NPV} = \dfrac{tn}{\text{All negative tests}} = \dfrac{tn}{tn + fn}$

- 95% confidence interval: $\bar{x} \pm 1.96 \dfrac{s}{\sqrt{n}}$

- 99% confidence interval: $\bar{x} \pm 2.58 \dfrac{s}{\sqrt{n}}$

- Formula for testing H_0 when $n \leq 30$: $t = \dfrac{\bar{x} - \mu}{\frac{s}{\sqrt{n}}}$ where $d.f. = n - 1$

- The t-statistic: $t = \dfrac{\sum(A-B)/n - \mu}{\sqrt{\dfrac{\sum(A-B)^2 - \dfrac{(\sum(A-B))^2}{n}}{n-1}}} \times \sqrt{n}$

- The correlation coefficient: $r = \dfrac{n\sum x\,y - (\sum x)(\sum y)}{\sqrt{n(\sum x^2)-(\sum x)^2}\ \sqrt{n(\sum y^2)-(\sum y)^2}}$

- Linear regression analysis: The formulas for m and b are:

$$m = \frac{n(\sum xy)-(\sum x)(\sum y)}{n(\sum x^2)-(\sum x)^2} \qquad b = \frac{(\sum y)(\sum x^2)-(\sum x)(\sum xy)}{n(\sum x^2)-(\sum x)^2}$$

- The standard error estimate: $\text{SEE} = \sqrt{\dfrac{\sum(y_m - y_c)^2}{n-2}}$

TEMPERATURE

- To calculate the temperature in Fahrenheit, given the temperature in Celsius, use one of the formulas below:

$$°F = \left(°C \times \frac{9}{5}\right) + 32° \qquad \text{or} \qquad °F = (°C \times 1.8) + 32°$$

- To calculate the temperature in Celsius, given the temperature in Fahrenheit, use the formula below:

$$°C = \frac{°F - 32°}{1.8}$$

APPENDIX D

West Nomogram

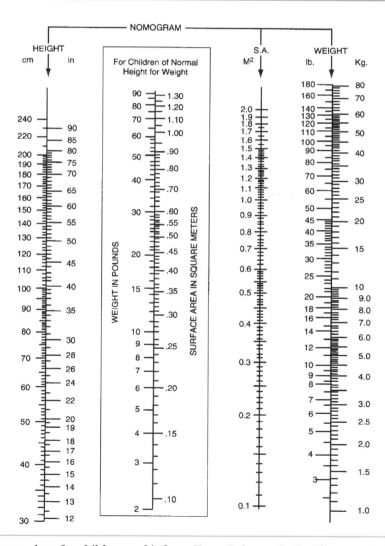

Source: West nomogram chart for children and infants. From Behram, R. E., Kliegman, R. M., and Jenson, H.B. (2004). *Nelson Textbook of pediatrics* (17th ed.). Philadelphia: Saunders. Reprinted with permission.

APPENDIX E

Answers to Odd-Numbered Questions

CHAPTER 1

Section 1.1

1. −5
3. −3
5. 11
7. −6
9. −50
11. 18
13. −3
15. −17
17. 5
19. −5
21. −15
23. 3
25. −20
27. −42
29. 81
31. 25
33. 14
35. −24

37. 40
39. −2
41. −5
43. −5
45. 8
47. −8
49. 10
51. −5
53. 0

Section 1.2

1. $\frac{7}{8}$
3. $\frac{1}{24}$
5. $\frac{5}{8}$
7. $\frac{5}{6}$
9. $\frac{5}{24}$
11. $\frac{25}{48}$
13. $1\frac{1}{6}$
15. $8\frac{1}{9}$
17. $4\frac{1}{4}$
19. $7\frac{11}{15}$

21. $4\frac{5}{24}$

23. $\frac{2}{15}$

25. $\frac{3}{10}$

27. $\frac{2}{15}$

29. $\frac{1}{6}$

31. $\frac{1}{12}$

33. $7\frac{7}{8}$

35. 11

37. $9\frac{1}{2}$

39. $4\frac{1}{72}$

41. 2

43. $-2\frac{2}{9}$

45. $1\frac{1}{6}$

47. 1

49. $1\frac{17}{28}$

51. $\frac{1}{16}$

53. $1\frac{1}{12}$

55. $1\frac{11}{12}$

57. $4\frac{23}{28}$

59. $\dfrac{\$450}{1\,\text{week}}$

61. $\dfrac{6{,}000\,\text{cells}}{1\,\text{mm}^2}$

63. $\dfrac{0.2\,\text{grams}}{1\,\text{liter}}$

65. $\dfrac{1}{24}$

67. $\dfrac{1}{4}$

69. $\dfrac{1}{8}$

71. $1\dfrac{1}{2}$

73. $\dfrac{13}{144}$

75. $\dfrac{1}{32}$

77. $1\dfrac{43}{147}$

Section 1.3

1. 0.05

3. 0.129

5. 0.0045

7. 0.08

9. 0.045

11. 11.3%

13. 3%

15. 40%

17. 125%

19. 12%

21. 0.9%

23. 75%

25. 60%

27. 64%

29. 80%

31. 25%

33. 250%

35. 175%

37. 225%

39. 11.625%

41. $8\frac{1}{3}$ %

43. 4.2%

45. $6\frac{2}{3}$ %

47. 10%

Chapter 1 Test

1. a) −1

   b) −7

   c) −15

   d) 7

   e) −1

   f) 54

   g) −21

h) −48

i) 5

j) −2

k) −5

3. 0.07

5. 30%

7. 11.2%

CHAPTER 2

Section 2.1

1. −4

3. 6

5. 5

7. 11

9. 15

11. 12

13. 21

15. 2

17. ½

19. 20

21. ½

23. ¼

25. $\frac{1}{1,600}$

27. $1\frac{1}{13}$

29. 6

31. 45

33. 24

35. 100

37. 15

39. $\frac{1}{288}$

41. $y = 15, x = 60$

43. $y = 8, x = 4$

45. $r = 6, A = 113.04$

Section 2.2

1. $c = \dfrac{A}{\epsilon l}$

3. $w = \dfrac{V}{lh}$

5. $c = A - b - d$

7. $h = 2\dfrac{A}{b}$

9. $a = 2\dfrac{R}{h} - b$

11. $x = \frac{1}{4}y + 3$

13. $y = x - 2$

15. $y = 3x - 2$

Section 2.3

1. $7\,\frac{8}{11}$

3. $1{,}333\,\frac{1}{3}$

5. 15

7. 60

9. ¼

11. $6\frac{1}{4}$

13. 210

15. 20

17. 150

19. 350

21. 900

23. $1{,}133\,\frac{1}{3}$

25. 20

27. 6 hr 40 min

29. 50

31. 60.8

33. 37.5

Section 2.4

1. 16%

3. 4%

5. 25%

7. 50

9. 605

11. 40

13. 75

15. 4

17. 60

19. 20%

21. 18

23. 94%

25. About 14 or 15

27. 37.6%

29. 87.5%

Section 2.5

1. $3^{11} = 177,147$

3. $10^6 = 1,000,000$

5. 512,000

7. x^3

9. $\dfrac{1}{y^9}$

11. $\dfrac{1}{x^8}$

13. x^{12}

15. $\dfrac{1}{x^{10}}$

17. $\dfrac{1}{x^{18}}$

19. x^3

21. $\dfrac{1}{x^6}$

23. $\dfrac{1}{y^4}$

25. $\dfrac{1}{10^6}$

27. $\dfrac{1}{10^{11}}$

29. 10

31. $\dfrac{1}{10^4}$

33. $\dfrac{1}{10^6}$

35. $\dfrac{1}{10^4}$

37. 10^7

39. 100,100

41. $11\frac{1}{100}$

43. $10\dfrac{1}{10}$

Section 2.6

1. 7

3. 16

5. 8

7. −16

9. 0

11. 1

13. 13

Section 2.7

1. 2

3. 5

5. 1

7. 1

9. 4

11. 1

13. 4

15. 3

17. 4

19. 1.1

21. 1.0

23. 8.3

25. 0.1

27. 99.9

29. 334.09

31. 87.29

33. 1,500.01

35. 0.91

37. 287.50

39. 9.6

41. 8.9

43. 25.6

Section 2.8

1. 2.0×10^{-5}

3. $0.28 = 2.8 \times 10^{-1}$

5. 1.23×10^{11}

7. $1.7 \times 10^1 = 1.7 \times 10$

9. 9.2×10^{-5}

11. 4.35×10^5

13. 650,200

15. 9,920

17. 900,000

19. 0.00055

21. 0.087

23. 0.000007

25. 7.564×10^{-9}

27. 2.0×10^{17}

29. 4.0×10^{-2}

31. 4.0×10^{-8}

33. 1

35. 3×10^{10}

37. 5.0×10^{14}

39. 1.6×10^{10}

Section 2.9

1. ft

3. ft^2

5. ft

7. ft

9. ft^3

11. ft^3

13. 6 grams per hour

15. milliliters per minute

17. grams

19. moles per liter

21. 57.6 cubic millimeters

Section 2.10

1. 1×10^8

3. 5×10^{18}

5. 0.01

7. 1,602,564.103

9. 0.01

11. 0.25

13. 400,000

Chapter 2 Test

1. $x = 18$

3. $x = 18$

5. $x = 6$

7. $a = 3r - b$

9. $x = 75$

11. 6.4%

13. 125

15. 1.5%

17. x^{19}

19. $\dfrac{1}{x^{30}}$

21. 3.0

23. 4

25. 4

27. grams per liter

29. 0.02

CHAPTER 3

Section 3.1

1. 2.55×10^{-5} g
3. 7.5×10^0 cm
5. 1.0×10^5 dag
7. 1.25×10^7 km
9. 6×10^2 mL
11. 1×10^5 mg
13. $1.51 \times 10^4 \, \mu$g
15. 5×10^0 dg
17. 1.2×10^{-2} km
19. 1.5×10^5 mL
21. 9.1×10^{-6} kg
23. 3,000 $^{mg}\!/_{L}$
25. 0.5 $^{g}\!/_{L}$
27. 2,700 $^{mg}\!/_{dL}$
29. 42 $^{mg}\!/_{mL}$
31. 0.3 $^{mg}\!/_{mL}$
33. 55 $^{g}\!/_{L}$

Section 3.2

1. 141.5 g
3. 1,435.2 mL
5. 8,613.1 lb
7. 9,096 mL
9. 8,050 m
11. 6.2×10^{-5} lb
13. 0.67 fl oz
15. 8.4 kg
17. 106.3 lb
19. 86.03 g
21. 18.8 liters
23. 5.31 gallons
25. 1,913.6 cm³

Section 3.3

1. 40 fl dr
3. $\frac{1}{4}$ fl oz
5. 42 fl oz
7. $1\frac{1}{2}$ tsp
9. 72 tsp
11. 480 mL
13. 50 tsp
15. 2.5 mL
17. 12 minims
19. 26 fl oz

Section 3.4

1. 302°F
3. 194°F
5. −13°F
7. 10°C
9. 65.$\overline{5}$°C
11. −34.$\overline{4}$°C
13. 273.15°K
15. 323.15°K
17. −23.15°C

Chapter 3 Test

1. a) 2.5×10^{-5} mL
   b) 1.0×10^4 nL
   c) 4×10^{-5} km
   d) 1.5×10^{-11} kg
   e) 6×10^{-3} mg
   f) 1.2 cg
   g) 0.2 $^{g}\!/_{L}$
   h) 2.5×10^{-3} $^{g}\!/_{dL}$
3. 720 cc
5. 0.$\overline{55}$ lb
7. 8 mL

CHAPTER 4

Section 4.1

1. $3\frac{1}{3}$

3. $6\frac{2}{3}$

5. The ratio of serum to saline is $\frac{2}{5}$, and the ratio of saline to total volume is $\frac{5}{7}$.

7. The ratio of urine to water is $\frac{4}{11}$, and the ratio of water to total volume is $\frac{11}{15}$.

9. The dilution is $\frac{1}{7}$, and the serum to total volume is also $\frac{1}{7}$.

11. The dilution is $\frac{2}{17}$, and the urine to total volume is also $\frac{2}{17}$.

13. $\frac{2}{5}$

15. $\frac{1}{11}$

17. To make this solution, we would take 162 mL urine and add it to 108 mL water to get a total solution of 270 mL.

19. To make this solution, we would take $31\frac{1}{4}$ mL urine and add it to $18\frac{3}{4}$ mL water to get a total solution of 50 mL.

21. $\frac{2}{14}$

23. 15 μL serum and 105 μL of diluent

25. 10 μL serum and 140 μL of diluent

27. Take 300 mL of concentrate and add it to 200 mL diluent to get a total of 500 mL solution.

29. 12.5 μL of serum

31. 2 μL of serum

33. 1.5%

35. 1%

37. 2

39. 1,050 mg/dL

41. 6

43. 20

Section 4.2

1. a) Tube 1: 5 mg/dL
   Tube 2: 5/2 mg/dL
   Tube 3: 5/4 mg/dL
   b) Solution dilution: 1/8 mg/dL
   c) Final concentration: 5/4 mg/dL

3. a) Tube 1: 5 mg/dL
   Tube 2: 1/2 mg/dL
   Tube 3: 1/20 mg/dL
   Tube 4: 1/200 mg/dL
   b) Solution dilution: 1/10,000 mg/dL
   c) 1/200 mg/dL

5. a) Concentration in tube 1 = 200 mg/dL
   Concentration in tube 2 = 50 mg/dL
   Concentration in tube 3 = 25/4 mg/dL
   Concentration in tube 4 = 25/64 mg/dL
   b) 1 part urine + 3 parts diluent
   c) 1/1,024 mg/dL
   d) 25/64 mg/dL

7. a) Concentration in tube 1 = 75 mg/dL
   Concentration in tube 2 = 75/2 mg/dL
   Concentration in tube 3 = 75/4 mg/dL
   b) 1/8 mg/dL
   c) 75/4 mg/dL

9. a) Concentration in tube 1 = 250 mg/dL
   Concentration in tube 2 = 125 mg/dL
   Concentration in tube 3 = 125/2 mg/dL
   Concentration in tube 4 = 125/4 mg/dL
   Concentration in tube 5 = 125/8 mg/dL

b) 1 part urine + 1 part diluent

c) 1/32 $^{mg}/_{dL}$

d) 125/8 $^{mg}/_{dL}$

11. a) 1/1,280 $^{mg}/_{dL}$

    b) 1/1,024 $^{mg}/_{dL}$

13. a) 1/10 $^{mg}/_{dL}$

    b) 1/16 $^{mg}/_{dL}$

15. 15 $^{mg}/_{dL}$

Section 4.3

1. 8

3. 32

Chapter 4 Test

1. Use 25 μL of sodium hydroxide and 275 μL of diluent to get the total of 300 μL.

3. $\dfrac{1}{9}$

5. $\dfrac{4}{19}$

7. To make this solution, take 450 mL of concentrate and add it to 150 mL of diluent to get a total of 600 mL of solution.

9. 0.8%

11. Concentration in tube 1: 28 $^{mg}/_{dL}$

Concentration in tube 2: 2.8 $^{mg}/_{dL}$

Concentration in tube 3: 0.28 $^{mg}/_{dL}$

The solution dilution is $\dfrac{1}{1,000}$.

The final concentration is 0.28 $^{mg}/_{dL}$.

13. Concentration in tube 1: 42 $^{mg}/_{dL}$

Concentration in tube 2: 4.2 $^{mg}/_{dL}$

Concentration in tube 3: 0.42 $^{mg}/_{dL}$

Concentration in tube 4: 0.042 $^{mg}/_{dL}$

1 part urine was added to 9 parts diluent.

The solution dilution is $\dfrac{1}{10,000}$.

The final concentration is 0.042 $^{mg}/_{dL}$.

CHAPTER 5

Section 5.1

1. a) quadrant II

    b) quadrant III

    c) quadrant IV

    d) quadrant I

    e) quadrant IV

    f) quadrant III

3. (0, 0)

Section 5.2

1. 4

3. –2

5. –1

7. –2

9. $m = 5$.

11. $\dfrac{10}{3}$

13. –1

15. –3

Section 5.3

1.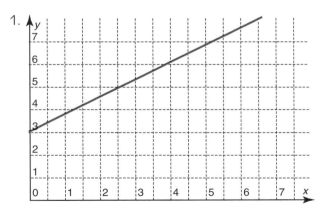

3.
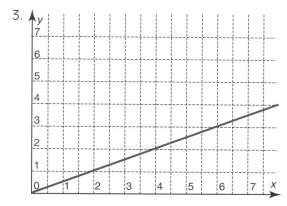

5.
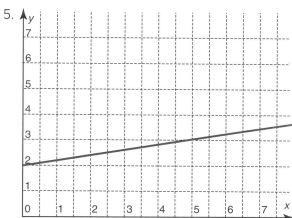

7.
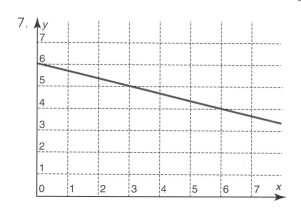

9.
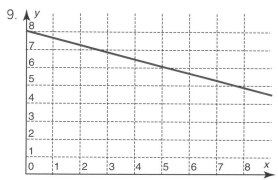

11.
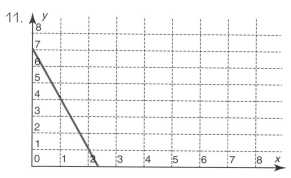

13.
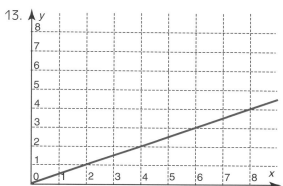

15.
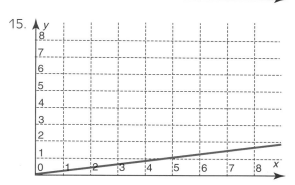

Section 5.4

1. When $t = 2$ the concentration is 20 mmol/L.

   When $t = 5$ the concentration is 50 mmol/L.

   When the concentration is 30 mmol/L, the time is 3 sec.

   When the concentration is 70 mmol/L, the time is 7 sec.

3. When $t = 4$ the population is about 1,080 (give or take).

   When the time is 3, the population is 600.

When the population is 200, the time is about 1.75 hours.

When the population is 1,200, the time is about 4.25 hours.

5. When the amount of reactant is 1, the absorbance is approximately 0.43.

When the amount of reactant is 3, the absorbance is approximately 0.66.

When the absorbance is 0.6, the approximate amount of reactant is 2.

When the absorbance is 0.5, the approximate amount of reactant is 1.25.

7. When the concentration is 300 $^{mg}\!/_{dL}$, the percent transmittance is approximately 10%. When T is 20%, the concentration is approximately 100 $^{mg}\!/_{dL}$.

Section 5.5

1. 1×10^9

3. When the concentration is 400, the absorbance will be 1.2. When the absorbance is 1.5, the concentration is 500 $^{mg}\!/_{dL}$.

5. When the concentration is 1.0, the absorbance will be 0.16. When the absorbance is 0.1, the concentration is 0.625 $^{mg}\!/_{mL}$.

7. When the volume is 4.5 cubic feet, the pressure is 10 lb per ft².

9. When the volume is 8 cubic feet, the pressure is 5 lb per ft².

11. a is 2.4 when c is 10

13. y is 60 when x is 10

15. y is 150 when x is 20

17. y is 78.4 when x is 9.8

Chapter 5 Test

1. 1.5

3. $m = 5$

5. $m = \dfrac{1}{3}$

7.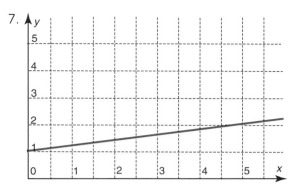

9.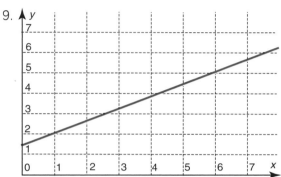

11. When $x = 1$, $y = 3$. When $x = -1$, $y = 1$. When $y = 3$, $x = 1$

13. 60 lb per ft²

15. $y = 20$

CHAPTER 6

Section 6.1

1. 400 mL

3. 233.33 mL

5. 700 mL

7. 0.5%

9. 0.75%

11. 270 mL

13. 166.67 mL

Section 6.2

1. Take 22.5 g NaOH and mix it with 102.5 grams of solution

3. Take 6.75 g NaCl and mix it with 68.25 grams of solution

5. Dissolve 37.5 grams of NaCl in 150 mL of diluent.

7. Dissolve 1 gram of NaCl in 50 mL of diluent.

9. Dissolve 21 grams of HCl in 150 mL of diluent.

11. Take 40 mL of alcohol and add it to 160 mL of water.

13. There are 49 mL of ethanol in 70 mL of a 70% v/v solution.

15. There are 1,200 mL of ethanol in 4,000 mL of a 30% v/v solution.

17. Take 12 mL of ethanol and add it to 88 mL of water.

19. There are 13.5 g of NaCl in 45 mL of a 30% w/v NaCl solution.

Section 6.3

1. 1.0

3. 3.0

5. 0.99 eqw

7. 0.4 eqw

9. 0.78 *g*

11. There are 1.75 g of this nitric acid in 2.50 mL of a 70% assay.

13. Take 168 mL of the 70% solution and dilute it up to 1,000 mL.

15. Take 98.5 mL of the 70% solution and dilute it up to 1,000 mL.

17. $1.20 \frac{\%}{mL}$

Chapter 6 Test

1. 1.2%

3. 0.59%

5. Take 5 g NaOH and mix it with 45 grams of solution.

7. 2.0

9. 0.30 eqw

CHAPTER 7

Section 7.1

1. 1

3. 7

5. a) 5.67

   b) 1.95

   c) 1.35

   d) 1.52

   e) 2.52

7. 2

9. 5

11. 9

Section 7.2

1. 0.141

3. 0.231

5. 0.420

7. 0.515

9. 0.499

11. $4.2 \times 10^{-5} \frac{mol}{L}$

13. $4.3 \times 10^{-5} \frac{mol}{L}$

15. $8.30 \times 10^{-5} \frac{mol}{L}$

17. $8.40 \times 10^{-5} \frac{mol}{L}$

19. 2.6×10^3

21. 2.7×10^3

23. 1.6×10^{-5} $\frac{mol}{L}$

25. 8.4×10^{-5} $\frac{mol}{L}$

Chapter 7 Test

1. 2.9542

3. −5

5. 8

7. 0.213

9. 0.376

11. 4.3×10^{-6} $\frac{mol}{L}$

CHAPTER 8

Section 8.1

1. 1,450 WBCs

3. $0.2\ mm^2$

5. 1,000 WBCs per cubic millimeter

7. 10,000 WBCs per cubic millimeter

9. 1,125 WBCs per cubic millimeter

11. 6,093,750 RBCs per cubic millimeter

13. 3,437,500 RBCs per cubic millimeter

15. 280,000 platelets per cubic millimeter

17. 237,500 platelets per cubic millimeter

Section 8.2

1. 82

3. 80

5. 27 pg

7. 31%

9. 27%

Section 8.3

1. 5,988

3. 7,604

5. hemoglobin: $8.6\frac{g}{dL}$, hematocrit: 30% − 33%

7. hemoglobin: $8.5\frac{g}{dL}$, hematocrit: 26% − 29%

Chapter 8 Test

1. $875 / mm^3$

3. 90

5. 25 pg

7. 36%

9. 6,404

CHAPTER 9

Section 9.1

1. 1,280 mg creatinine in sample

   1.28 g/day 1.11 mL/min

3. 1,445 mg in total

   1.45 g/day

5. 405 mg protein in sample

   810 mg/day

7. 1,330 mg creatinine in sample

   1.33 g/day

9. 192 mg creatinine in sample

   0.77 g/day

Section 9.2

1. $119.6\frac{mL}{min}$

3. $113.8\frac{mL}{min}$

5. $148.4\frac{mL}{min}$

7. $130.8\frac{mL}{min}$

9. $19.6\frac{mL}{min}$

11. 29.5 $\frac{mL}{min}$

13. 28.5 $\frac{mL}{min}$

Chapter 9 Test

1. 245 mg in sample; 490 $\frac{mg}{day}$

3. 276 mg in sample; 828 $\frac{mg}{day}$

5. 39.5 $\frac{mL}{min}$

CHAPTER 10

Section 10.1

1.

Class	Frequency
1–8	14
9–16	21
17–24	11
25–32	6
33–40	4
41–48	4

3.

Class	Frequency
0–1	12
2–3	8
4–5	6
6–7	4

5.

Class	Frequency
0–19	11
20–39	9
40–59	10
60–79	8
80–99	7

7.

Class	Frequency
0–4	7
5–9	10
10–14	5
15–19	8

Section 10.2

1.

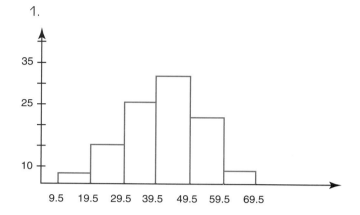

3.

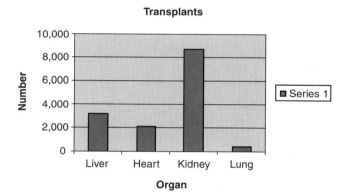

5.

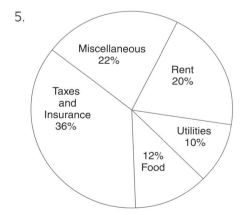

7. The bar chart is:

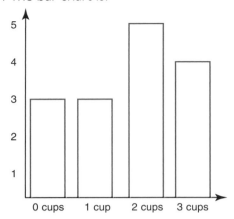

The pie chart would be:

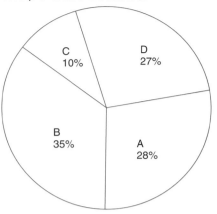

9. The pie chart is:

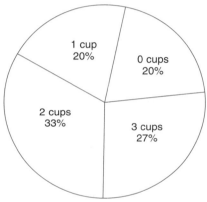

Chapter 10 Test

1. Histograms, frequency polygons, bar graphs, and pie graphs.

3. The bar chart would be:

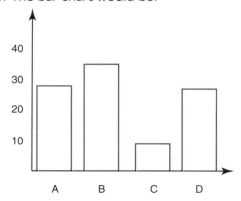

CHAPTER 11

Section 11.3

1. a) 85.93
   b) 85
   c) 85
   d) 94.69
   e) 9.73
   f) 11%
   g) 76.20 – 95.66;　66.47 – 105.39;
      56.74 – 115.12

3. a) 190.80
   b) 176.5
   c) no mode
   d) 3126.18
   e) 55.91
   f) 29%
   g) 134.89 – 246.71;　78.98 – 302.62;
      23.07 – 358.53
   h) 8
   i) 9
   j) All the data values

5.

	Set 1	Set 2
a)	Mean = 61.00	Mean = 61.50
b)	Median = 61	Median = 61.5
c)	Mode = 61	No mode
d)	Variance = 2	Variance = 21.90
e)	Standard deviation = 1.41	Standard deviation = 4.68
f)	CV = 2.3%	CV = 7.6%
g)	Set 1 is more precise.	

7.

	Set 1	Set 2
a)	Mean = 15.38	Mean = 15.00
b)	Median = 15.5	Median = 14
c)	Mode = 12	Mode = 13
d)	Variance = 10.27	Variance = 15.43
e)	Standard deviation = 3.20	Standard deviation = 3.93
f)	CV = 20.8%	CV = 26.2%
g)	Set 1 is more precise.	

9.

	Method A	Method B
a)	Mean = 153.00	Mean = 150.00
b)	Median = 154	Median = 150
c)	Mode = 154	No mode
d)	Variance = 39.00	Variance = 134.00
e)	SD = 6.24	SD = 11.58
f)	CV = 4.1%	CV = 7.7%
g)	Method A is more precise.	

Section 11.4

1. a) 68.3%

   b) 95.5%

   c) 99.7%

   d) 4.5%

   e) 0.3%

   f) 31.7%

3. a) ±1 SD range: 212.5–237.5

   ±2 SD range: 200–250

   ±3 SD range: 187.5–262.5

   b) 68.3%, 95.5%, and 99.7%, respectively

   c) 31.7%, 4.5%, and 0.3 %, respectively

5. a) ±1 SD range: 74.2–85.8

   ±2 SD range: 68.4–91.6

   ±3 SD range: 62.6–97.4

   b) 68.3%, 95.5%, and 99.7%, respectively

   c) 31.7%, 4.5%, and 0.3%, respectively

Section 11.6

1.

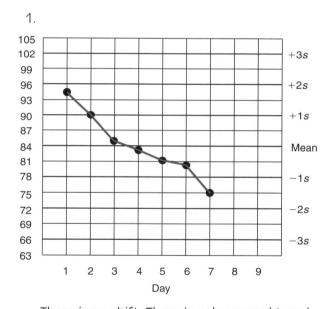

There is no shift. There is a downward trend. Because there is a trend, the work process is out of control and results should not be reported.

3.

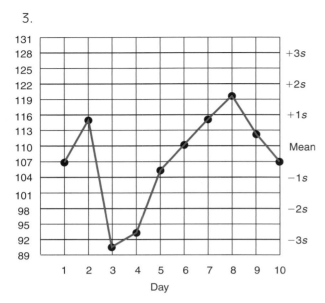

There is an upward trend. There is no shift. There is also a plot below −3*s*. Thus, we reject the run and do not report these results.

5.

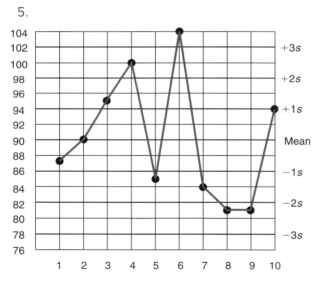

By inspection we see on days 8 and 9 the points lie below −2*s*. We also see that on day 6 the plot is above +3*s*. Therefore, this warrants the conclusion that the assay procedure needs to be analyzed to correct any problems and should not be used for patient diagnosis at this point.

7.

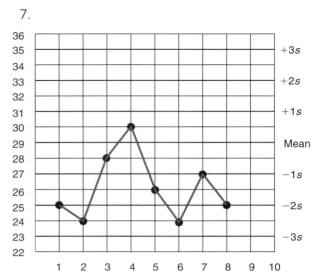

By inspection we see on days 2 and 6 the points lie below −2*s*. Therefore, this warrants the conclusion that the assay procedure needs to be analyzed to correct any problems. It may be that the instrument just needs to be calibrated, but from the information we have here, the run should be rejected.

9. None of the Westgard multirules has been violated. Therefore, the results should be reported.

11. We see rule 2_{2s} is violated across materials on day 6; therefore, the assay procedure needs to be analyzed to correct the problem.

13. We see rule R_{4s} is violated across materials on day 3; therefore, the assay procedure needs to be analyzed to correct the problem.

15. We see rule 2_{2s} is violated across materials on day 6; therefore, the assay procedure needs to be analyzed to correct the problem.

17. A warning goes up because of day 7 level I. However, no other Westgard rules have been violated; therefore, the results should be reported.

19. We see rule 2_{2s} is violated across materials on day 1; therefore, the assay procedure needs to be analyzed to correct the problem.

Section 11.7

1. We can see on days 15 and 16, for both levels, the standard deviation is less than –2. Therefore, rule 4_{1s} was violated and we should not report the results.

3. In level I the value is more than 3 standard deviations away from the mean. Therefore, rule 1_{3s} was violated and we should not report the results.

5. We see on day 17 the standard deviation is more than +3 for both levels. Thus, Rule 1_{3s} was violated and the assay procedure needs to be analyzed to correct the problem.

Chapter 11 Test

1.

	Set A	Set B
a)	mean = 6.00	mean = 10.00
b)	median = 5.5	median = 9.5
c)	mode = 2	mode = 9
d)	$s = 3.74$	$s = 1.93$
e)	CV = 62.3%	CV = 19.3%
f)	Method B is more precise.	

3. 95.5%

5. –3.5 and rule 1_{3s} has been violated.

7. We see rule 2_{2s} is violated across materials on day 8.

CHAPTER 12

Section 12.1

1. Sensitivity = 0.947, specificity = 0.778

3. Sensitivity = 0.789, specificity = 0.762

5. PPV = 0.978, NPV = 0.980

Section 12.2

1. 95%: 93–97
   99%: 92.4–97.6

3. 95%: 298.9–301.1
   99%: 298.5–301.5

Section 12.3

1. 2.508

3. 2.787

5. t lies in the rejection region, so reject the null hypothesis; therefore, at the 99% confidence level we can say the average salary is less than $50,000.

7. t lies in the rejection region so reject the null hypothesis; therefore, at the 99% confidence level we can say the average time is greater than 25.

9. There is not a significant statistical difference between their means, so this implies there is not a significant statistical difference between the two instruments.

11. There is not a significant statistical difference between their means, so this implies there is not a significant statistical difference between the two values of the two instruments.

Section 12.5

1. Because r is close to zero, there is not much of a correlation; therefore, we should not proceed with a linear regression analysis.

3. Because r is close to +1, there is a strong positive correlation and it would be appropriate to continue with a linear regression analysis.

5. Because $r = 0.998$, which is close to 1, there is a strong positive correlation and it would be appropriate to do a regression analysis. The equation for the line of best fit is $y = 0.997x + 4.182$. The SEE = 1.2306.

7. Because $r = 0.962$, which is close to 1, there is a strong positive correlation and it would be appropriate to do a regression analysis. The equation for the line of best fit is $y = 1.144x - 4.957$. The SEE = 1.4426.

Chapter 12 Test

1. Diagnostic sensitivity $= \dfrac{tp}{tp + fn}$

   Diagnostic specificity $= \dfrac{tn}{tn + fp}$

3. $\bar{x} \pm 1.96 \dfrac{s}{\sqrt{n}}$; $\bar{x} \pm 2.58 \dfrac{s}{\sqrt{n}}$

5. Yes, there is a strong positive correlation and it would be appropriate to do a linear regression analysis.

GLOSSARY

abscissa the x-coordinate on a Cartesian graph *(Chapter 5)*

absolute zero a theoretical temperature that is supposedly the coldest temperature in the universe *(Chapter 3)*

accuracy the accuracy of a number tells about the quantity of significant digits in the number; in general, the more significant digits a number has, the more accurate the measurement *(Chapter 2)*

acid a substance that donates hydrogen ions; substances with a pH lower than 7.0 are considered acids *(Chapter 7)*

area the amount of surface within a given boundary *(Chapter 2)*

area factor a factor that must be included when counting cells if an area other than one square millimeter was used in the counting process *(Chapter 8)*

associative property of addition a property of addition in which the regrouping of the addends does not change the outcome of the operations: $(a + b) + c = a + (b + c)$ *(Chapter 2)*

associative property of multiplication a property of multiplication in which the regrouping of the factors does not change the outcome of the operations: $(a \times b) \times c = a \times (b \times c)$ *(Chapter 2)*

Avogadro's number the number of particles in a mole; this number is approximately 6.02×10^{23} *(Chapter 6)*

base the portion of an exponential that is raised to an exponent *(Chapter 2)*

base a substance that can receive a hydrogen ion; substances with a pH higher than 7.0 are considered bases *(Chapter 7)*

bimodal describes a data set that has two numbers that appear the same amount of time and more than any of the other numbers *(Chapter 11)*

Cartesian plane a plane with a rectangular coordinate system that associates each point in the plane with a unique pair of numbers in an ordered pair of the form (x, y); the x value is the horizontal coordinate and the y value is the vertical coordinate *(Chapter 5)*

Celsius a temperature scale in which water freezes at $0°$ and boils at $100°$ *(Chapter 3)*

class an established range of values *(Chapter 10)*

class boundaries to find the boundaries of a class, add 0.5 to the upper class limit and subtract 0.5 from the lower class limit *(Chapter 10)*

coefficient of variation (CV) the standard deviation expressed as a percentage of the mean *(Chapter 11)*

coefficient of x the number in front of x in a linear equation $y = mx + b$ *(Chapters 2, 5)*

colorimetry the science of colors; a colorimeter is an instrument that measures the depth of the color of a given solution as compared with the depth of the color of some standard solution *(Chapter 7)*

commutative property of addition a property of addition in which the sum stays the same when the order of the addends is changed: $a + b = b + a$ *(Chapter 2)*

commutative property of multiplication a property of multiplication in which the product stays the same when the order of the factors is changed: $a \times b = b \times a$ *(Chapter 2)*

concentrate a concentrated solution *(Chapter 4)*

concentration the amount of a particular substance in a given volume *(Chapter 4)*

confidence interval an interval of values that comes from sample information and gives a percentage that measures the level of confidence *(Chapter 12)*

controls measurements known to be accurate *(Chapter 11)*

coordinate plane a plane marked with two perpendicular number lines, used to graph ordered pairs of numbers *(Chapter 5)*

corrected count index a method for measuring response to the transfusion of platelets *(Chapter 8)*

correlation coefficient a numerical value that identifies the strength of relationship between variables *(Chapter 12)*

creatinine a protein produced by the body that enters the bloodstream; the rate at which the kidney clears the plasma of creatinine is often used to measure renal clearance *(Chapter 9)*

cross products the numerator of the first ratio times the denominator of the second and the denominator of the first proportion times the numerator of the second; the cross products of a proportion are always equal *(Chapter 2)*

degrees of freedom (d.f.) one less than the number of data values *(Chapter 12)*

denominator the bottom number in a fraction *(Chapter 1)*

density measure of how much matter is in a given volume or the amount of mass per volume *(Chapter 6)*

depth factor a factor that must be included when counting cells if an amount other than one cubic millimeter was used in the counting process *(Chapter 8)*

descriptive statistics a branch of statistics that involves the collection of data followed by summarizing and describing the characteristics of that data *(Chapter 11)*

diagnostic sensitivity the probability that all patients who are infected will test positive *(Chapter 12)*

diagnostic specificity the probability that all patients who are not infected will not test positive *(Chapter 12)*

diluent a solvent *(Chapter 4)*

dilution factor reciprocal of the dilution *(Chapters 4, 8)*

dilutions represent parts of concentrate in total volume *(Chapter 4)*

dimensional analysis a method of manipulating unit measures algebraically to determine the proper units for a quantity computed algebraically *(Chapter 3)*

distributive property property that establishes a relationship between multiplication and addition such that multiplication distributes across the addition: $a(b + c) = ab + ac$ *(Chapter 2)*

electrolyte a substance that carries electrical current by the migration of ions *(Chapter 7)*

empirical rule a handy quick estimate of the spread of the data given the mean and standard deviation of a data set that follows the normal distribution *(Chapter 11)*

enzyme kinetics the study of the rate at which enzymes react *(Chapter 5)*

equivalent weight molecular weight divided by valence *(Chapter 6)*

exponent a number or symbol placed above and to the right of another number or symbol indicating the number of times that that value is to be multiplied by itself *(Chapter 2)*

Fahrenheit a temperature scale in which water freezes at 32° and boils at 212° *(Chapter 3)*

fn *false negatives* are the number of patients who are infected but test negative *(Chapter 12)*

fp *false positives* are the number of patients who are not infected but test positive *(Chapter 12)*

frequency distribution a way of organizing data that shows how often certain data appears *(Chapter 10)*

frequency distribution table a table used to organize data to show how often certain data values appear within a particular range *(Chapter 10)*

Gaussian distribution most commonly observed probability distribution whose shape resembles that of a bell; also known as normal distribution *(Chapter 11)*

glomerular filtration rate (GFR) measures how well the kidneys remove and filter substances *(Chapter 9)*

hematocrit the percentage of (packed) red blood cells that makes up the blood *(Chapter 8)*

hematology the study of the science of blood *(Chapter 8)*

hemoglobin the oxygen-carrying protein that gives red blood cells their color *(Chapter 8)*

histogram a graph that presents data by using vertical bars, with the height of each bar equivalent to the frequency of the class *(Chapter 10)*

household system a measurement system used for dispensing medication in the household *(Chapter 3)*

improper fraction a fraction whose numerator is larger than the denominator; all improper fractions are greater than 1 *(Chapter 1)*

in control If about 1 in 22 of the control values fall outside the established range of controls we usually consider the work process to be reliable and say the test run is in control *(Chapter 11)*

inferential statistics a branch of statistics that involves the process of gathering a portion of the data, called a sample, from an entire population and using the information from the sample to make a general conjecture about some characteristic of the entire population *(Chapter 11)*

ion a positively or negatively charged atom or molecule *(Chapter 7)*

ionization when an electrically neutral atom or molecule is transformed into either a positively or negatively charged atom or molecule *(Chapter 7)*

Kelvin a temperature measurement scale used in the scientific community; zero K represents absolute zero and corresponds to $-459°$ Fahrenheit or $-273°$ Celsius *(Chapter 3)*

least common denominator the least common multiple of the denominators in two or more fractions *(Chapter 1)*

line of best fit a straight line used as a best approximation of a summary of all the points in a scatter plot *(Chapter 12)*

linear equation any equation whose graph is a straight line *(Chapter 5)*

linear function a function whose graph is a straight line *(Chapter 5)*

logarithm base 10 defined as $y = \log x$ if and only if $x = a^y$ *(Chapter 7)*

lower class limit the smallest data value in a class (or sometimes a value slightly less), used in the construction of a frequency distribution table *(Chapter 10)*

mean a common measure of central tendency that is found by adding up all the data values and dividing that result by the total number of data values *(Chapter 11)*

median the middle value of an entire data set *(Chapter 11)*

mixed number a number expressed as a whole number together with a fraction *(Chapter 1)*

mode the number in a data set that appears most frequently *(Chapter 11)*

molarity number of moles of solute per unit of volume of solution *(Chapter 6)*

mole amount of an element or compound equal to its molecular or atomic weight in grams *(Chapter 6)*

natural logarithm a logarithm whose base, instead of 10, is about 2.718 *(Chapter 7)*

negative exponent rule when an exponential is raised to a negative exponent, it can be rewritten as 1 over the exponential with a positive exponent *(Chapter 2)*

normal distribution most commonly observed probability distribution whose shape resembles that of a bell; also known as Gaussian distribution *(Chapter 11)*

normality the number of equivalent weights per unit volume *(Chapter 6)*

numerator the top number in a fraction *(Chapter 1)*

ordered pair a pair of numbers in which the order is specified, used to locate a point in a coordinate plane *(Chapter 5)*

ordinate the *y*-coordinate on a Cartesian graph *(Chapter 5)*

origin the point of intersection of coordinate axes; where the values of the coordinates are zero *(Chapter 5)*

out of control If more than 1 in 22 fall outside the established range of controls we assume there are errors, check the work process to detect and correct those errors, and say the test run is out of control *(Chapter 11)*

outliers values that deviate from the mean by an extreme amount *(Chapter 11)*

PEMDAS an acronym useful for remembering the order of operations; the P stands for parentheses, E for exponents, M for multiplication, D for division, A for addition, and S for subtraction *(Chapter 2)*

percent per 100 *(Chapter 1)*

percent transmittance percentage that tells how much light can shine through a solution *(Chapter 5)*

percent volume per unit volume mL of concentrate divided by 100 mL of solution *(Chapter 6)*

percent weight per unit volume grams of solute divided by 100 mL of solution *(Chapter 6)*

percent weight per unit weight grams of solute divided by 100 grams of solution *(Chapter 6)*

pH a measure of the acidity or basicity (alkalinity) of a material when dissolved in water; expressed on a scale from 0 to 14 *(Chapter 7)*

population the entire aggregation of items from which samples can be drawn *(Chapter 11)*

power rule an exponential rule that tells us to multiply the exponents when an exponential is raised to a power *(Chapter 2)*

precision the precision of a number is determined by the place value of the last significant digit *(Chapter 2)*

product rule an exponential rule that tells us to add the exponents when exponentials are multiplied *(Chapter 2)*

proper fraction a fraction whose denominator is larger than the numerator *(Chapter 1)*

proportion two ratios are said to be in proportion with each other if they are equivalent *(Chapter 2)*

quality control process used to make sure laboratory results are precise and dependable *(Chapter 11)*

quotient rule an exponential rule that tells us to subtract the exponents when exponentials are divided *(Chapter 2)*

rate a ratio that compares the relationship of two quantities that each have different units *(Chapter 2)*

ratio the quotient of two quantities *(Chapter 2)*

raw data collected data that has not yet been organized *(Chapter 10)*

reciprocal two numbers are said to be reciprocals of each other if the product of the two numbers is 1 *(Chapter 2)*

rejection region when the value of a t-statistic falls in this region the null hypothesis is rejected *(Chapter 12)*

renal clearance refers to how fast the kidneys clear the blood of a material *(Chapter 9)*

sample a portion of data from an entire population *(Chapter 11)*

scientific notation a method of representing a number as a product of a number between 1 and 10 and a power of 10; a shorthand way of writing very large or very small numbers *(Chapter 2)*

serial dilutions a series of dilutions *(Chapter 4)*

shift when six or more consecutive plots all fall on/above or on/below the mean line *(Chapter 11)*

significance level the probability of rejecting a set of assumptions when they are in fact true *(Chapter 12)*

significant digits give information about the accuracy of a measurement *(Chapter 2)*

simultaneous equations two different equations that are interrelated *(Chapter 2)*

slope the amount by which the value along the vertical axis increases as the result of a change in one unit along the horizontal axis; calculated by dividing the change in the vertical axis (the "rise") by the change in horizontal axis (the "run") *(Chapter 5)*

slope-intercept form convenient form in which to write linear equations: $y = mx + b$ *(Chapter 5)*

solution dilution the final dilution for a system *(Chapter 4)*

specific gravity ratio of the density of a liquid to the density of pure water at some specific temperature *(Chapter 6)*

spectrophotometry the science of measuring the absorption of light by using a spectrophotometer; a spectrophotometer measures the intensity of the light after it travels through a solution *(Chapter 7)*

standard curve a graph that is typically used to help determine the concentration of some substance *(Chapter 5)*

standard deviation a measure of the spread or dispersion of a set of data *(Chapter 11)*

standard error estimate the standard deviation of the measured values about the predicted values

standard form the basic form of any linear equation: $Ax + By = C$ *(Chapter 5)*

substrate a substance that an enzyme is working on *(Chapter 5)*

titer estimation of the amount of a substance in a solution *(Chapter 4)*

tn *true negatives* are the number of patients who are not infected and also test negative *(Chapter 12)*

tp *true positives* are the number of patients who are infected and test positive *(Chapter 12)*

transmittance the fraction of light transmitted through a sample *(Chapter 7)*

trend when six or more consecutive plots all fall in one direction, specifically upward or downward *(Chapter 11)*

unit one pint of whole blood *(Chapter 8)*

unit fraction a fraction that equals 1 *(Chapter 1)*

unit rate a rate where the numerical value in the denominator is 1 *(Chapter 1)*

upper class limit the largest data value in a class, used in the construction of a frequency distribution table *(Chapter 10)*

urinalysis the inspection of urine *(Chapter 9)*

variance measure of how the values in a distribution are spread around the expected value *(Chapter 11)*

volume the amount of space a three-dimensional object encloses *(Chapter 2)*

Westgard multirules a multiple rule design to determine whether a method is in or out of control *(Chapter 11)*

x-axis the horizontal number line in a coordinate plane *(Chapter 5)*

y-axis the vertical number line in a coordinate plane *(Chapter 5)*

y-intercept the value of y when the line or curve intersects or crosses the y-axis *(Chapter 5)*

y varies directly with x if, when y increases x also increases or when y decreases x also decreases *(Chapter 5)*

y varies inversely with x if, when x increases y decreases or visa versa *(Chapter 5)*

z-score number that tells how far a measurement is from the mean in terms of standard deviations *(Chapter 11)*

REFERENCES

Blaisdell, E. A. (1993). *Statistics in practice*. Fort Worth, TX: Saunders College Publishing.

Bluman, A. G. (2001). *Elementary statistics* (4th ed.). New York: McGraw Hill.

Campbell, J. M., & Campbell, J. B. (Eds.). (1997). *Laboratory mathematics, medical and biological applications* (5th ed.). St. Louis, MO: Mosby.

Carman, R. A., & Saunders, H. M. (1992). *Mathematics for the trades: A guided approach* (6th ed.). Upper Saddle River, NJ: Prentice-Hall.

D'Agostino, R., Sr., Sullivan, L., & Beiser, A. (2004). *Introductory applied biostatistics*. Thomson Brooks/Cole.

Doucette, L. J. (1997). *Mathematics for the clinical laboratory*. Philadelphia: W. B. Saunders Company.

K/DOQI clinical practice guidelines for chronic kidney disease: Evaluation, classification, and stratification. Part 5: Evaluation of laboratory measurements for clinical assessment of kidney disease. Guideline 4: Estimation of GFR. (2002). Retrieved April 17, 2006, from http://www.kidney.org/professionals/kdoqi/guidelines_ckd/p5_lab_g4.htm

Tiger, S., Kirk, J. K., & Solomon, R. J. (2000). *Mathematical concepts in clinical science*. Upper Saddle River, NJ: Prentice-Hall.

The United States National Library of Medicine. (n.d.). Retrieved May 18, 2006, from www.nlm.nih.gov

Westgard, J. O. (2000). *QC—The idea*. Retrieved November 15, 2006, from http://www.westgard.com/lesson11.htm

Westgard, J. O. (2000). *QC—The multirule interpretation*. Retrieved November 15, 2006, from http://www.westgard.com/lesson18.htm

INDEX